ORAL
HEALTH
SOURCEBOOK

Health Reference Series

Volume Thirty

RK
61
.O66
1997

ORAL
HEALTH
SOURCEBOOK

*Basic Information about Diseases and
Conditions Affecting Oral Health including
Cavities, Gum Disease, Dry Mouth, Oral
Cancers, Fever Blisters, Canker Sores, Oral
Thrush, Bad Breath, Temporomandibular
Disorders, and other Craniofacial Syndromes
along with Statistical Data on the Oral Health
of Americans, Oral Hygiene, Emergency First
Aid, Information on Treatment Procedures
and Methods of Replacing Lost Teeth*

Edited by
Allan R. Cook

Omnigraphics, Inc.

Penobscot Building / Detroit, MI 48226

Bibliographic Note

Since this page cannot legibly accommodate all the copyright notices, the Bibliographic Note section of the Preface constitutes an extension of the copyright notice.

Edited by
Allan R. Cook

Peter D. Dresser, Managing Editor, Health Reference Series
Karen Bellenir, Series Editor, Health Reference Series

Omnigraphics, Inc.

Matthew P. Barbour, Production Manager
Laurie Lanzen Harris, Vice President, Editorial
Peter E. Ruffner, Vice President, Administration
James A. Sellgren, Vice President, Operations and Finance
Jane J. Steele, Marketing Consultant

Frederick G. Ruffner, Jr., Publisher

Copyright © 1998, Omnigraphics, Inc.

Library of Congress Cataloging-in-Publication Data

```
Oral health sourcebook : basic information about diseases and
   conditions affecting oral health ... / edited by Allan R. Cook.
       p.   cm. -- (Health reference series ; v. 30)
   Includes bibliographical references and index.
   ISBN 0-7808-0082-6 (lib. bdg. : alk. paper)
   1. Dentistry--Popular works.  2. Mouth--Diseases.  3. Mouth--Care
and hygiene.   I. Cook, Allan R.   II. Series.
RK61.O66  1997
617.5'22--dc21                                              97-28301
                                                                CIP
```

∞

Printed in the United States of America

Table of Contents

Part III: Gum Disease

Part IV: The Oral Cavity, Including the Tongue, Lips, and Throat

Part V: The Jaw and Other Structural Problems

Part VI: Braces, Implants, and Dentures

Part VII: Special Needs and Concerns

Part VIII: Dental Emergencies

Preface

About This Book

Oral diseases and disorders are perhaps the most universal of all afflictions. An estimated 99.5 percent of Americans will have experienced dental caries (cavities) by the time they reach age 65, and some 10 million of them will have lost all their teeth. Half of all Americans over age 55 wear some form of partial or complete denture and 60 percent of them complain of improper fit or function. And the process starts early. In 1996, some 45 percent of all school-aged children had dental caries in their permanent teeth, and 38 percent of children aged 2-9 had caries in their primary (baby) teeth. Half of these had not been treated for the tooth decay.

High cost seems to be the primary barrier to treatment. In 1992, expenditures for dental care topped $38.7 billion. By the year 2000, that number is expected to rise to $62.3 billion.

Other oral disorders stemming from genetic, chronic and immune disorders also affect millions of Americans yearly. Oropharyngeal cancer alone strikes approximately 30,000 Americans yearly and kills 8,000.

This book contains basic information for the layperson on a wide range of common oral disorders and conditions and offers simple and inexpensive methods of promoting oral health. Patients, family members, and the interested general public will find useful tips for maintaining a regimen of oral hygiene, responding to dental emergencies, and identifying oral conditions that require medical attention.

Bibliographic Note

This volume contains individual publications issued by the following government agencies: National Institute of Dental Research (NIDR); National Institute of Aging (NIA); National Institutes of Health (NIH); Wisconsin Department of Health and Social Services, Division of Health and Social Services; Arizona Department of Health Services, Office of Oral Health; New York State Dental Sealant Program; *Public Health Reports*; Food and Drug Administration (FDA); *FDA Consumer*; Centers for Disease Control; U.S. Department of Health and Human Services; *NCRR Reporter*; and the Maine Department of Human Services, Office of Dental Health.

The volume also includes non-government, non-copyrighted materials reprinted with acknowledgment from the following sources: Johnson & Johnson Consumer Products, Inc.; and The Kaiser Foundation, National AIDS Treatment Information Project.

In addition it uses copyrighted materials reprinted with permission from the following sources: the American Academy of Periodontology; the American Association of Endodontists; *American Health*; the American Heart Association; the Boston, MA HIV Dental Ombudsman Program, Division of Public Health, Boston Department of Health and Hospitals; the BoWoW Kids; the Cleft Palate Foundation; *Consumer Reports*; Consumers Union; *FACES*: The National Association for the Craniofacially Handicapped; the *Journal of the American Dental Association* (JADA); *Mayo Clinic Health Letter*; the Tennessee Craniofacial Center; and the United Scleroderma Foundation.

All copyrighted material is reprinted with permission. Document numbers where applicable and specific source citations are provided on the first page of each chapter. Every effort has been made to secure all necessary rights to reprint the copyrighted material. If any omissions have been made, contact Omnigraphics to make corrections for future editions.

How To Use This Book

This book is divided into parts and chapters. Parts focus on broad areas of interest and chapters on specific topics within those areas.

Part I: *Oral Health* outlines the general concerns of oral health and gives some advice on basic oral hygiene. It also provides statistical information on the oral health of Americans and programs to promote improvements.

Part II: *Teeth* looks specifically at the teeth and their care, considering specifically ways to fight tooth decay and repair cavities.

Part III: *Gum Disease* focuses on the gums as anchors for teeth and examines some common conditions that can lead to early tooth loss.

Part IV: *The Oral Cavity Including the Tongue, Lips, and Throat* broadens the examination to include the rest of the oral cavity and presents some major concerns including cancer, thrush, Xerostomia, and Sjögren's Syndrome.

Part V: *The Jaw and Other Structural Problems* looks at the underlying structure of bones and joints and some common temporomandibular disorders and other craniofacial syndromes and their treatments.

Part VI: *Braces, Implants, and Dentures* considers the options for straightening and stabilizing misaligned teeth and for replacing lost teeth.

Part VII: *Special Needs and Concerns* addresses the oral concerns of patients with heart disease, cancer, diabetes and other conditions. It also outlines the current recommendations for infection control in dentistry.

Part VIII: *Dental Emergencies* identifies the probable source of tooth pain and gives specific first-aid suggestions for dental emergencies.

Index: gives page references and cross-references for key words and phrases used in the various articles.

Acknowledgments

Many people and organizations have contributed the material that comprises this volume. The editor gratefully acknowledges the assistance and cooperation of the American Academy of Periodontology; the American Association of Endodontists; *American Health*; the American Heart Association; the Boston, MA HIV Dental Ombudsman Program, Division of Public Health, Boston Department of Health and Hospitals; the BoWoW Kids; the Cleft Palate Foundation; *Consumer Reports*; Consumers Union; *FACES*: The National Association for the

Craniofacially Handicapped; Johnson & Johnson Consumer Products, Inc.; the *Journal of the American Dental Association* (JADA); The Kaiser Foundation, National AIDS Treatment Information Project; *Mayo Clinic Health Letter*; and the Tennessee Craniofacial Center; the United Scleroderma Foundation. Special thanks to Margaret Mary Missar for her patient search for the documents that make up this volume, Karen Bellenir for her technical assistance and advice, Bruce the Scanman and special assistant Mike for their textual recycling and Valerie Cook for her sharp-eyed verification.

Note from the Editor

This book is part of Omnigraphics' *Health Reference Series*. The series provides basic information about a broad range of medical concerns. It is not intended to serve as a tool for diagnosing illness, in prescribing treatments, or as a substitute for the physician/patient relationship. All persons concerned about medical symptoms or the possibility of disease are encouraged to seek professional care from an appropriate health care provider.

Part One

Oral Health

Chapter 1

Perspectives on Dental Science

Dental Science—Dental Health

Dental science has matured from a narrow concern with teeth and gums to encompass all the oral tissues, their normal metabolism, function, and pathology, as well as the behaviors associated with the cause and prevention of disease and the maintenance of oral health. This expanded domain of research is manifest in current studies of oral viral infections, genetic anomalies, bone and joint diseases, oral cancers, acute and chronic pain conditions, salivary gland dysfunctions, and public, provider, socio-environmental, and cultural dimensions of oral health and disability.

These investigations have led to some remarkable recent achievements, notably in the development of an *in vitro* system to measure the invasiveness of tumor cells and the development of new anti-metastatic drugs, the isolation of protein growth factors for bone, the identification of the precise region of immunoglobulin receptors responsible for hypersensitivity reactions, new experimental vaccines against oral herpes virus infections, and anti-inflammatory and anti-enzymatic agents to counter the destructive effects of chronic inflammatory reactions.

NIH Publication No. 88-1868. National Institute of Dental Research, 1988. *NIDR at 40.*

3

A Look to the Future

In the course of four decades, research has made enormous strides in our understanding of oral diseases, as well as in methods to prevent them. Without question, dentistry has moved further down the road of prevention than any other health discipline. The next 40 years also can be expected to bring their share of surprises in new discoveries, new treatments—and new diseases.

New directions in research will contribute to a major task that the NIDR has undertaken for well into the 1990s: the development of a Research and Action Program which will unite biomedical and behavioral scientists, the dental profession, industry, and the general public in working toward the elimination of toothlessness and the prevention of diseases and disorders of the mouth.

In perhaps another 40 years, the major oral diseases which have plagued mankind since ancient times will be under control. Scientific advances will allow dentists to expand their role to address the full range of diseases and disorders that affect the oral and facial tissues. Dentists will strengthen their partnership with other biomedical specialists and, by virtue of their broader diagnostic and therapeutic scope and skills, these physicians of the mouth will be able to maintain the health of the teeth and associated tissues over a lifetime.

Research Highlights

The NIDR supports more than 1,000 research and training programs at some 200 institutions worldwide; another hundred projects are under way in NIDR's own laboratories on the NIH campus. NIDR-supported scientists are working on periodontal diseases, caries, salivary disorders, craniofacial anomalies, and behaviors that affect oral health. They are looking at bone and other mineralized tissues, at the immune responses that figure in oral health and disease, at viruses that invade oral tissues. New technologies and information emerging from dental research laboratories are refining our understanding and treatment of oral tissues—and of the human organism as a whole. The following examples of NIDR-sponsored research give some idea of the range and importance of dental science today.

Periodontal Diseases

The discovery three decades ago that the periodontal diseases are infectious in nature set the stage for today's intensive research attack against these age-old disorders. The focus now is on identifying the bacteria responsible for periodontal destruction, clarifying host-bacterial interactions, understanding the pathological process more fully, and determining the role of genetic and environmental factors in the natural history of periodontal disease.

Regenerating Periodontal Tissues. As periodontal disease progresses, bacteria attack and destroy the connective tissue fibers and bone supporting the tooth. Eventually, the tooth loosens and falls out. New lines of research suggest it may be possible to rebuild the supporting tissues and restore tooth attachment. This approach depends on allowing the preferential migration of periodontal ligament cells to the site of periodontal destruction. These cells and their progeny have the potential of generating new bone, new fibers, and new hard tissue around the root of the tooth, thereby enabling the tooth to regain its firm anchorage in the jaw.

Chemically Modified Tetracycline. Recent work has shown that in addition to its antibiotic properties, tetracycline inhibits production of collagenase, an enzyme that destroys collagen. It is collagen destruction that leads to the gradual deterioration of supporting tissues in periodontal disease and other connective tissue disorders. Concerns that long-term use of tetracycline might induce development of resistant strains of bacteria have limited its use in periodontal treatment. Now, NIDR grantees have modified the drug, removing its antibiotic properties while conserving its anti-collagenase activity. The chemically modified tetracycline should be safe and effective for long-term use in treating periodontal diseases and other collagen-related disorders, such as rheumatoid arthritis.

Overcoming Problems of Diagnosis. One problem dentists face in trying to control periodontal diseases is the lack of simple methods for distinguishing active from quiescent states in disease progression. Typically, serial x-rays are used to record bone loss over time. In order to reverse the disease process, however, intervention must be introduced early, before significant bone loss has occurred. Also, there is a need to identify individuals at risk for the severe and rapidly progressive forms of periodontal disease, some of which may be hereditary.

The advent of more sophisticated radiological, biochemical, and genetic diagnostic methods is helping to resolve this problem. Digitized subtraction radiography and nuclear medicine techniques introduced recently can detect subtle changes in bone, providing a sensitive measure of periodontal disease activity. Also coming into use are molecular biology tools that can detect signs of inflammation and immune responses at selected sites in the mouth.

These investigations are providing insight into the pathological processes of periodontal destruction, especially the more severe genetic forms.

Blocking Bacterial Attachment. Attachment of harmful bacteria to host tissues is prerequisite to the initiation of most infectious diseases. Scientists have discovered that many bacteria implicated in periodontal disease attach to oral tissues, or to bacteria already affixed to the tissues, through the interaction of proteins called adhesins and receptors for these proteins located on the surfaces of oral tissues or bacteria.

Already, investigators have characterized the adhesin molecules and their receptors on several species of disease-causing bacteria, and are determining the amino acid sequences of the proteins. This basic research on bacterial attachment and colonization has a number of possible clinical applications. Down the road, it may be possible to use adhesins to diagnose periodontal disease or to raise antibodies that would interfere with bacterial attachment to oral tissues. It might also be possible to block bacterial colonization by introducing adhesins from harmless oral bacteria into a diseased periodontal pocket; the adhesins would bind to receptors on gum tissues or bacteria, making these receptors unavailable to new disease-causing bacteria.

Caries

Most technologically advanced countries have experienced significant declines in the prevalence of tooth decay since the advent of fluoride several decades ago. Nevertheless, there remain individuals who, for unknown reasons, are highly susceptible to dental caries. It is estimated that 20 percent of school children account for 80 percent of the tooth decay in U.S. youngsters.

Identifying High-Risk Individuals. Until recently, the techniques available for identifying caries-prone individuals have been generally inadequate. Investigators now have devised better sampling techniques and are using genetic probes and monoclonal antibodies to detect specific organisms or molecules of interest. The availability of safe, accurate techniques for identifying caries-susceptible children will make it possible to reduce the risk factors for those individuals, thereby preserving their teeth. At the same time, these highly refined diagnostic approaches will enhance our understanding of the natural history of dental caries and the events that lead to alterations in oral ecology.

Caries Resistance. The study revealed that 40 percent of the first-degree relatives of caries-free adults were also completely free of tooth decay. The investigator attributed this finding to differences in the salivary components of caries-free and caries-susceptible individuals. Something in the saliva of caries-free adults may inhibit production of the acids that destroy tooth enamel, for example, or it may be that the saliva of caries-resistant adults is more effective at buffering and neutralizing the acids before they can attack the enamel.

Fluoride. Fluoride remains the most effective weapon available in the fight against tooth decay. Not only does it protect tooth enamel against bacterial acids, fluoride also reverses the early stages of decay by aiding in remineralization of the teeth. Today almost 7,000 communities nationwide—over half the U.S. population—fluoridate their drinking water. In addition, approximately 13 million children participate in school-based fluoride mouth-rinsing programs.

NIDR continues to monitor the oral health effects of fluoride. An Institute-funded study recently found that children develop almost 50 percent fewer cavities during their junior high school years if they participated in fluoride mouth-rinsing programs from kindergarten through sixth grade. Studies such as this help school, community, and dental leaders develop effective public health strategies for fighting tooth decay.

Restoratives

While progress toward disease prevention moves full speed ahead, the need remains to provide safe, effective, and reliable treatment for the millions of people who suffer from the broad range of dental disorders. Today, dental scientists are developing restorative materials and techniques that will allow dentists to repair decayed teeth with minimal cavity preparation and less removal of healthy tooth substance than are required for traditional amalgam restorations.

New Bonding Materials. New synthetic materials that can bond directly to tooth enamel are transforming restorative dentistry by reducing the need for drilling. Until recently, however, the new materials have not been as successful for treating lesions that affect the dentin—the softer mineralized tissue underlying enamel. Now NIDR grantees have perfected techniques that have doubled and tripled the strength of the bonds between the synthetics and dentin. Once the mechanisms and nature of the process are understood better, it should be possible to vary components in order to develop bonding materials reliable enough for use in the dental office. Potential uses include the treatment of cervical and root lesions, repairs of tooth crowns, and as protective coatings on tooth root surfaces exposed by gum recession.

Sealing in Decay. In the early 1970s, dental researchers developed acrylic sealants that could be painted onto teeth to seal out decay. Now they are finding that one approach to treating small caries lesions is to seal in the decay. A sealed composite restoration is placed on an early caries lesion, with no cavity preparation or removal of the lesion. Clinical tests have shown no sign of disease progression up to four years after placement.

Saliva

Human salivary glands secrete about a quart of saliva daily. This natural liquid—composed of water and about 30 other ingredients—protects, maintains, and even repairs oral tissues. In addition, saliva is an essential component of the digestive process. Salivary enzymes initiate the breakdown of starches and macromolecules in food, and saliva lubricates food so it can be swallowed easily. Saliva also acts as a solvent for the tastable elements in food, allowing these molecules to bathe and excite the cells in taste buds lining the tongue.

Saliva and Taste. Recent work by NIDR scientists has changed our thinking about the role of saliva in taste. It was believed that saliva nourished the taste buds and was necessary for their growth. Without saliva, it was thought, we could not taste food. The NIDR researchers now have found that taste cells may continue to function normally despite a chronic absence of saliva. They tested a group of patients with complete salivary gland dysfunction and found that the patients could taste normally if they used water to dissolve their food. This finding demonstrates that saliva does not contain unique factors essential for taste bud growth and survival, but plays a key part in taste by dissolving food and delivering it to the taste buds.

Treating Dry Mouth. Other NIDR researchers are developing better treatments for patients suffering from dry mouth. This condition—characterized by a decrease in salivary flow and a change in the composition of saliva—is not a disease, but a common side effect of many medications and medical treatments. It is also a symptom of certain disorders, including Sjögren's syndrome. Patients with dry mouth are at risk for developing rampant caries; in severe cases, they experience difficulty eating, swallowing, and even speaking. NIDR scientists are using small doses of pilocarpine—a drug that opens blocked secretory channels—to restore salivary flow. Clinical trials show that when pilocarpine is taken three times daily, it can significantly restore salivary flow in patients who have some functional salivary gland tissue.

Craniofacial Malformations

A quarter of a million babies—7 percent of all infants born in the United States each year—have some mental or physical defect that is evident at birth or later on. Common among these defects are craniofacial malformations, defined as any structural, functional, or biochemical abnormality of the head or face.

Dental researchers have made important contributions to the field of craniofacial anomalies through genetic and cell biology studies of the various hereditary defects involving the head and face. The most common of these disorders are cleft lip and cleft palate. Scientists believe these and other structural abnormalities of the jaw and facial bones are caused by a combination of genetic and environmental factors.

Genetic Basis for Cleft Lip. Oriental populations have a higher incidence of cleft lip and cleft palate than do other ethnic groups. In a recent study of these craniofacial defects in Chinese families, NIDR grantees reported preliminary findings indicating that cleft lip—with or without cleft palate—may be caused by a single gene in this population. The gene seems to put a fetus at risk of developing the defect if the fetus is exposed to specific environmental factors. The researchers now are trying to identify this gene and to define its structure. This knowledge will aid in detecting people who are carriers of the gene.

Pain

With more than one-fourth of all chronic pain localized in the orificial region, it is not surprising that dental scientists are at the forefront of pain research. At the NIH, the dental institute heads the country's first multidisciplinary pain clinic devoted entirely to research. There, NIDR staff—in collaboration with scientists from other NIH institutes—investigate the causes, measurement, and treatment of a variety of acute and chronic pain conditions.

Relieving Post-operative Pain. Investigators recently found that patients who take a nonsteroidal anti-inflammatory drug such as ibuprofen before having their third molars extracted experience significant reductions in post-operative pain. Patients who receive ibuprofen or similar drugs secrete higher levels of the hormone beta-endorphin, which is associated with pain reduction. Follow-up studies are looking at the effects of various drugs on beta-endorphin release and the role of the hormone in modifying pain perception.

Relieving the Pain of Neuropathies. Clinical investigators have affirmed the usefulness of tricyclic antidepressants in the treatment of painful peripheral neuropathies. They have found that the drug amitriptyline relieves atypical facial pain as well as pain associated with diabetes and shingles. Myofascial pain can be controlled by the combination of ibuprofen and diazepam, an anti-anxiety drug, they found. Other studies are exploring pharmacological and non-pharmacological methods for enhancing the analgesia produced by activating the brain's own pain-suppressing systems.

Mineralized Tissues

The past decade has seen great strides in research on mineralized tissues. Earlier studies of bones and teeth have paid off in important discoveries about collagen, tooth enamel, and the factors that regulate growth, maintenance, and repair of the body's hard tissues. With these findings has come increased understanding of the destructive processes at work in a broad range of bone diseases. Clinical researchers are using this basic information to develop new therapies for systemic disorders as well as new approaches for the diagnosis and treatment of dental diseases.

Regenerating Bone. NIDR grantees are trying to isolate and produce the naturally generated compounds that promote the growth and repair of cartilage and bone. The hope is that one day these compounds can be used to correct bone- or cartilage-related birth defects. One research group has isolated a protein from bone that induces cells drawn to a fracture site to develop into cartilage cells. The cartilage is then transformed into bone. The researchers are now assessing the most effective way of applying the protein—called chondrogenic-stimulating activity (CSA) protein—to broken bones to facilitate healing. Once a CSA delivery system is perfected, researchers may be able to use the protein together with other compounds to reconstruct cartilage or bone in children born with deformed jaws, shortened limbs, facial asymmetries, and other anomalies. The compounds could also be used to regenerate bone in children or adults who have had large sections of bone removed in the course of cancer therapy.

Soft Tissue Diseases

The mouth is a complex assemblage of mineralized tissues—teeth and jaw bones—and varied soft tissues, including the lips, gums, tongue, palate, and salivary glands. The problems affecting the oral soft tissues are as diverse as the tissues themselves, ranging in severity from self-healing mouth ulcers to highly malignant oral cancers.

Cancers of the mouth are very serious, often growing quickly and invading other tissues. Oral cancers account for 9,000 deaths annually in the United States. The major cause of death in patients with oral cancer—or any type of cancer—is metastasis, or the spread of tumor cells to healthy tissues.

Understanding Metastasis. Researchers in NIDR's intramural program are devoting considerable effort to understanding the events involved in the spread of cancer. It is known that basement membranes—tough structures that underlie epithelia and surround blood vessels and many other tissues of the body—form a major barrier to tumor cell invasion. Most tumor cells cannot penetrate this barrier, and do not metastasize. Malignant cells, however, are able to attach to and degrade basement membranes, giving the cancer cells access to the circulation and healthy tissues.

The NIDR investigators have identified the precise site on basement membranes to which malignant cells attach: a five-amino-acid peptide within the protein laminin, a major component of basement membranes. They synthesized the peptide and tested its ability to block tumor metastasis in laboratory mice. A group of control mice injected with highly malignant melanoma cells developed numerous lung metastases. Mice who received the peptide along with the melanoma cells, however, developed few or no lung metastases. The researchers concluded that the synthetic peptide competed with laminin

11

for the laminin receptors on the tumor cells, thereby blocking the attachment of the cells to basement membranes. Instead of metastasizing, the melanoma cells died in the circulation.

The same group of researchers has developed a simple, rapid *in vitro* assay for measuring the invasiveness of tumor cells. The assay measures the ability of cells to cross a synthetic basement membrane gel, which was developed by the NIDR scientists. The assay is already being tested for its potential to assess the malignancy of human tumors. At one Midwestern medical school, for example, an oncologist is using the assay to predict whether prostate tumors can metastasize — information that is critical in deciding how aggressively to treat the disease. The assay is also being used at NIDR and elsewhere to rapidly screen drugs for their ability to block the metastatic potential of tumors. This application could lead to the development of new anti-cancer treatments.

Smokeless Tobacco. Using smokeless tobacco increases the risk of oral cancer and, according to a recent study, may increase the risk of periodontal disease. Investigators report that periodontal ligament cells taken from extracted third molars are severely limited in growth or even destroyed when exposed to high concentrations of smokeless tobacco extract. Periodontal ligament cells are the cells responsible for the attachment of teeth to bone. According to recent estimates, about 10 million Americans use smokeless tobacco, almost a third of whom are under age 21.

Behavioral Studies

Behavioral and social science research at the NIDR focuses not only on strategies for promoting oral health, but also on the behavioral contributors to oral disease. Behaviors can play a role in the etiology of many oral diseases, including oral cancer and certain orificial pain syndromes. Studies have shown that temporomandibular joint (TMJ) disorders may be correlated with stress, and some current interpretations of the etiology of TMJ dysfunction emphasize the role of psychological factors leading to chronic orificial muscular hyperactivity.

TMJ Studies. Patients with TMJ pain or dysfunction often suffer from other pain conditions and physical illnesses as well, researchers have found. In one study, investigators assessed the role of psychosocial risk factors in a group of TMJ patients. During monthly interviews, they collected information on the patients' stress level, social support, general health, emotional state, and other variables. They found that TMJ patients tend to be distressed individuals beleaguered by many physical illnesses and injuries as well as pain. A second study looked at TMJ patients enrolled in a health maintenance organization. More than half the patients suffering from jaw pain also reported back pain, 41 percent reported headaches, 25 percent reported abdominal pain, and 18 percent reported chest pain.

For the first time, epidemiological studies are providing information on the prevalence of TMJ disorders among North American populations. These studies are producing important leads on characteristics differentiating individuals who seek care from those who do not. Significantly, disorders of the TMJ and associated muscles of mastication have been identified as the major source of non-dental pain in the orificial region. Demands for treatment of these disorders are increasing. Encouraging preventive behaviors research has shown us how to prevent many oral problems; the challenge is getting people to adopt preventive behaviors. Behavioral scientists are focusing on ways to increase adherence to preventive dental regimens. In a recent study, brushing and flossing behaviors were evaluated. At the beginning of the study, only 14 percent of the participants practiced regular, effective flossing. Some behavioral interventions, such as those using social supports (for example, small group instructional sessions involving college roommates in systematic reminder and mutual reinforcement programs to sustain flossing) were not effective in the long run. More promising results are reported from interventions using multiple educational and behavioral components, such as self-monitoring, performance contracts, and periodic feedback on gingival health.

AIDS

Since it was first reported in the United States in 1981, acquired immunodeficiency syndrome (AIDS) has had a significant impact on the nation's health and health policy. The high mortality and increasing incidence of AIDS have prompted a massive marshaling of resources to counteract the disease. NIDR investigators are conducting basic, clinical, and epidemiological studies to learn more about the natural history of AIDS and, in particular, its oral manifestations and their clinical management.

HIV and Saliva. The human immunodeficiency virus (HIV)—the virus that causes AIDS—has been recovered from human saliva, but very infrequently. The consensus among researchers is that the virus is not secreted from salivary glands, but rather is a contaminant from blood or gum fluids mixing with the saliva in the mouth. Now NIDR scientists have found in preliminary studies that human salivary glands secrete a factor that actually blocks the AIDS virus from infecting cells. Their finding may help explain why the disease is not transmitted orally. The researchers collected saliva samples from a small group of healthy men not in any known risk group for AIDS. They collected whole saliva, and they collected secretions directly from the major salivary glands. Both whole saliva and submandibular/sublingual gland secretions rendered HIV unable to infect lymphocytes—immune cells which are major targets for HIV—whereas parotid gland secretions in general provided little or no protection against the virus. The experiments showed that the inhibitory activity of saliva comes from the salivary glands, not from any contaminant in the mouth. The researchers now are expanding these preliminary studies and are trying to identify the inhibitory factor.

Early Oral Signs of AIDS. Dental researchers have documented the frequent occurrence of HIV-related infections in the mouth, in many cases before the development of full-blown AIDS. These infections include oral Kaposi's sarcoma; oral candidiasis, herpes virus, and papillomavirus infections; unusually severe forms of gingivitis and periodontal disease; and hairy leukoplakia, a condition characterized by patches of whitish corrugated tissue seen most often on the tongue. In other work, studies of salivary secretions of HIV-infected individuals in good health have shown there may be specific changes in salivary components early in the course of infection. If confirmed, these signs may be important diagnostic markers for AIDS.

AIDS and Monocytes. NIDR scientists have established that monocytes—cells of the immune system that identify and kill infectious agents—can themselves be infected by HIV, which seriously impairs the cells' defense functions. The loss of a potent monocyte population leaves the AIDS patient more susceptible to opportunistic infections. The Institute is continuing basic immunological studies on the role of the monocyte in AIDS.

Developing AIDS Treatments. Several treatments for AIDS are under development at the NIDR. One involves the production of human monoclonal antibodies to HIV using blood drawn from healthy subjects who have been inoculated with the new HIV subunit vaccine.

14

Other experimental therapies include the synthesis of proteins that can bind to the same receptor on T4 cells (major targets of HIV infection) to which HIV attaches, thereby blocking viral attachment. The synthetic proteins, linked to antiviral drugs, might also gain access to infected cells and destroy the AIDS virus while sparing the cell.

NIDR-Army Collaboration. A collaborative epidemiological project that adds an oral component to a Walter Reed Army Institute of Research longitudinal study is being expanded. Army personnel who test positive for HIV may enter a study in which they are examined periodically and classified into one of several stages of HIV infection. The dental component allows monitoring of saliva and oral tissue changes over time, and permits analysis of data relating to risk factors, systemic changes, and other variables associated with HIV infection.

Caries Prevalence among U.S. School Children

"Look Ma, no cavities."

That was the headline in newspapers across the country in June 1988, when NIDR officials announced the results of a nationwide survey of children's oral health. The survey revealed that half of U.S. school children, ages 5 to 17, have no tooth decay. Only a generation ago, dental caries was rampant in this country, affecting virtually all school-age children.

Evidence that one out of two youngsters is caries free comes from the National Survey of Oral Health in U.S. School children: 1986-87, a follow-up to a similar survey conducted in 1980. In both studies, NIDR-trained dentists performed oral examinations on 40,000 children at almost a thousand schools located throughout the United States. The sample populations were chosen to represent the approximately 43 million school children in the country.

Caries Decline Continues. The new survey showed that American children have 36 percent less dental caries today than they did at the beginning of the decade. That decline follows a similar drop in the prevalence of tooth decay during the 1970s.

It also showed that 49.9 percent of all children have no decay in their permanent teeth. In 1980, 36.6 percent of U.S. schoolchildren were caries free. An estimated 28 percent had no tooth decay in the early 1970s.

Not only are fewer children getting cavities today, but those who do are getting fewer of them. In 1980, children had an average of almost five decayed, missing, or filled surfaces (DMFS) on their permanent teeth (out of 128 possible surfaces). In 1987, they had an average of only three DMFS. The average number of decayed or filled surfaces on the deciduous teeth of 5- to 9-year-olds dropped from more than five in 1980 to fewer than four in 1987.

Fluoride Credited. The NIDR survey did not address the question of what is causing the decline in dental caries, but Institute epidemiologists believe the widespread use of fluoride—in community water supplies, toothpastes, and other forms—is mainly responsible. Improved diet and oral hygiene, combined with preventive services in the dental office, are also playing a role in caries reduction.

Significantly, decay on the smooth surfaces of teeth—the surfaces that benefit most from fluoride—is disappearing, the survey results showed. Today, two-thirds of caries is found on the occlusal, or chewing, surfaces of teeth. Decay on occlusal surfaces could be virtually eliminated, NIDR officials say, by the combined use of fluorides and adhesive sealants.

The survey findings revealed that interproximal caries, or decay on the surfaces between adjoining teeth, is approaching eradication. The prevalence of interproximal caries dropped 54 percent between 1980 and 1987, while the prevalence of decay on occlusal surfaces and the exposed smooth surfaces of teeth dropped 32 percent.

Regional Differences Noted. While the country as a whole experienced a decline in the prevalence of dental caries, regional differences noted since the 1940s again emerged in the 1987 survey. Children in the Northeast and Pacific Coast regions continue to have the highest prevalence of tooth decay, while youngsters in the Southwest have the least caries. The reasons behind these consistent geographic disparities remain an epidemiologic puzzle.

Other findings of the new survey are that females have slightly more decay than males—a pattern seen in earlier studies, and that the level of dental care has improved somewhat since 1980. Today, 82 percent of DMFS are filled, about 13 percent are decayed, and 4 percent are missing. Seven years ago, 76 percent of DMFS were filled, 17 percent were decayed, and 7 percent were missing.

A comparison of two NIDR national surveys of children's oral health shows that the declines in tooth decay at the beginning of the decade are continuing. Today, half of U.S. school children ages 5 to 17 have never had a cavity.

Focus Shifts to High-Risk Groups. Despite the dramatic declines in tooth decay over the past two decades, caries will probably never be completely eradicated, NIDR epidemiologists say. There remain individuals in all segments of society who are caries prone, as well as persons who are unable or unwilling to perform appropriate self-care or to seek dental services regularly. The recent successes against tooth decay in children will allow the dental research community to channel its efforts toward these high-risk populations, and to the oral health needs of older Americans.

The Oral Health Status of American Adults

Quietly, almost unnoticed, modern dentistry has changed the face of America. The new American face has healthier teeth, and more of them. Toothlessness has been almost eliminated among middle-aged adults, and caries is on the decline, at least in people under age 35. Americans visit their dentist regularly for preventive checkups and enjoy a high level of dental care. Those are the findings of the National Survey of Oral Health in U.S. Employed Adults and Seniors, conducted by the NIDR in 1985. The survey was the most comprehensive of its kind, and the first to look at the prevalence of root caries and periodontal disease in detail.

Few Working Adults Toothless. Over the course of a year, NIDR-trained dentists conducted oral examinations on almost 21,000 adults aged 18 to 103. The examinations took place at 800 business establishments and 200 senior centers located throughout the continental United States. The sample population, divided into employed adults aged 18-64 and non-employed seniors aged 65 and older, was chosen to represent more than 100 million working adults and 4 million older Americans.

The survey showed that half of all working adults aged 18 to 64 had lost at most one tooth. Very few—only 4 percent—were toothless. Unfortunately, toothlessness remains a major problem among Americans aged 65 and older. Forty-one percent of the older people were missing all their teeth, and only 2 percent still had all 28 teeth (third molars were not included in this survey).

Caries Still a Problem. Both younger and older adults continue to suffer from decay on the crowns of teeth, with a slightly higher rate in females than in males. Employed adults had an average of 23 decayed or filled coronal surfaces (out of 128 possible surfaces in people with all their teeth), and seniors had an average of 20. (Older people would be expected to have fewer DFS, because they have fewer teeth left.) Almost 95 percent of the coronal lesions in both groups had been filled—an extraordinarily high level of dental care.

Decay of tooth roots was three times more extensive in seniors than in working adults. Root caries was found in 21 percent of the employed adults and 63 percent of the seniors. In both groups, only about half of the lesions had been filled. Root caries was more prevalent in men than in women—a reversal of the trend seen with coronal caries.

Assessing Periodontal Health. The majority of the adults surveyed showed signs of periodontal disease, with increasing prevalence and worsening of symptoms with age. Two measures were used to assess periodontal health: gums were gently probed at 28 sites to check for bleeding, and the sites were examined for loss of attachment of supporting tissues from the teeth.

Gingival bleeding was noted in 43 percent of the working adults and 47 percent of the seniors. Seventy-seven percent of the working adults and 95 percent of the older group had at least one site with periodontal attachment loss measuring 2 millimeters or more. More severe periodontal destruction—attachment loss of 4 mm or more— was found in 24 percent of the employed adults and 68 percent of the older persons. Fewer than 8 percent of working adults and 34 percent of seniors had attachment loss of 6 mm or more. In both age groups, males had a higher rate of periodontal destruction than did females.

Level of Dental Care High. The survey revealed that Americans are going to the dentist. Eighty percent of the employed adults and 76 percent of the seniors who still had teeth had visited a dentist within the past two years. Almost 60 percent of the employed group and half of the seniors said the main reason for their last visit was prevention and checkup. Only 29 percent of the edentulous seniors had seen a dentist in the past two years; not surprisingly, more than 70 percent said the main reason for their last visit was prosthodontics.

Adults' Dental Health Improving. While the older segments of our society continue to suffer high rates of dental disease, the overall picture from the survey is one of continuing improvement in the oral health status of American adults. Comparison of the new data to those of surveys conducted in 1960-62, 1971-74, and 1981 clearly demonstrate that people are keeping their teeth longer today. The prevalence of coronal caries has declined during the past decade, at least in people under age 35. With the results of both the 1985 adult survey and the 1987 children's survey in hand, NIDR now has reliable data on the oral health of some 150 million Americans aged 5 to 85-plus.

Chapter 2

The Mouth as the Body's Mirror

The mouth: Lovers kiss with it, babies coo with it, fighters curl it in rage, winners lift it up in victory, and the doctor looks into it.

In fact, approximately 20 percent of visits to the doctor are because of mouth or throat complaints. But by peering into the mouth, the doctor may discover more than a strep infection or a canker sore. It is a truism in medical circles that the mouth is the mirror of the body. "The mouth is affected by many bodily processes," says Jerome Goldstein, M.D., executive vice president of the American Academy of Otolaryngology—Head and Neck Surgery.

When the doctor asks you to stick out your tongue and say "aah," he or she may discover tell-tale clues that reflect underlying disorders elsewhere in the body. Stories are legendary of physicians who looked carefully at a patient's tongue and cleverly diagnosed disorders in other areas of the body.

Donald R. Haggerty, D.D.S., M.D., a medical officer with the Food and Drug Administration, recalls a patient who complained of a persistent bad taste in her mouth. Haggerty discovered multiple telangiectasis (little red spots formed by dilated blood vessels) in her mouth. Further evaluation revealed difficulty in swallowing and cold hands, leading to a diagnosis of a particular connective tissue disease—a serious chronic disease of the skin and internal organs.

Other disorders may also signal their presence by oral symptoms. Gums that have grown over the teeth may mean a patient has leukemia. A red or furry tongue may indicate scarlet fever; a tongue covered

FDA Consumer, Dec 89-Jan 90.

21

with brownish sores, typhoid fever; and a pale, smooth glossy tongue, pernicious anemia. A fine black line that appears on the gums is an important diagnostic sign of chronic lead poisoning, while spongy gums signal chronic mercury poisoning.

A doctor can also find diagnostic clues to Addison's disease (a disease of the adrenal glands that afflicted the late President John F. Kennedy), diabetes mellitus, vitamin B deficiency, scurvy, Sjögren's syndrome (an autoimmune disorder described in the February 1989 *FDA Consumer* article "Eyes Too Dry to Cry: How Sjögren's Syndrome Makes the Body a 'Desert'" Reprinted in this volume), inflammatory bowel disease, and multiple sclerosis by examining the oral cavity. Foul breath may indicate a lung abscess. Pain in the jaw may mean a patient is suffering from angina. And an extended tongue that bends to one side may indicate a stroke.

"The mouth is a valuable reflection of what's going on elsewhere in the body," says Goldstein.

Common Complaints

Although the condition of the mouth can provide a wealth of information about disorders elsewhere in the body, in most cases, complaints about the mouth or throat are usually more mundane. Following are some of the most common reasons people visit the doctor for mouth problems.

Fever Blisters or Cold Sores: Painful little blisters about the size of a dime that usually form on the lips, cold sores are caused by herpes simplex virus type-one or HSV-1. (Genital herpes is caused by a cousin, known as HSV-2.) Most people have been infected by the virus (40 percent of Americans acquire the virus by age 30), but it lies dormant in the body, flaring up from time to time with a cold or fever, exposure to excessive sunlight, or during periods of stress. People with cold sores should avoid kissing others and making skin contact with newborns or people with weakened immune systems—who are particularly vulnerable to infection.

There is no cure for cold sores; they must run their course. Keeping the affected area clean or using a protective cream may help relieve the pain. Over-the-counter products usually contain astringents that dry tissues, but these products do not necessarily speed healing. People who are susceptible to cold sores brought on by sun exposure should use a sunscreen on their lips. Persons experiencing recurring cold sores should consult their doctors. One drug for treating herpes, Zovirax (acyclovir), is available by prescription as either an ointment or capsule.

Canker Sores: Not to be confused with cold sores, these sores are ulcers that occur in the mucous membrane inside the mouth. They can range from the size of a pinhead to the size of a quarter and may appear alone or in clusters. Most canker sores heal within two weeks, although recurrent canker sores may afflict some people. One out of every two people will have at least one episode during their lifetimes.

The cause of canker sores remains a mystery, although stress may be a factor. For example, college students are most often afflicted before exam time. Certain foods, such as nuts, or sweet and acidic foods may cause canker sores. They may also result from deficiencies of folic acid, iron, or vitamin B12. Even genetics play a role; a predisposition to canker sores runs in families.

There is no treatment that speeds healing, but antiseptic mouthwashes may prevent their spread. "Washing the infected area with hydrogen peroxide may also relieve the symptoms," says Jean Rippere, a microbiologist with FDA.

Xerostomia (dry mouth): There are many disorders that can cause a dry mouth, such as diabetes, anemia, Sjögren's syndrome, infection of the salivary glands, stress, even aging. Treatment falls into two categories: saliva substitutes and saliva stimulators. Demulcents such as glycerin solution soothe and coat the dry area. And a simple remedy such as sugarless lemon drops may temporarily stimulate some salivary flow. For some persons, a dry throat may simply be the result of not drinking enough water. The remedy, of course, is to drink more water.

Sore Throats: A sore throat is a common medical complaint that can be caused by allergies or irritations such as industrial pollutants, tobacco smoke, dry heat during the cold winter months, and cheering too loudly at a sports event.

- **Viruses and Infections.** The most common causes of sore throats are viral illnesses (such as the "flu," the "common cold," or mononucleosis) or bacteria (such as *Streptococcus*). A viral sore throat can be a symptom of measles, chicken pox, or whooping cough. Antibiotics can be used to treat bacterial infections

23

but have no effect against sore throats caused by viral illness. The body heals itself of a viral infection by building up antibodies that destroy the virus.

Such over-the-counter remedies as throat lozenges or anesthetic sprays may bring some relief. Increasing liquid intake (warm tea with honey is a favorite), gargling with warm salt water, and using a humidifier or mild pain relievers may also offer temporary relief.

- **Bacterial infections.** Bacterial infections in the nose and sinuses can cause sore throats because mucus drains down into the throat, carrying the infection with it. One of the more serious kinds of bacterial infection is caused by *Streptococcus* bacteria. As many as 1 out of 10 Americans develops "strep throat" every year, and 40 million adults will see a doctor for it, according to the American Academy of Otolaryngology. Complications of streptococcal infections include tonsillitis, pneumonia, scarlet fever, and ear infections. A strep test approved by FDA a few years ago for use in a doctor's office detects an infection in about 15 minutes rather than the 24 hours usually required for a throat culture. Antibiotics can be administered if the test results are positive.

FDA is currently evaluating over-the-counter mouth remedies to make sure the ingredients are safe and effective. "If we discover that some ingredients do not live up to their billing or are unsafe, we will request that the manufacturer reformulate the product," said FDA's Rippere.

Role of Emotions

Not only does the mouth reflect what is happening elsewhere in the body, but changing the posture of the mouth can elicit bodily changes. Even a mere smile or frown can affect the nervous system. Researchers from the University of Michigan and the University of California Medical School at San Francisco have shown that lifting the corners of the lips in a smile or puckering the lips in a frown can affect the temperature of the blood flowing to the brain and change heart and breath rate.

In a series of experiments, participants were told to arrange their face and mouth in different poses. But the volunteers were not told what emotion they were mimicking or even that the study was testing the relationship between facial expressions and emotions. Volunteers reported feeling the emotion their expressions portrayed. For instance, when volunteers puckered their lips and mouthed the word "few" they reported feeling depressed or "down" even though they didn't know they were expressing a "down" mood. In other words, facial expressions are not only a sign of an emotion but actually contribute to the feeling itself.

Although people may pay little heed to their mouths except when something goes wrong, the importance of the mouth cannot be underestimated. Its condition provides clues to disease elsewhere in the body, and its posturings can affect a person's emotions so that just as the eyes are a window to the soul, so the mouth is a mirror of the body.

—by Judy Folkenberg

Judy Folkenberg is a member of FDA's public affairs staff.

Chapter 3

Oral Hygiene—Not Just for Kids: Taking Care of Your Teeth and Mouth

A healthy smile is a bonus at any age. Too often older people—especially those who wear false teeth (or dentures)—feel they no longer need dental checkups. If you haven't learned the basics of oral health care, it is not too late to start. And even if you have, it's a good time to review.

Tooth Decay (Cavities)

Tooth decay is not just a children's disease; it can happen as long as natural teeth are in the mouth. Tooth decay is caused by bacteria that normally live in the mouth. The bacteria cling to teeth and form a sticky, colorless film called dental plaque. The bacteria in plaque live on sugars and produce decay-causing acids that dissolve minerals on tooth surfaces. Tooth decay can also develop on the exposed roots of the teeth if you have gum disease or receding gums (where gums pull away from the teeth, exposing the roots).

Just as with children, fluoride is important for adult teeth. Research has shown that adding fluoride to the water supply is the best and least costly way to prevent tooth decay. In addition, using fluoride toothpastes and mouthrinses can add protection. Daily fluoride rinses can be bought at most drug stores without a prescription. If you have a problem with cavities, your dentist or dental hygienist may

NIH Publication. National Institute on Aging. *Age Page: Taking Care of Your Teeth and Mouth,* 1994.

give you a fluoride treatment during the office visit. The dentist may prescribe a fluoride gel or mouthrinse for you to use at home.

Gum (Periodontal) Disease

A common cause of tooth loss after age 35 is gum (periodontal) disease. These are infections of the gum and bone that hold the teeth in place. Gum diseases are also caused by dental plaque. The bacteria in plaque causes the gums to become inflamed and bleed easily. If left untreated, the disease gets worse as pockets of infection form between the teeth and gums. This causes receding gums and loss of supporting bone. You may lose enough bone to cause your teeth to become loose and fall out.

You can prevent gum disease by removing plaque. Thoroughly brush and floss your teeth each day. Carefully check your mouth for early signs of disease such as red, swollen, or bleeding gums. See your dentist regularly—every 6 to 12 months—or at once if these signs are present.

Cleaning Your Teeth and Gums

An important part of good oral health is knowing how to brush and floss correctly. Thorough brushing each day removes plaque. Gently brush the teeth on all sides with a soft-bristle brush using fluoride toothpaste. Circular and short back-and-forth strokes work best. Take the time to brush carefully along the gum line. Lightly brushing your tongue also helps to remove plaque and food debris and makes your mouth feel fresh.

In addition to brushing, using dental floss is necessary to keep the gums healthy. Proper flossing is important because it removes plaque and leftover food that a toothbrush cannot reach. Your dentist or dental hygienist can show you the best way to brush and floss your teeth. If brushing or flossing results in bleeding gums, pain, or irritation, see your dentist at once.

An antibacterial mouthrinse, approved for the control of plaque and swollen gums, may be prescribed by your dentist. The mouthrinse is used in addition to careful daily brushing and flossing.

Some people (with arthritis or other conditions that limit motion) may find it hard to hold a toothbrush. To overcome this, the toothbrush handle can be attached to the hand with a wide elastic band or may be enlarged by attaching it to sponge, styrofoam ball, or similar object. People with limited shoulder movement may find brushing easier if the handle of the brush is lengthened by attaching a long piece of wood or plastic. Electric toothbrushes are helpful to many.

Other Conditions of the Mouth

Dry mouth (xerostomia). Dry mouth is common in many adults and may make it hard to eat, swallow, taste, and speak. This condition happens when salivary glands fail to work properly as a result of various diseases or medical treatments, such as chemotherapy or radiation therapy to the head and neck area. Dry mouth is also a side effect of more than 400 commonly used medicines, including drugs for high blood pressure, antidepressants, and antihistamines. Dry mouth can affect oral health by adding to tooth decay and infection.

Until recently, dry mouth was regarded as a normal part of aging. We now know that healthy older adults produce as much saliva as younger adults. So if you think you have dry mouth, talk with your dentist or doctor. To relieve the dryness, drink extra water and avoid sugary snacks, beverages with caffeine, tobacco, and alcohol—all of which increase dryness in the mouth.

Cancer therapies. Cancer therapies, such as radiation to the head and neck or chemotherapy, can cause oral problems, including dry mouth, tooth decay, painful mouth sores, and cracked and peeling lips. Before starting cancer treatment, it is important to see a dentist and take care of any necessary dental work. Your dentist will also show you how to care for your teeth and mouth before, during, and after your cancer treatment to prevent or reduce the oral problems that can occur.

Oral cancer (mouth cancer). Oral cancer most often occurs in people over age 40. The disease frequently goes unnoticed in its early, curable stages. This is true in part because many older people, particularly those wearing full dentures, do not visit their dentists often enough and because pain is usually not an early symptom of the disease. People who smoke cigarettes, use other tobacco products, or drink excessive amounts of alcohol are at increased risk for oral cancer. It is important to spot oral cancer as early as possible, since treatment works best before the disease has spread. If you notice any red or white patches on the gums or tongue, sores that do not heal within two weeks, or if you have difficulty chewing or swallowing, be sure to see a dentist.

29

A head and neck exam, which should be a part of every dental checkup, will allow your dentist to detect early signs of oral cancer.

Dentures

If you wear false teeth (dentures), keep them clean and free from food that can cause stains, bad breath, and gum irritation. Once a day, brush all surfaces of the dentures with a denture-care product. Remove your dentures from your mouth and place them in water or a denture-cleansing liquid while you sleep. It is also helpful to rinse your mouth with a warm saltwater solution in the morning, after meals, and at bedtime.

Partial dentures should be cared for in the same way as full dentures. Because bacteria tend to collect under the clasps of partial dentures, it is especially important to clean this area.

Dentures will seem awkward at first. When learning to eat with false teeth, select soft non-sticky food, cut food into small pieces, and chew slowly using both sides of the mouth. Dentures may make your mouth less sensitive to hot foods and liquids, and lower your ability to detect harmful objects such as bones. If problems in eating, talking, or simply wearing dentures continue after the first few weeks, see your dentist about making adjustments.

In time, dentures need to be replaced or readjusted because of changes in the tissues of your mouth. Do not try to repair dentures at home since this may damage the dentures which in turn may further hurt your mouth.

Dental Implants

Dental implants are anchors that permanently hold replacement teeth. There are several different types of implants, but the most popular are metal screws surgically placed into the jaw bones. If there isn't enough bone, a separate surgical procedure to add bone may be needed. Because bone heals slowly, treatment with implants can often take longer (four months to one year or more) than bridges or dentures. If you are considering dental implants, it is important to select an experienced dentist with whom you can discuss your concerns frankly beforehand to be certain the procedure is right for you.

Professional Care

In addition to practicing good oral hygiene, it is important to have regular checkups by the dentist whether you have natural teeth or dentures. It is also important to follow through with any special treatments that are necessary to ensure good oral health. For instance, if you have sensitive teeth caused by receding gums, your dentist may suggest using a special toothpaste for a few months. Teeth are meant to last a lifetime. By taking good care of your teeth and gums, you can protect them for years to come.

Additional Dental Health Information

More information about general dental care is available from:

National Institute of Dental Research (NIDR)
Building 31, Room 2C35
31 Center Dr MSC 2290
Bethesda MD 20892-2290
301-496-4261

NIDR publishes information on oral research and general dental care. Some publications available are:

Fever Blisters and Canker Sores
Fluoride to Protect the Teeth of Adults
Rx for Sound Teeth
What You Need to Know About Periodontal (Gum) Disease

National Oral Health Information Clearinghouse
1 NOHIC Way
Bethesda, MD 20892-3500
301-402-7364

NIDR also offers publications on oral health for special care patients through the National Oral Health Information Clearinghouse. Special care patients are people whose medical conditions or treatments affect oral health. Publications available include:

Dry Mouth (Xerostomia)
Chemotherapy and Oral Health
Periodontal Disease and Diabetes—A Guide for Patients

Radiation Therapy and Oral Health
TMD (Temporomandibular Disorders)
What You Need to Know About Oral Cancer

American Dental Association (ADA)

211 East Chicago Avenue
Chicago, IL 60611
800-621-8099

ADA distributes educational materials on dental health and sponsors the National Senior Smile Week.

National Agricultural Library Food & Nutrition Information Center

Room 304
10301 Baltimore Blvd.
Beltsville, MD 20705-2351
301-504-5719

The Food Nutrition Center offers the bibliography *Nutri-Topics Series: Nutrition and Dental Health*. This bibliography lists information available to consumers.

National Institute on Aging (NIA)

P.O. Box 8057
Gaithersburg, MD 20898-8057
800-222-2225
800-222-4225 (TTY)

NIA publishes fact sheets on various health-related topics of interest to older people and their families. For a complete listing of publications, call or write to the above address.

Chapter 4

Anesthesia and Sedation in the Dental Office

Introduction

Pain is a major factor that brings patients to the dental office, while fear and anxiety about pain are common reasons patients fail to seek dental care. The magnitude of this public health problem is indicated by the fact that there are 35 million Americans who avoid dental treatment until forced into the office with a toothache. The control of pain and anxiety is therefore an essential part of dental practice.

To accomplish this objective, various techniques are used, including psychological approaches, local anesthetics, and various types and combinations of sedative and general anesthetic agents. The choice of the most appropriate modality for a particular situation is based on the training, knowledge, and experience of the dentist; the nature, severity, and duration of the procedure; the age and physical and psychological status of the patient; the level of fear and anxiety; and the patient's previous response to pain control procedures.

The use of sedative and anesthetic techniques in the dental office represents a unique situation when compared with their use in the hospital environment. Dental patients are ambulatory and generally in good health, the procedures are usually shorter, the depth of anesthesia or level of sedation is often less, and it is the fear and apprehension of the patient rather than the nature of the procedure that

NIH Publication Consensus Development Conference Statement Volume 5 Number 10, April 22-24, 1985.

frequently dictates the use of these techniques. These differences often are not clearly understood. As a result, the use of sedation and anesthesia in the dental office has sometimes been unduly criticized.

Despite the record of safety that has been established by the dental profession, problems have occurred and questions have been raised regarding the training necessary for the safe and effective use of sedation and general anesthesia, the indications and contraindications for the use of these techniques in different age groups, the appropriate agents to be used to provide the greatest margin of safety, and the proper management and monitoring of the patient. To resolve some of these questions, the National Institute of Dental Research of the National Institutes of Health (NIH) along with the Food and Drug Administration and the NIH Office of Medical Applications of Research convened a Consensus Development Conference on Anesthesia and Sedation in the Dental Office on April 22-24, 1985

After listening to a series of presentations by experts in the relevant basic and clinical science areas, a consensus panel composed of individuals knowledgeable in medical and dental anesthesiology, oral and maxillofacial surgery, pediatric dentistry, general dentistry, dental education, pharmacology, behavioral science, biostatistics, epidemiology, and the public interest considered all of the material presented and agreed on answers to the following questions:

- What are the differences between general anesthesia, deep sedation, and conscious sedation?

- What are the indications and contraindications for the use of general anesthesia and sedation in children, adults, and the geriatric population?

- What are the appropriate agents and techniques for general anesthesia and sedation?

- What are the risks associated with the use of general anesthesia and sedation?

- What facilities, equipment, personnel, and training are needed for managing and monitoring patients?

- What are the directions for future research?

What are the differences between general anesthesia, deep sedation, and conscious sedation?

Drugs that depress the central nervous system produce a progressive dose-related continuum of effects. Small doses produce light sedation. In this state, the patient remains conscious, with some alteration of mood, relief of anxiety drowsiness, and sometimes analgesia. As the dose is increased, or as other drugs are added, greater central nervous system depression occurs, resulting in deepening of sedation and sleep from which the patient can be aroused. Finally, when consciousness is lost and the patient cannot be aroused, light general anesthesia begins. General anesthesia can be deepened by additional drug administration. The amount of training, experience, and skill needed to safely produce and manage central nervous system depression increases with the degree of depression involved.

The degree and duration of central nervous system depression required varies with the procedure being performed and with the special requirements of the patient; these may be altered during the procedure as operative requirements change. Only a brief period of central nervous system depression may be necessary to permit the performance of procedures such as administration of a local anesthetic or the uncomplicated extraction of a tooth.

Pharmacologic approaches used for relief of pain and anxiety in dentistry, in addition to local anesthesia, include sedation and general anesthesia. These are defined as follows:

- Sedation describes a depressed level of consciousness, which may vary from light to deep. At light levels, termed conscious sedation, the patient retains the ability present before sedation to independently maintain an airway and respond appropriately to verbal command. The patient may have amnesia, and protective reflexes are normal or minimally altered. In deep sedation, some depression of protective reflexes occurs, and although more difficult, it is still possible to arouse the patient.

- General anesthesia describes a controlled state of unconsciousness, accompanied by partial or complete loss of protective reflexes, including the inability to independently maintain an airway or respond purposefully to verbal command.

When sedative or anesthetic drugs are used, the exact technique can be further described by specifying route of administration, agents used, and their dosage.

What are the indications and contraindications for the use of general anesthesia and sedation in children, adults, and the geriatric population?

The selection of a particular drug or drugs to allay apprehension, anxiety, fear, and pain ultimately rests on the clinical judgment of the dentist. A comprehensive medical history is essential in making this decision. Laboratory tests should be selected on the basis of necessity, specificity, sensitivity, and cost. Consideration of the patient's preference and risk/benefit ratios should influence the method of treatment. Sedation and general anesthesia should only be used when there are adequate facilities and appropriately trained personnel.

The decision to use a particular technique in a certain age group is based on the following:

Adults. For the anxious adult patient, sedation provides a calming effect, and the addition of local anesthesia provides relief of pain or discomfort.

Sedation may also be indicated to minimize stress in the presence of certain medical conditions (e.g., hypertension) and for complex procedures requiring an extended period of operating time. The chief contraindication to the use of sedative techniques is the presence of a medical condition that significantly increases the risk to the patient.

General anesthesia for healthy (ASA class I or II) patients may be indicated when there is greater complexity of the procedure, higher levels of preoperative anxiety, or a greater need for a pain-free operative period. A contraindication to local anesthesia might also require that a general anesthetic be administered.

General anesthesia in an office setting may be contraindicated in patients who are not healthy (ASA class III or IV). These individuals demand special consideration, which may require treatment in the hospital or a similar setting.

Geriatric Parents. The indications for use of sedation or general anesthesia for the geriatric patient are basically the same as for other adults. However, advancing age brings marked changes in pharmacodynamics and pharmacokinetics as well as an increase in medical problems. Chronic use of multiple prescription and over-the-counter drugs is frequently encountered, thus increasing the risk of adverse drug interactions. Contraindications to the use of sedation or general anesthesia for older patients are based almost entirely on the nature and severity of such risk factor.

Pediatric Patients. The dentist's need for a cooperative and quiescent patient for the rendering of high-quality care is a prime indication for the use of sedation or general anesthesia in some children. These modalities tend to reduce fear and anxiety and assist the uncooperative child to accept and continue to receive regular dental care. Pediatric patients with extensive and complicated treatment needs, with acute pain and/or trauma, as well as those who are physically disabled or mentally retarded, may require sedation or general anesthesia. At times, the very young child (up to three years of age) and those with limited or compromised ability to comprehend and communicate also are candidates for such procedures.

Additionally, there may be an indication for sedation or general anesthesia when the child would be better served by increasing the length of the appointment time and thus reducing the number of visits to accomplish the required treatment.

Although the presence of a severe, compromising medical condition is generally a contraindication to sedation, some patients in this category may benefit from its use. These children should be managed in close cooperation with the physician involved in their medical care.

While not necessarily contraindicated in the dental office, general anesthesia in the very young child often is best managed in the hospital or a similar setting, especially for lengthy restorative procedures. In all children, severe, compromising medical conditions contraindicate general anesthesia in the dental office.

What are the appropriate agents and techniques for general anesthesia and sedation?

The drug groups used for sedation or general anesthesia in the dental office are essentially the same as those used in the hospital setting. These groups include benzodiazepines (e.g., diazepam), barbiturates (e.g., pentobarbital), alcohols (e.g., chloral hydrate), the opioid analgesics (e.g., meperidine, fentanyl), antihistamines (e.g., diphenhydramine, hydroxyzine), phenothiazines (e.g., promethazine), and nitrous oxide/oxygen.

Drugs that in low dosage produce sedation, but are generally recognized as general anesthetics, are the halogenated inhalation agents (e.g., enflurane), ultra-short-acting barbiturates (e.g., thiopental, methohexital), and the dissociative agent ketamine. Accessory agents are the antimuscarinics (e.g., atropine, glycopyrrolate), which are useful in sedation and general anesthesia, and the neuromuscular blocking agents (e.g., curare, succinylcholine), which are useful only in general anesthesia.

The routes of drug administration used in the dental office include oral, inhalation, submucosal, intramuscular, intravenous, and rectal. The selection of the route of administration and agents to be used depends on the dentist's expertise and experience and the ability to optimally accomplish the treatment plan. The dentist should utilize psychological approaches as much as possible to minimize drug dosage and thus ensure the safest levels of pharmacologic central nervous system depression. Careful attention must be given to the very young, the elderly, and the special patient. These considerations will ensure that management of each patient will be highly individualized.

What are the risks associated with the use of general anesthesia and sedation?

Reliable national estimates of mortality or morbidity associated with the use of general anesthesia and sedation in the dental office are not available for the United States. The most valid data, derived from a population-based study in Great Britain, indicate a mortality rate of 1:250,000 general anesthetic administrations for the period 1970-1979. Two large surveys of oral and maxillofacial surgeons in the United States suggest lower estimates of risk, ranging from 1:350,000 to 1:860,000; however, the validity of these latter estimates cannot be evaluated because of questions about the survey methods, completeness of data collection, and the degree to which the findings can be generalized.

The British study indicates that treatment with local anesthesia with or without conscious sedation carries less risk than treatment with deep sedation or general anesthesia. Risks may increase in the medically compromised, the elderly, and the very young.

Data concerning morbidity are extremely limited and do not permit the calculation of rates. A general impression suggests that an increased morbidity and mortality are associated with greater duration of anesthesia and complexity of the dental procedure.

Confounding effects of medication being taken by the patient may increase the risks associated with sedation and general anesthesia. A consultation with the patient's physician may be advisable prior to the administration of sedative or general anesthetic agents.

Another important consideration in risk assessment relates to the choice and dosage of specific sedative and anesthetic agents. The use of any effective drug is almost always associated with some undesirable effects. For example, opioid drugs in therapeutic dosage cause respiratory depression and may cause airway obstruction. The use of central nervous system depressants for conscious sedation, especially when used in combinations, requires careful titration and close monitoring to avoid unanticipated deep sedation or general anesthesia.

Special caution is advised when considering anesthetic care for the patient who may develop malignant hyperthermia. A high index of suspicion based on the patient's family history indicates the need for further evaluation and management in the hospital.

For the medically compromised patient, the benefits of using sedation to relieve stress sometimes clearly outweigh the risk of aggravating the medical condition.

What facilities, equipment, personnel, and training are needed for managing and monitoring patients?

Facilities and Equipment. The effectiveness of all techniques used for control of pain and anxiety is significantly enhanced by a quiet environment. The facility should be properly equipped with suction and monitoring equipment, emergency drugs, and equipment capable of delivering oxygen under positive pressure. A protocol for management of emergencies should be developed, and emergency drills should be carried out and documented.

Gas delivery machines should have an oxygen fail-safe system, and should be checked and calibrated periodically. All emergency equipment and drugs should be maintained on a scheduled basis. An adequate, supervised recovery space should be available.

Monitoring. For conscious sedation, the chart should contain documentation that heart rate, blood pressure, respiratory rate, and responsiveness of the patient were checked at specific intervals, including the recovery period. In addition, for deep sedation or general anesthesia, use of the precordial stethoscope for continuous monitoring of cardiac function and respiratory rate is a minimal requirement; an intravenous line, electrocardiographic monitoring or pulse oximetry, and temperature monitoring in children are desirable. Postoperative instructions and precautions should be discussed at the time that the preoperative consent is obtained and should be reinforced in printed form at the time of discharge.

Personnel. For conscious sedation, the practitioner responsible for treatment of the patient and/or administration of the drugs must be appropriately trained in the use of this modality. The minimum number of people involved should be two, i.e., the dentist or other licensed professional and an assistant trained to monitor appropriate physiologic parameters.

For deep sedation or general anesthesia, at least three individuals, each appropriately trained, are required. One is the operating dentist, who directs the deep sedation or general anesthesia. The second is a person whose responsibilities are observation and monitoring of the patient; if this person is an appropriately trained professional, he or she may direct the deep sedation or general anesthesia. The third person assists the operating dentist.

Training. Training for the use of conscious sedation techniques should conform to the American Dental Association's Guidelines for Teaching the Comprehensive Control of Pain and Anxiety in Dentistry, Parts I and III. The didactic background and clinical experiences can be provided at the predoctoral, postdoctoral, and continuing education levels. The curriculum should be sequenced to build on the basic science education, knowledge of physical evaluation, an understanding of psychological approaches, and the didactic material specific to each modality. The techniques should be taught to the level of clinical competence.

Training for deep sedation and general anesthesia requires a minimum of one year of advanced study or its equivalent as described in Part II of the American Dental Association's Guidelines for Teaching the Comprehensive Control of Pain and Anxiety in Dentistry. This training should have a dental orientation to assure the ability to apply the entire spectrum of pain and anxiety control to the needs of the dental patient.

What are the directions for future research?

There is a critical need for a comprehensive approach to research in dental anesthesiology. Major areas that should be explored include epidemiology, clinical trials of drug safety and efficacy, behavioral approaches to pain and anxiety control, pharmacokinetics, pharmacodynamics, and drug interactions.

Comprehensive data on the indications for dental anesthesia, the most efficacious drug regimens, and the morbidity and mortality rates will permit a more effective use of available sedative and anesthetic modalities. In addition, definitive clinical research in pediatric, adult, and geriatric populations is essential.

The panel specifically recommends research in the following areas:

- Epidemiology

  1. Data on the number and type of sedative and anesthetic procedures by geographic region and type of practice.

  2. Information on specific drugs and dosages currently being used in each type of practice for conscious sedation, deep sedation, and general anesthesia.

  3. Morbidity and mortality rates by demographic characteristics, preoperative status, type of sedation or anesthesia, and specific drugs. There is a need for development of statistically sound models for such studies. State, regional, and national data would be useful.

- Drug Efficacy Studies

  1. There is a need for well-controlled, randomized, double-blind safety and efficacy studies. There should be continued development of methods to quantitate onset, peak effects, duration of effects, and recovery from sedation and anesthesia. Oral, parenteral, and inhalation regimens should be evaluated.

  2. Studies should address the risk/benefit ratio of single and combination drug regimens. Emphasis should be on the dose-response effects of each regimen and on the contribution of each drug in combination therapy.

  3. Studies should include the pediatric, adult, and geriatric populations, with special emphasis on the risks unique to each group.

- Monitoring of Patients

  1. Studies are needed to determine the type and amount of monitoring best suited for the various sedation and anesthesia regimens. These studies should consider the cost-effectiveness of monitoring equipment and the necessary criteria for early intervention for drug toxicity.

  2. Better methods are needed for early detection of malignant hyperthermia to permit more rapid therapeutic intervention for this sudden and potentially fatal complication.

- Behavioral and Other Nonpharmacologic Approaches

  1. Behavioral approaches and other techniques used alone or in conjunction with pharmacologic pain control need to be systematically studied.

  2. Barriers to the use of psychologic approaches need to be identified and remedial programs developed.

- Environmental Risk Assessment

  1. Special studies should address the hazards of anesthetic agents to the professional personnel and office staff. This is particularly important with gaseous or volatile anesthetics.

- New Drugs

  1. There should be continuing efforts to develop new and better drugs for sedation and general anesthesia.

  2. Specific reversal agents for each class of drugs should also be sought. Drugs such as the opioid antagonists and soon-to-be available benzodiazepine antagonists should be evaluated for use in dentistry as they are being developed.

- Resources

  1. It is particularly important that there be a critical mass of trained clinical and basic science researchers. It is necessary to assess whether there are adequate personnel to implement comprehensive teaching and research programs.

Conclusions

The use of all effective drugs carries some degree of risk, however small. Available evidence suggests that use of sedative and anesthetic drugs in the dental office by appropriately trained professionals has a remarkable record of safety. However, even this record can be improved as scientific knowledge of dental anxiety and pain control is expanded, as strong training programs at all levels of professional education are developed, and as appropriate guidelines governing requirements for dental office personnel, facilities, and equipment are promulgated and adopted.

Chapter 5

Healthy Teeth for Happy Smiles

Healthy Primary (Baby Teeth)

Fluoride in drinking water is most important for a lifetime of healthy teeth. The first step toward healthy teeth is to ask your dentist or doctor if your baby's drinking water has enough fluoride. If it does not, you should give your baby fluoride each day from birth.

Proper use of the bottle is the next step in preventing dental problems.

- Bottles are used to feed babies who are not yet able to drink from a cup.

- Feed only formula, breast milk or water from a bottle.

- Offer the bottle only at feeding times. Do not let baby carry a bottle around at other times. A bottle is not a toy or pacifier.

- Sleeping times are not feeding times. Do not put baby to bed with a bottle.

- Putting the baby to bed with a bottle may increase the chance of tooth decay and ear infection.

Adapted from *Healthy Teeth for Healthy Smiles*, Developed by California Department of Health Services. Department of Health and Social Services, Division of Health, Wisconsin Department of Health and Social Services, P. O. Box 309, Madison. Wisconsin. 53701. POH 4078 (Rev. 2/92).

Baby Bottle Tooth Decay

The baby who goes to bed with a bottle can get painful tooth decay. This is called "baby bottle tooth decay."

- The sugar in formula, milk, juice and sweetened drinks can decay the teeth if it stays in baby's mouth during sleep.

- Do not add sugar, syrups, sweeteners, soft drinks, or honey to the bottle or pacifier.

- If baby needs a bottle at night, fill with plain water; or offer a blanket, stuffed animal, or favorite toy at sleep time instead of a bottle.

- "Baby bottle tooth decay" can be very serious.

Good Nutrition

Nutritious foods and beverages are needed for healthy teeth and gums.

- Encourage good eating habits. Choose a variety of foods from each of the food groups. Set regular meal and snack times. Good snacks: popcorn, cheese, fruit, dry cereal (low sugar).

- When your child is thirsty, offer water. Avoid sweet drinks such as soda pop, Hi-C®, Kool-aid®, Tang® and fruit punch.

- Brush after eating, especially after eating those foods which stick to the teeth.

- Help your child control a "sweet tooth." Avoid candy, cookies, cake, pastries, Jello, doughnuts, granola bars, baby desserts, raisins/dried fruit, peanut butter, syrup, honey, jelly/jam, crackers, soft bread.

Protect Teeth with Fluoride and Sealants

- Fluoride will help strengthen teeth and protect them from decay. If water in your area does not contain enough fluoride, ask your dentist or doctor about giving your child fluoride drops or tablets.

- Sealants will prevent decay on the biting parts of back teeth. A thin, plastic coating will seal out food and germs that cause decay. Ask your dentist or dental hygienist if your child needs sealants.

Time for a Cup

When your baby is able to sit well, begin offering water from a small cup.

- Be patient . . . it will take your baby time to learn to drink from a cup.

- As baby gets used to drinking from a cup, offer formula, breast milk or juice in a cup.

- Take bottles away gradually. Most babies will not want to give up the bottle all at once.

- Babies should be drinking from a cup by their first birthday.

- By eighteen months of age, the bottle should no longer be used.

Teething: What to Expect

Eruption of Teeth

Usually between six and seven months of age, your infant's baby (primary) teeth will begin to appear. Although this is the first visible sign of teeth, they began forming before your child was born. The first teeth to appear probably will be the front teeth, either on the top or bottom.

By age two to three years, your child probably will have all 20 baby (primary) teeth.

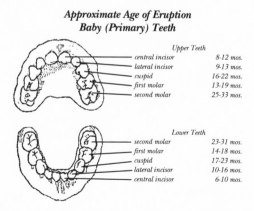

Approximate Age of Eruption
Baby (Primary) Teeth

Upper Teeth	
central incisor	8-12 mos.
lateral incisor	9-13 mos.
cuspid	16-22 mos.
first molar	13-19 mos.
second molar	25-33 mos.

Lower Teeth	
second molar	23-31 mos.
first molar	14-18 mos.
cuspid	17-23 mos.
lateral incisor	10-16 mos.
central incisor	6-10 mos.

Figure 5.1.

Signs of Teething

Teething may or may not be associated with the following:

- Biting or chewing on anything, including fingers.

  Offer a clean, smooth object such as a rubber or plastic ring to help cut teeth and relieve possible gum soreness. This is preferable to using food as a pacifier.

- Drooling, excess salivation.

  Use a bib to help keep clothes clean and dry. The salivary glands are just beginning to function to help your child digest solid foods.

- Restlessness, fussiness, loss of appetite.

  Don't urge your child to eat just because he/she is crying. He will eat when he/she is hungry. Your child may need extra love and attention during teething.

Your baby is changing and growing in many other ways at the same time teething happens. Parents who see fever, stuffy or runny nose, cough, rash, or changes in bowel movements at the same time as teething may think it's all due to teething. These conditions are probably not related to the teething, but should be reported to your baby's doctor if they continue.

Care of Teeth Begins Early in Life

Birth to 1 year

- Wipe baby's gums and teeth with damp cloth or gauze daily.
- Ask your dentist or doctor about giving your child fluoride to build strong teeth.

1 to 2 years

- Gently brush child's teeth with a soft toothbrush after meals and at night.
- First dental visit for oral exam and preventive health education no later than 12 months of age.

2 to 3 years

- Take child to dentist for fluoride and sealant preventive care.

- Brush and floss child's teeth after meals and before bed.

- Begin to teach child to brush teeth with soft brush using a very small dab (pea-sized) of fluoridated toothpaste.

- Avoid sweet snacks.

3 to 4 years

- Take child to dentist regularly for fluoride and sealant preventive care.

- Help child brush and floss teeth after meals and before bed.

- Avoid sweet snacks.

- Encourage brushing after eating.

6 years and up

- Remind child to brush and floss after meals and before bed.

- Encourage brushing after eating sweets or sticky foods.

- Take child to dentist regularly for fluoride and sealant preventive care.

Chapter 6

Primer on Oral Hygiene

Brushing Your Teeth

Your teeth are meant to last a lifetime. Tooth decay or cavities, and periodontal disease, also known as gum disease, can be avoided or reduced by the daily removal of plaque.

Plaque is made up of germs that live on your teeth, all the time. It is important to remove this plaque daily to prevent these germs from making acid and other products that can cause cavities and harm your gums and the bone around your teeth.

If you spend less than three minutes brushing your teeth, probably all the plaque is not being removed. Also, a toothbrush with worn-out bristles cannot clean your teeth properly. Try to replace your toothbrush at least every three to four months.

A dental home care plan should include:

- daily toothbrushing with a soft toothbrush that is not worn out or frayed
- using dental floss daily to clean the areas your toothbrush cannot reach that are between your teeth and under the gumline
- using a toothpaste or mouthrinse with fluoride
- eating balanced meals and limiting foods high in sugar

Adapted from ORAL Health Fact Sheets from the Arizona Department of Health Services, Office of Oral Health and the New York State Dental Sealant Program.

To brush away the plaque on your teeth, follow these steps:

1. Start by brushing the sides of your teeth that touch your cheek. Angle your tooth brush so it is up against your teeth and gums and jiggle the toothbrush back and forth in small strokes. Do only a few teeth at a time, and do it several times in each spot.

2. When you have completed the cheek side of your top and bottom teeth brush the side that faces your tongue on the top and bottom teeth in the same way.

3. Brush the flat, chewing surfaces of your top and bottom teeth. These surfaces have many deep grooves where germs can "hide out." Brush your tongue when you finish brushing your teeth to help your mouth feel fresher. To maintain the health of your teeth and gums, clean in between your teeth with dental floss after toothbrushing.

Flossing Your Teeth

Dental health begins with good oral hygiene. Proper toothbrushing helps to remove the germs that live on your teeth (called plaque), from the outside, inside and chewing surfaces of your teeth. But plaque will still remain on your teeth unless dental floss is also used.

Flossing will remove plaque from between your teeth, especially in those hard-to-reach areas under the gumline. By combining the use of dental floss with toothbrushing to thoroughly remove plaque each day, you will be able to help prevent cavities and an infection in your gums called periodontal disease or gum disease.

How to Floss: First wrap an 18-inch piece of floss around the middle finger of each hand. Hold about an inch of floss tightly between your thumb and forefinger.

Gently slide the floss between the teeth. Be certain not to snap the floss in, or you may hurt your gums. Press the floss against one side of the tooth and move the floss up and down the tooth several times, being sure to reach under the gumline.

Floss both sides of every tooth. When you move on to the next tooth, be sure to use a clean section of the floss.

Your gums may bleed slightly the first few days you use dental floss. They will become healthier if you keep flossing. If it is hard for you to use floss, try a floss holder that you can buy at a drug store or pharmacy. It is recommended that you regularly visit a dental office to maintain the health of your teeth and gums.

Baby Bottle Tooth Decay

What is Baby Bottle Tooth Decay?

When an infant or small child develops several cavities, usually on the top front teeth, this is called Baby Bottle Tooth Decay. These cavities may look like dark pits, holes or broken teeth and may cause toothaches and make it hard for the child to eat.

What Causes Baby Bottle Tooth Decay?

It happens when liquids that contain sugar are left in a baby's mouth for long or frequent periods of time. Even breast milk and formula contain sugar.

How Can You Protect Your Child's Teeth?

Your child should NOT:

- go to bed with a bottle filled with milk, formula, juices or sweetened drinks
- sleep at night at the breast
- drink from a bottle throughout the day
- use a pacifier if it is dipped in honey, syrup or anything sweet, such as jello water, soda pop, fruit juices, Kool-aid, sugar water, milk or formula.

Your child SHOULD:

- start drinking from a cup at six months of age and be weaned from their bottle by one year of age
- go to bed without a bottle. If your child must have a bottle to sleep, fill it with plain water. You may need to mix the drink in the bottle with water, a little more water each night, until your child is drinking plain water
- have their teeth cleaned after each feeding with a clean washcloth, gauze pad, or a soft infant toothbrush. It is very important to clean your baby's teeth before bedtime.

Are Baby Teeth Important?

Baby teeth are important for chewing of food, proper speech, and they also give your child a nice appearance and good self image. If they are lost too early, the permanent teeth can come in crowded or out of line. Be sure your child visits a dentist before two years of age. Your early efforts will be the key to your child's future dental health.

Fluoride to Prevent Tooth Decay

What is Fluoride?

Fluoride is a mineral your body needs to grow and be healthy. Fluoride makes teeth and bones strong, and it protects your teeth against decay. It can be found naturally in all soil, plants, animals and water.

How Does Fluoride Help Your Teeth?

Fluoride is needed for infants and children, when teeth are still forming under the gums. The fluoride swallowed at this time, in water or from vitamins that contain fluoride, deposits itself into the outer part of the tooth and makes the tooth stronger and better able to fight decay.

Fluoride also works after the teeth erupt, and are present in your mouth. At this time, fluoride from water, food, toothpaste, mouthrinses, and fluoride treatments received in a dental office, wash over the teeth and help to prevent decay or even stop small areas of decay that have already started. The fluoride minerals make the outer surface of the teeth stronger.

What is the Best Way to Get Fluoride?

Even though natural fluoride is found in food, plants, animals and water, the amount is usually too low to provide the best protection from decay. Many communities add a small amount of fluoride to their water supply so the best protection will be provided. This is called water fluoridation. Drinking fluoridated water from birth can reduce decay by 40 to 65 percent.

If a community does not have the benefits of water fluoridation, a dentist or physician can write a prescription for a vitamin with fluoride, in tablet form or drops. For best results, these tablets or drops should be taken from 6 months of age through 14 years of age.

Many schools that do not have enough fluoride in their drinking water supply offer a fluoride mouthrinse program. The children that participate in this program swish with a fluoride mouthrinse once a week in their classroom. This program has been shown to reduce decay by 35 percent.

Another way to get fluoride is through dental products such as toothpastes or mouthrinses that have the seal of the American Dental Association on their label. These products are good for children and adults, whether or not they drink fluoridated water.

Dental Sealants

In the past, we commonly treated tooth decay after a cavity had developed. This usually involved drilling away decayed portions of the tooth and filling the cavity with a decay-resistant material.

Today, we know that there are effective ways to prevent tooth decay, such as regular brushing and flossing. Fluorides, either through community water fluoridation or fluoride supplement programs, have been shown to reduce decay significantly. And, a new material, called a pit and fissure sealant, can provide more protection against tooth decay when used in combination with brushing and flossing, proper diet and fluorides.

What is a Sealant?

Tooth decay is frequently found on the chewing surfaces of back molar teeth. These surfaces have indentations, called "pits" and "fissures." Since these pits and fissures are so tiny, and since the tooth enamel is very thin in these areas, they make ideal spots in which decay-causing bacteria can become trapped.

A sealant is a thin, plastic coating that is applied as a liquid to the chewing surface of a tooth. This coating adheres to the tooth and hardens to form a protective barrier that seals the pits and fissures of the tooth surface. The sealant is a barrier against decay-causing bacteria.

How is a Sealant Applied?

The procedure is simple and painless. No tooth material is removed. Applying sealants may be done by a dental hygienist or dentist. First, the teeth are cleaned. Then the teeth to be sealed are dabbed with a conditioner, a very mild acid solution similar in strength to vinegar or lemon juice. This roughens the tooth surface slightly so that the sealant will bond to it. After the tooth is prepared, the sealant is painted onto the tooth with a droplet applicator. It flows into the pits and grooves and hardens in about 60 seconds. After sealing, bacteria cannot reach the pits and grooves and cause decay. Applying sealants requires no drilling or removal of the tooth surface.

Who Should Receive Sealants?

Children, with newly-erupted first or second molar teeth, can benefit most from sealants. First molar teeth generally appear at about six years of age. Second molar teeth usually appear at the age of 12. To work effectively, sealants should be applied as soon as possible after the molars erupt, and before the teeth have had a chance to decay.

What Are the Benefits of Sealants?

By forming a thin covering over the pits and fissures, sealants keep out plaque and decrease the risk of decay.

How Long Will a Sealant Last?

A single application of a sealant can last as long as five years or even longer. Since the sealant may wear off, or become loose, it must be checked periodically and reapplied, if necessary.

Are Sealants Visible?

Since sealants are only applied to back teeth, they can't be seen when a child smiles or talks. A sealant may be clear, white or tinted.

Will Sealants Make the Teeth Feel Different?

A sealant may be slightly noticeable until normal chewing wears it into place. Since sealants are very thin and only fill the pits and fissures, they will not cause a change in the bite.

Are Sealants Expensive?

The cost of sealing teeth will vary, but it is usually less than the cost of having a tooth filled.

Are Sealants Safe?

Yes. The ingredients in sealant materials are, for the most part, the same as those used in tooth-colored filling materials.

Sealants have been approved by the American Dental Association and have been proven to be safe and effective. They are recommended by the National Institute of Dental Research, the American Public Health Association, the American Association of Public Health Dentistry, the American Dental Hygienists' Association and numerous other organizations.

Can Decay Occur Beneath Sealants?

Sealants prevent decay-causing bacteria from getting oxygen and nutrients. As a result, decay is not likely to progress, even if some bacteria are trapped under the sealant.

Do Sealants Eliminate the Need for Other Preventive Measures?

No. Sealants are only a part of a child's total dental health care. For complete protection against tooth decay, your child should:

- use fluorides, as directed by the dentist—either in fluoridated water, fluoride supplements, topical fluoride treatments or fluoride mouthrinses and toothpastes;

- brush at least twice a day;

- floss every day;

- eat well-balanced meals; and

- visit the dentist every six months

Why Is Sealing a Tooth Better than Waiting for Decay and Filling a Cavity?

Sealants help to keep teeth healthy by protecting them from decay. Decay destroys parts of the tooth. Each time a tooth is filled or a filling is replaced, more tooth is lost. Silver fillings last about 6 to 8 years before they need to be replaced. Using sealants saves time and money and helps to keep teeth healthy.

How Can I Learn More?

To learn more about sealants, talk to your dentist, contact your local health department, or write:

Dental Sealant Program
Bureau of Dental Health
N.Y.S. Health Department
Corning Tower, Empire State Plaza
Albany, NY 12237

Periodontal Disease

Periodontal disease, also known as gum disease, is an infection that attacks the bone and gums that support your teeth. It is the most common cause of tooth loss in adults.

Bacteria in your mouth, called plaque, is the major cause of periodontal disease. Other things can contribute to periodontal disease such as the general condition of your teeth, your nutrition and general health, habits and emotional stress.

If the bacteria is not removed regularly by brushing and flossing, it can harden into tartar, also called calculus. The rough surface of this calculus will help more bacteria to stay close to your teeth and under the gumline.

This bacteria makes products that can harm your gums and the bone around your teeth.

Periodontal disease is painless, and in the early stages it is difficult to detect. Common early warning signs of periodontal disease may include bad breath and tender or swollen gums that bleed when you brush and floss your teeth.

Periodontal disease can be prevented with proper dental care from an early age, including brushing, flossing and regular dental visits for treatment from a dental hygienist and dentist. Caught in the early stages, periodontal disease is easy to treat.

You can keep your teeth and mouth healthy for a lifetime. Ask your dental hygienist and dentist to evaluate the health of your gums.

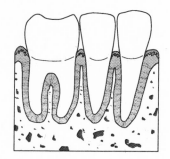

Figure 6.1. This is how gums and bone look in a healthy mouth.

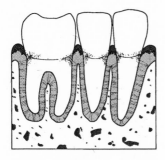

Figure 6.2.*Notice how tartar, also known as calculus, has started to build up on these teeth. Bacteria live on its rough surface.*

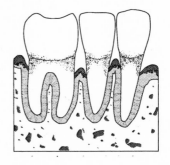

Figure 6.3.*The bacteria on the calculus has caused these teeth to lose some of their bony support and has also caused the gums to shrink away from the teeth.*

Tobacco Facts

The nicotine found in cigarettes and in spit tobacco is a powerful, addictive drug that acts on several parts of the body. Once addicted, it becomes difficult, but not impossible, to quit using spit tobacco or to stop smoking.

The use of tobacco products is not only addicting, but is directly related to a number of health problems and diseases. A few of the oral health problems smokers or spit tobacco users can develop are:

- black hairy tongue
- gum disease and loss of teeth
- brown, stained teeth
- gum ulcers
- ground-down teeth
- bad breath
- receding gums
- cancer of the esophagus
- cancer of the palate
- cancer of the tongue
- cancer of the lip
- cancer of the cheek

Some of the harmful ingredients found in tobacco are:

- nicotine
- fertilizer
- arsenic
- cyanide
- dead bugs
- manure
- pesticides
- soot
- formaldehyde
- dirt

At least 19 different types of cancer-causing substances, called nitrosamines, are found in tobacco products.

Oral cancer is serious. When it spreads to the lymph nodes in the neck, it is often deadly.

Spit tobacco is NOT a harmless alternative to smoking. It is just as hazardous to your health as cigarettes. Protect your health—avoid all tobacco products.

The risk of developing lung cancer is ten times greater for smokers than non-smokers. Also, breathing second-hand smoke (someone else's smoke) can be as dangerous as smoking.

Once you stop using tobacco products, within 20 minutes your blood pressure, pulse rate and skin temperature will return to normal. Within 8 hours, high levels of carbon monoxide in your blood will return to normal, and within a few weeks, your circulation will improve, your sense of taste and smell will improve, you will have fewer colds and more energy. IT'S NEVER TOO LATE TO STOP.

Quitting Spit Tobacco

Before You Quit:

- Change to a brand you don't like
- Postpone your first chew of the day by 1 hour for a few days, then by 2 hours, then by 3 hours, etc.
- Set a date for quitting

When You Quit:

- Get rid of all your tobacco
- Tell everyone you know that you are quitting
- Have sugarless gum available for when you have the urge to chew
- Save the money you would have spent on tobacco and treat yourself to something you wouldn't usually purchase

When You Have the Urge to Use Tobacco, Do One of These Activities Instead:

- Take a walk or exercise with a friend
- Drink a glass of water

If You Feel You Need More Assistance With Quitting:

- Talk to your dental professional or physician
- Call the American Cancer Society at 1-800-227-2345
- Call the Arizona Lung Association at (602)458-7505

After You Quit:

- Don't worry if you are more sleepy or irritable than usual; these symptoms should go away.
- When you're in a tense situation, try to keep busy. Tell yourself that chewing won't solve the problem.
- Don't give up. YOU ARE WORTH IT.

Oral Cancer

Oral cancer will be found in an estimated 30,000 Americans this year, and will cause close to 8,000 deaths. Only half of those people with the disease will live more than five years.

Who Is at Risk for Developing Oral Cancer?

People who use tobacco and excessive alcohol increase their risk of oral cancer. People who spend a great deal of time in the sun may also have a higher risk for lip cancer.

More than 90 percent of all oral cancers are found in people over the age of 45, but oral cancer can happen at any age. Men develop oral cancer twice as often as women, and it occurs more often in African-Americans than in whites.

What Are the Symptoms of Oral Cancer?

If it is found and treated early, deaths from oral cancer can be reduced. Changes in your mouth that may be the start of oral cancer often can be seen and felt easily. A person can find these changes by doing a monthly exam of their mouth. Look for these signs, which are some of the warning signs of oral cancer:

- A sore in your mouth that bleeds easily and does not heal
- A lump or thick spot in your cheek that can be felt with your tongue
- A white or red patch on your gums, tongue, or anywhere in your mouth
- Soreness or a feeling that something is caught in your throat
- Difficulty chewing or swallowing your food
- Difficulty moving your jaw or tongue
- Numbness of your tongue or other parts of your mouth
- Swelling of your upper or lower jaw that causes your dentures to fit poorly or hurt your mouth

These signs are not sure signs of cancer. They can also be caused by many other conditions. It is important to see a dentist or physician if any of these problems last more than 2 weeks. Pain is usually NOT a sign of oral cancer. Annual visits to a dental office are recommended for a professional oral cancer examination.

Caring for Your Dentures;

It is important to clean your mouth and denture daily so your mouth will stay healthy. It isn't enough to soak your dentures in water or a denture cleaner. They must be brushed with a soft toothbrush, or a toothbrush made especially for dentures.

Be sure to brush and massage your gums daily with a soft toothbrush, and brush any remaining natural teeth you may have.

- Do not clean a denture with boiling water.

- Clean all the surfaces of your denture, both inside and outside, with a denture brush and denture cleaner that you can buy at a drug store. Do not use an abrasive cleaning powder like Ajax or Comet.

- When cleaning a denture, hold it over a bowl of water between your thumb and forefinger. If it slips out of your hand, it will land in the water and not break.

- If a denture smells, it can be soaked in a solution of 1 teaspoon of bleach (Clorox) in one cup of water. Soak the denture for 30 minutes. Rinse the denture well before putting it back in your mouth.

- Take your denture out of your mouth for at least 8 hours every day. When it is out of your mouth, keep the denture in a bowl of water or diluted mouthwash.

- Do not try to adjust a denture with sandpaper or files. They will ruin the denture. Do not use denture liners or denture adhesives.

Go to the dentist for the following:

- Your regular fitting appointments after you get a denture
- When you have mouth sores that last for more than 1 week
- When your dentures become loose in your mouth
- One time a year to check the health of your mouth and the fit of your denture.

Chapter 7

Snack Smart for Healthy Teeth

What's wrong with sugary snacks, anyway?

Sugary snacks taste so good, but they aren't so good for your teeth or your body. The candies, cakes, cookies, and other sugary foods that kids love to eat between meals can cause tooth decay. Some sugary foods have a lot of fat in them too.

Kids who consume sugary snacks eat many different kinds of sugar every day, including table sugar (sucrose) and corn sweeteners (fructose). Starchy snacks can also break down into sugars once they're in your mouth.

Did you know that the average American eats about 147 pounds of sugars a year? That's a big pile of sugar. No wonder the average 17-year-old in this country has more than three decayed teeth.

How do sugars attack your teeth?

Invisible germs called bacteria live in your mouth all the time. Some of these bacteria form a sticky material called plaque on the surface of the teeth. When you put sugar in your mouth, the bacteria in the plaque gobble up the sweet stuff and turn it into acids. These acids are powerful enough to dissolve the hard enamel that covers your teeth. That's how cavities get started. If you don't eat much sugar, the bacteria can't produce as much of the acid that eats away enamel.

National Institute of Dental Research. Website.

How can I "snack smart" to protect myself from tooth decay?

Before you start munching on a snack, ask yourself what's in the food you've chosen. Is it loaded with sugar? If it is, think again. Another choice would be better for your teeth. And keep in mind that certain kinds of sweets can do more damage than others. Gooey or chewy sweets spend more time sticking to the surface of your teeth. Because sticky snacks stay in your mouth longer than foods that you quickly chew and swallow, they give your teeth a longer sugar bath.

You should also think about when and how often you eat snacks. Do you nibble on sugary snacks many times throughout the day, or do you usually just have dessert after dinner? Damaging acids form in your mouth every time you eat a sugary snack. The acids continue to affect your teeth for at least 20 minutes before they are neutralized and can't do any more harm. So, the more times you eat sugary snacks during the day, the more often you feed bacteria the fuel they need to cause tooth decay.

If you eat sweets, it's best to eat them as dessert after a main meal instead of several times a day between meals. Whenever you eat sweets—in any meal or snack—brush your teeth well with a fluoride toothpaste afterward.

When you're deciding about snacks, think about:

- the number of times a day you eat sugary snacks
- how long the sugary food stays in your mouth
- the texture of the sugary food (chewy? sticky?)

If you snack after school, before bedtime, or other times during the day, choose something without a lot of sugar or fat. There are lots of tasty, filling snacks that are less harmful to your teeth—and the rest of your body—than foods loaded with sugars and low in nutritional value.

Snack Smart

Low-fat choices like raw vegetables, fresh fruits, or whole-grain crackers or bread are smart choices. Eating the right foods can help protect you from tooth decay and other diseases. Next time you reach for a snack, pick a food from the list inside or make up your own menu of non-sugary, low-fat snack foods from the basic food groups.

How Can You Snack Smart? Be Choosy.

Pick a variety of foods from these groups:

Fresh fruits and raw vegetables

- berries
- oranges
- grapefruit
- melons
- pineapple
- pears
- tangerines
- broccoli
- celery
- carrots
- cucumbers
- tomatoes
- unsweetened fruit and vegetable juices
- canned fruits in natural juices

Grains

- bread
- plain bagels
- unsweetened cereals
- unbuttered popcorn
- tortilla chips (baked, not fried)
- pretzels (low-salt)
- pasta
- plain crackers

Milk and dairy products

- low or non-fat milk
- low or non-fat yogurt
- low or non-fat cheeses
- low or non-fat cottage cheese

Meat, nuts and seeds

- chicken
- turkey

- sliced meats
- pumpkin seeds
- sunflower seeds
- nuts

Others (these snacks combine foods from the different groups)

- pizza
- tacos

Remember to:

- choose sugary foods less often
- avoid sweets between meals
- eat a variety of low or non-fat foods from the basic groups
- brush your teeth with fluoride toothpaste after snacks and meals

Note to Parents

The foods listed in this chapter have not all been tested for their decay-causing potential. However, knowledge to date indicates that they are less likely to promote tooth decay than are some of the heavily sugared foods children often eat between meals.

Candy bars aren't the only culprits. Foods such as pizza, breads, and hamburger buns may also contain sugars. Check the label. The new food labels identify sugars and fats on the Nutrition Facts panel on the package. Keep in mind that brown sugar, honey, molasses, and syrups also react with bacteria to produce acids, just as refined table sugar does. These foods also are potentially damaging to teeth.

Your child's meals and snacks should include a variety of foods from the basic food groups, including fruits and vegetables; grains, including breads and cereals; milk and dairy products; and meat, nuts, and seeds. Some snack foods have greater nutritional value than others and will better promote your child's growth and development. However, be aware that even some fresh fruits, if eaten in excess, may promote tooth decay. Children should brush their teeth with fluoride toothpaste after snacks and meals. (So should you.)

Please note: These general recommendations may need to be adapted for children on special diets because of diseases or conditions that interfere with normal nutrition.

Chapter 8

Toward Improving the Oral Health of Americans

Introduction

Dental and oral diseases may well be the most prevalent and preventable conditions affecting Americans. More than 50 percent of U.S. children, 96 percent of employed U.S. adults, and 99.5 percent of Americans 65 years and older have experienced dental caries (also called cavities). Millions of Americans suffer from periodontal diseases and other oral conditions, and more than 17 million Americans, including 10 million Americans 65 years or older, have lost all of their teeth. Preventive dental services are known to be effective in preventing and controlling dental diseases. Unfortunately, groups at highest risk for disease—the poor and minorities—have lower rates of using dental care than the U.S. average.

Cost is the principal barrier to dental care for many Americans. Of the $38.7 billion spent for dental services in 1992, public programs, including Medicaid, paid for less than 4 percent of dental expenditures. More than 90 percent of care was paid for either out-of-pocket by dental consumers or through private dental insurance.

Americans are at risk for other oral health problems as well. Oropharyngeal cancer strikes approximately 30,000 Americans each year and results in an estimated 8,000 deaths annually. Underlying medical or disabling conditions, ranging from rare genetic diseases to more common chronic diseases, affect millions of Americans and can lead to oral health problems. Among persons with compromised

1993, *Public Health Reports*.

immune systems, oral diseases and conditions can have a significant impact on health.

Oral diseases and conditions, though nearly universal, can be prevented easily and controlled at reasonable cost. Prevention and early, regular primary dental care are the best strategies to improve the oral health and quality of life of all Americans.

Jonathan Kozol, in his 1991 book, *Savage Inequalities: Children in America's Schools*, describes a picture unseen by most policy makers, but all too common for those who have worked in public programs serving poor, minority, and under-served populations (1).

Although dental problems don't command the instant fears associated with low birth weight, fetal death or cholera, they do have the consequences of wearing down the stamina of children and defeating their ambitions. Bleeding gums, impacted teeth and rotting teeth are routine matters for the children I have interviewed in the South Bronx. Children get used to feeling constant pain. They go to sleep with it. They go to school with it. Sometimes their teachers are alarmed and try to get them to a clinic. But it's all so slow and heavily encumbered with red tape and waiting lists and missing, lost or canceled welfare cards, that dental care is often long delayed. Children live for months with pain that grown-ups would find unendurable. The gradual attrition of accepted pain erodes their energy and aspirations. I have seen children in New York with teeth that look like brownish, broken sticks. I have also seen teenagers who were missing half their teeth. But, to me, most shocking is to see a child with an abscess that has been inflamed for weeks and that he has simply lived with and accepts as part of the routine of life.

Millions of Americans suffer from diseases and conditions of the oral cavity that result in decreased economic productivity through lost work and school days, needless pain, increased costs, loss of self-esteem, and death. Oral diseases and conditions, including dental caries (also known as cavities), periodontal diseases, and tooth loss afflict more persons than any other single disease in the United States. Americans cannot be truly healthy unless they are free from the burden of oral diseases.

The purpose of this chapter is to review the epidemiology of dental and oral diseases, including dental caries, periodontal diseases, tooth loss, and oral cancer, and the impact that these diseases and conditions have on Americans. It will describe the need for, and use of, dental services and current expenditures for those services. Finally, it will identify the current gaps in services that need to be addressed to improve the nation's oral health.

Epidemiology of Oral Diseases

Oral Diseases among Children

Dental caries may well be the most common disease of U.S. children, affecting more than 50 percent of children 5 to 17 years old (see Figure 8.1) (2). Dental caries is a progressive disease process. Unless restorative treatment is provided, the carious lesion will continue to destroy the tooth, eventually resulting in pain, acute infection, and costly treatment to restore the tooth or have it removed. Fortunately, with early professional intervention, caries can either be prevented or treated easily at minimal cost.

During the past 20 years, on average, there has been a dramatic decline in the level of dental caries among school age children (2). Many reasons have been suggested for this decline, including

- community water fluoridation (3),
- increased use of toothpastes containing fluorides (4),
- use of fluoride supplements and mouthrinses (5),
- increased availability of fluoride in foods and bottled liquids processed with fluoridated water (6), and
- changes in diet (for example, decreased sugar consumption) (7).

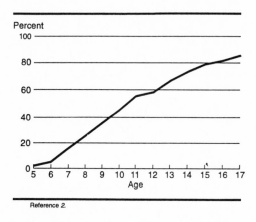

Reference 2.

Figure 8.1. Percentage of U.S. children 5-17 years of age who have experienced dental caries, 1986-97.

Although many herald this improvement, millions of children still have significant levels of dental caries. Seventy-five percent of children's dental caries are concentrated in 25 percent of the population (2). Higher disease levels generally are found among minorities, children from poor and low-income families, and children whose parents have less than a high school education. Among American Indian and Alaska Native children ages six to eight years, 88 percent have experienced dental caries. By age 15, the disease rate increases to 91 percent in this group.

Age (years)	Mean DMFT	Percent D of DMFT	Percent M of DMFT	Percent F of DMFT
		White Americans		
All ages ...	1.97	11.7	0.8	87.5
5	0.04	76.2	0.0	23.8
6	0.09	54.1	0.0	45.9
7	0.28	38.3	0.1	61.7
8	0.52	25.9	0.7	73.4
9	0.75	21.7	0.7	77.7
10	1.06	17.9	0.8	81.3
11	1.54	14.0	0.7	85.4
12	1.73	15.5	0.5	84.0
13	2.41	13.5	0.6	85.9
14	3.05	10.1	0.6	89.2
15	3.65	11.0	1.0	88.0
16	4.18	8.0	0.9	91.1
17	4.86	6.6	1.0	92.4
		African Americans and other minorities		
All ages ...	1.99	27.2	3.2	69.6
5	0.07	66.7	0.0	33.3
6	0.11	28.7	0.0	71.3
7	0.34	36.0	0.0	64.0
8	0.48	36.7	0.0	63.3
9	0.82	31.5	2.8	65.7
10	1.28	29.4	2.5	68.0
11	1.43	29.7	2.0	68.3
12	2.03	32.7	2.4	64.9
13	2.43	32.2	3.4	64.4
14	3.03	25.6	3.8	70.6
15	3.70	25.4	2.9	71.7
16	4.23	23.5	3.3	73.2
17	5.33	24.6	4.2	71.2

Table 8.1. *Mean and percent components of decayed (D), missing (M), and Filled (F) permanent teeth for children ages 5-17 years, United States, 1986-87[1].*

When dental caries in permanent teeth does occur among children, minority children are less likely to have their disease treated than white children, and they have more permanent teeth extracted as a consequence (see Table 8.1) (2). The level of untreated dental disease among American Indian and Alaska Native children is much higher than that for other minority children (according to the Dental Branch, Indian Health Service, Public Health Service, Rockville, MD, February 1993).

Fluoridation and the use of other fluorides have been successful in decreasing the prevalence of dental caries on the smooth surfaces of teeth. Unfortunately, these efforts have much less effect on dental caries that occur in the pits and fissures of teeth (particularly on the biting surfaces of teeth) where more than 85 percent of dental caries now occur (2). Dental sealants (a plastic coating placed on the biting surfaces) applied by a dental professional are an effective, proven preventive intervention for this type of decay. To be effective, however, dental sealants must be applied early, periodically assessed, and re-applied as necessary. Unfortunately, the utilization rate of dental sealants among all children, regardless of ethnic or racial background or income level, is significantly less than the national health promotion and disease prevention target level of 50 percent (8).

As of 1989, only 10.9 percent of American children had sealants applied (9). The mean charge for dental sealants among a dentally insured population in 1988 was $17.80 (standard deviation $3.74) (10). Many poor Americans are unable to afford this relatively inexpensive preventive dental care. Approximately 5.3 percent of children ages 5 to 17 years from families whose incomes are less than $10,000 have dental sealants, compared with more than 21 percent of children in families with incomes in excess of $35,000 (see Figure 8.2). For children ages 9 to 11, only 6 percent of African American children and 10.3 percent of Hispanic and other minority children have dental sealants, compared with 21 percent of white American children.

Children whose parents and caregivers have less than a high school education or whose parents and caregivers are American Indians or Alaska Natives appear to be at markedly increased risk for developing baby bottle tooth decay (also called nursing caries), a severe form of caries that can destroy primary teeth. This type of dental caries is caused by frequent or prolonged use of baby bottles that contain milk, sugared water, fruit juice, or other sugary beverages during the day or night. The prevalence of baby bottle tooth decay has been estimated at 53 percent among rural American Indian and Alaska Native Head Start children and as high as 11 percent in some urban areas (11, 12).

Children who experience baby bottle tooth decay are at increased risk for dental disease throughout their lives. The psychological trauma, health risks, and costs associated with restoration of these grossly carious teeth for children affected by baby bottle tooth decay can be substantial, often requiring general anesthesia. Dietary counseling and intervention by dental and other professionals provide the best means of preventing this serious oral disease (8).

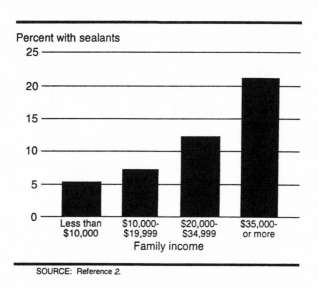

SOURCE: Reference 2.

Figure 8.2. Use of dental sealants among U.S. children 5-17 years of age by family income, 1989.

Oral Disease among Adults

While the overall oral health of adults is improving, dental caries, gingivitis, and periodontal diseases continue to affect most adult Americans. A recent national survey found that 96 percent of employed adults in the United States, nearly 100 million persons, had experienced dental caries (13).

The number of decayed or filled teeth is greater for white Americans than for African Americans and other minorities (10.3 decayed or filled teeth for whites versus 6.8 decayed or filled teeth for African Americans). However, the percent of diseased teeth with untreated decay is greater among African Americans than white Americans at all ages (see Table 8.2).

Gingivitis and adult-onset periodontitis, two diseases that involve the supporting tissue of teeth, affect nearly half of all employed Americans between 18 and 64 years of age (13). Untreated periodontal diseases can lead to tooth mobility, poor esthetics, decreased ability to eat, chew, or speak; and tooth loss. One measure of periodontal diseases is recession, exposure of tooth root surfaces due to a loss of gum tissue. More than 45 percent of employed adults 55 to 64 years of age had moderate recession. Another measure of periodontal disease is the depth of pockets between the teeth and supporting tissue. Almost 20 percent of employed adults 55 to 64 years of age have periodontal pockets 4 millimeters or greater, indicating a moderately compromised status of the supporting periodontal tissue.

Age (years)	Mean DFT	Percent D of DFT	Percent F of DFT
White Americans			
All ages	10.316	6.84	93.16
18–19	7.374	12.79	87.21
20–24	7.990	12.91	87.09
25–29	9.159	10.12	89.88
30–34	10.269	7.87	92.13
35–39	11.422	3.92	96.08
40–44	12.198	5.10	94.90
45–49	12.174	4.53	95.47
50–54	11.607	3.96	96.04
55–59	11.075	4.10	95.90
60–64 or older	10.267	3.94	96.06
African Americans			
All ages	6.839	22.14	77.86
18–19	5.587	52.28	47.72
20–24	6.731	26.46	73.54
25–29	7.723	23.48	76.52
30–34	6.689	20.83	79.17
35–39	7.098	18.44	81.56
40–44	8.407	14.51	85.49
45–49	6.182	22.27	77.73
50–54	6.452	21.15	78.85
55–59	4.986	20.60	79.40
60–64 or older	4.163	43.93	56.07

[1] Reference *13*.

Table 8.2. *Mean and percent components of decayed (D) and filled (F) teeth (T) for employed persons by race, United States, 1985–86*[1].

Untreated periodontal disease can lead to the loss of the supporting tissue from the tooth, exposing the roots of the teeth. Deprived of their protective tissue, root surfaces are more susceptible to dental caries than the crowns of teeth. Because the degree of recession generally increases with age, the rate of decay on the roots of teeth is greater among older Americans. As Table 8.3 illustrates, by 64 years of age, 54 percent of all employed Americans had experienced dental caries on at least one root surface (13). The mean number of root surfaces affected by decay among white and African Americans is approximately the same; however, African Americans have a larger percentage of root surfaces with untreated disease (see Table 8.4).

The end result of untreated dental caries and periodontal disease is tooth loss. Figure 8.3 shows that the percent of Americans who have lost all of their teeth increases dramatically after 45 years of age. In 1989, more than 7.2 million Americans (4.8 percent) between the ages of 18 and 64 were edentulous (9). The poor suffer disproportionately

Age (years)	Percent with at least 1 D or F root surface
All ages	21.16
18–19	6.64
20–24	6.30
25–29	9.41
30–34	13.67
35–39	18.30
40–44	25.26
45–49	33.36
50–54	42.14
55–59	42.83
60–64 or older	54.42

[1] Reference *13*.

Table 8.3. *Percent of dentate employed persons with at least one decayed (D) or filled (F) root surface by age group, United States, 1985–86*[1].

from tooth loss. Among both employed and unemployed adults 55 to 64 years of age whose annual income was below the Federal poverty threshold, 35.5 percent were edentulous. Fortunately, the rate of tooth loss among Americans is declining, resulting in improved esthetics and increased ability to eat and speak. This increase in the number of retained teeth has significant implications for preventive and primary oral health service needs. As figure 8.4 shows, almost twice as many teeth are projected to be at risk nationally for dental disease in 2030 as in 1972 (14). This shift is due to both a decrease in the number of teeth lost to disease, as well as an increase in the population. The largest increase in retained teeth is among persons older than 45 years.

Age	Mean DFS	Percent D of DFS	Percent F of DFS
White Americans			
All ages	1.025	39.62	60.38
18–19	0.176	58.68	41.32
20–24	0.358	59.23	40.77
25–29	0.627	64.13	35.87
30–34	0.788	49.87	50.13
35–39	0.757	28.53	71.47
40–44	1.309	43.78	56.22
45–49	1.448	35.41	64.59
50–54	1.742	31.86	68.14
55–59	1.850	28.19	71.81
60–64 or older	2.644	29.81	70.19
African Americans			
All ages	0.927	70.26	29.74
18–19	0.445	100.00	0.00
20–24	0.326	84.44	15.56
25–29	0.421	70.73	29.27
30–34	0.496	64.38	35.62
35–39	1.008	54.21	45.79
40–44	0.896	43.81	56.19
45–49	1.507	76.03	23.97
50–54	1.735	74.28	25.72
55–59	1.336	69.19	30.81
60–64 or older	3.992	91.41	8.59

[1] Reference 13.

Table 8.4. *Mean and percent components of decayed (D) and filled (F) root surfaces (S) in employed persons by race, United States, 1985–86[1].*

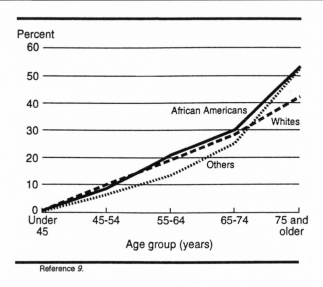

Figure 8.3. *Percentage distribution of edentulous population by race, United States, 1989.*

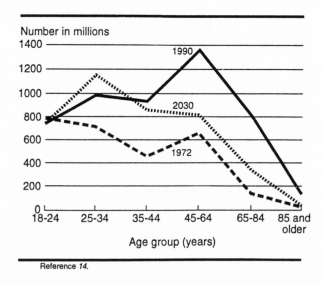

Figure 8.4. *Number of Teeth at risk for dental disease among U.S. adult population by age group, 1972, 1990, and 2030.*

Oral Disease and the Elderly

Dental caries, gingivitis, and periodontal disease affect almost all Americans older than 65 (13). More than 99 percent of the elderly had evidence of dental decay, missing teeth, or filled teeth in 1985. More than 56 percent of Americans older than 65 years had at least one decayed or filled root surface.

Tooth loss among the elderly is significant. A national survey conducted in 1989 found that 5 million Americans (28 percent) 65 to 74 years and 4.8 million Americans (43 percent) 75 years and older were edentulous (9). People with incomes above $35,000 were more likely to have kept their teeth, as the following survey data show (9):

	Percent edentulous	
Income	*65–74*	*75 and older*
Less than $10,000	46.1	56.3
$10,000–$34,999	28.8	40.4
$35,000 or more	12.0	30.3

Between 1986 and 1989, the percent of Americans between 55 and 64 years who were edentulous decreased by almost 3 percent, a significant decrease in such a short time (9, 15). This positive trend means that future cohorts of persons older than 65 years should have more teeth and, given adequate access to care, better oral health.

Gingivitis and periodontitis affect a majority of Americans older than 65 who have teeth (13). More than 86 percent of this age group had at least one tooth with moderate or severe recession, increasing the likelihood of root caries. More than 22 percent of the elderly had periodontal pockets 4 millimeters deep or greater.

Oral Cancer

In 1992, an estimated 30,000 new cases of oropharyngeal cancer were diagnosed, and more than 8,000 deaths occurred as a result of this disease (16). Oropharyngeal cancer is more common than leukemia, Hodgkin's disease, melanoma of the skin, and cancers of the brain, cervix, ovary, liver, pancreas, bone, thyroid gland, testes, or stomach. It is the 6th most common cancer found among U.S. men and the 12th most common among U.S. women. Figure 8.5 shows the estimated number of new cases of cancer and number of cancer deaths by type of cancer in 1992 (16). Use of tobacco products, including smokeless tobacco, and alcohol are associated with more than 70 percent of all oral cancer lesions (17). Oropharyngeal cancer is most frequent in men older than 40, but it can be found in teenagers with a history of smokeless tobacco use.

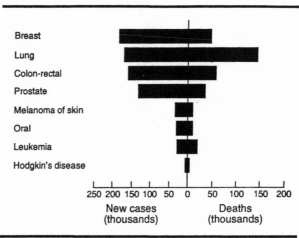

NOTE: Incidence estimates are based on rates from the National Cancer Institute Surveillance, Epidemiology, and End Results (SEER) Program, 1986-88.

Figure 8.5. *Estimated number of new cancer cases and number of cancer deaths by type of cancer.*

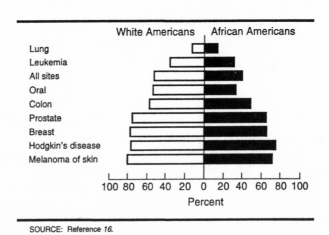

SOURCE: Reference 16.

Figure 8.6. *Relative 5 years' survival by site of cancer and by race, United States, 1981–87.*

Figure 8.6 illustrates the differences between white and African Americans in the relative percent of persons surviving five years for selected types of cancer (16). For African Americans, the relative five years'survival rate for oropharyngeal cancer is only 31 percent, compared with 54 percent for white Americans. This 23 percent is the largest difference for all types of cancers, as the following data show:

Cancer site	*(Percent five years' survival rate for white Americans) minus (percent five years' survival rate for African Americans.)[1]*
All sites	15
Lung	2
Hodgkin's disease	3
Leukemia	7
Colon	11
Melanoma of the skin	12
Prostate	13
Breast	15
Oral	23

[1]*Based on cancer mortality data from 1982-88.*

A significant portion of this difference in survival can be attributed to delayed detection and treatment of the cancer (16).

Those who are treated for oral cancer frequently face significant functional problems, disfigurement that decreases quality of life, and an increased risk of developing new oral cancers, as well as other types of cancer. Annual visits to an oral health professional greatly increase the probability of early detection and successful treatment outcomes.

Impact of Oral Health Problems

Millions of Americans are at high risk for oral health problems because of underlying medical or disabling conditions, ranging from very rare genetic diseases to more common chronic diseases like arthritis and diabetes (18). These conditions not only impact the person's quality of life (that is, their ability to eat, speak, taste, and swallow), but also they can be a significant source of pain and discomfort. For example, diabetics often experience more severe periodontal disease and delayed wound healing, affecting both their oral health and general health.

Congenital anomalies, like cleft lip and palate, often require extensive surgical repair. Several genetic diseases affect oral health, such as the ectodermal dysplasias, in which essential components of skin and teeth fail to develop properly; scleroderma, a genetic and autoimmune condition affecting the skin, which leads to limited mouth opening; osteogenesis and dentinogenesis imperfecta, in which bones and teeth are poorly developed and subject to fracture; and epidermolysis bullosa, which is characterized by severe blistering of skin and mucous membranes leading to loss of essential body fluids and sometimes fatal secondary infections.

Among persons with compromised immune systems, the presence of oral disease has been linked to opportunistic, infections. People who are human immunodeficiency virus (HIV) seropositive or have acquired immunodeficiency syndrome (AIDS) are likely to demonstrate a variety of oral complications associated with their disease. These complications primarily affect the soft tissues of the mouth and include painful oral candidiasis and potential life-threatening fungal infections ("thrush") of the esophagus, hairy leukoplakia (white, raised lesions on the lateral borders of the tongue), herpes (multiple, severe cold sores), and Kaposi's sarcoma, a type of cancer affecting blood vessels (19, 20). Many HIV-seropositive persons experience very aggressive forms of destructive periodontal diseases, which can significantly compromise their nutritional status and may require hospitalization.

Routine dental examinations can play an important role in the initial diagnosis of HIV infection and in the management of AIDS. In many instances, oral manifestations associated with HIV infection may be an initial presentation of the disease. Because effective drug regimens are now available that can delay the onset of AIDS after the initial HIV infection has occurred, early diagnosis and treatment are imperative. Dental professionals can and do make such diagnoses and refer persons for appropriate medical evaluations (21).

Untreated oral infections and dental treatment without adequate antibiotic prophylaxis are associated with infective endocarditis, an infection of the valves of the heart that can occur in people with defective heart valves (22-24). Infective endocarditis has a 50 percent mortality rate and is increasing in prevalence, and the elderly are at high risk. Morbidity and costs associated with heart valve replacement after infective endocarditis are substantial.

Similarly, those elderly with prosthetic joints (for example, hip, knee, and shoulder joints) are at risk for costly infections of those joints due to oral bacteria from untreated oral disease. The etiologic bacteria enter the bloodstream from the oral cavity and initiate an infection around the artificial joint (25-27). This may necessitate replacement of the infected joint. As the U.S. population ages, more and more hip, knee, and shoulder replacements will be required, potentially increasing the number of complications secondary to untreated oral diseases.

Untreated dental disease also complicates the treatment of patients undergoing organ and bone marrow transplants, sometimes resulting in death (28, 29). Dental disease also has been associated with severe complications including pneumonia, urinary tract infections, fever, and septicemia.

Poor oral health and untreated oral diseases and conditions can have a significant impact on quality of life. Oral and facial pain affects a substantial proportion of the general population. Studies to determine the number of persons experiencing oral pain have found that, at any given time, between 29 percent and 50 percent of those surveyed reported some dental and oral pain (30-36). In these same surveys, the percentage of people who reported moderate to severe dental pain ranged from 9 percent to 26 percent (30,32-34). The type of pain experienced by people varied by population groups. Among the elderly, dry mouth pain (xerostomia) and denture pain were common. Temporomandibular joint pain was common among young women. Patients seeking emergency dental care were often in pain from acute dental and oral infections (34,37-41).

Dental disease also has an impact on the economic productivity and on the ability of American children to learn. In 1989, more than 164,175,000 hours were missed from work (an average of 1.48 hours per employed U.S. adult), and more than 51,679,000 hours of school were lost (117,000 hours missed per 100,000 school age children) because of dental treatment and problems (42). Many of those who missed work or school hours could least afford it, including younger workers, minorities, low-wage earners, and those with severe dental disease.

Dental treatment may be delayed, ultimately requiring more extensive and costly treatment and resulting in restricted activity days and bed days. In 1991, for example, U.S. school age children experienced more than 4,794,000 restricted activity days (7.3 days per 100 school age children) and 2,200,000 bed days (3.36 days per 100 school age children) as a result of dental conditions (43). Americans 18 to 64 years of age reported more than 8 million restricted activity days (5.2 days per 100 adults) in 1991 and 3.9 million bed days (2.56 days per 100 adults).

Expenditures, Costs, and Sources of Payment

In 1992, an estimated $38.7 billion was spent on dental services, representing about 5.3 percent of all expenditures for personal health care in the United States, up from only $2 billion in 1960 (44, 45a). By the year 2000, an estimated $62.3 billion will be spent for dental services (see Table 8.5). While total expenditures for dental services continue to increase, the level of spending for dental services as a percent of personal health care continues to decline. Since 1960, this proportion has fallen from more than 8 percent to 5.3 percent in 1992. This trend is projected to continue, so that by the year 2000, dental expenditures will represent about 4 percent of personal health expenditures.

Growth in the price of dental services has out-paced the consumer price index for urban areas (CPI-U) for all goods and services since the early 1980s, but the growth continues to be lower than the CPI for physician and hospital services (see Table 8.6) (46). In part, this trend has resulted in the decrease in relative spending for dental services. It is estimated that the inflation of dental services will continue to outpace the inflation of all goods and services for the next 10 to 15 years (47).

In 1987, an average of $295 was spent for dental services for those Americans with a dental expense (48). More than 90 percent of these

Year	Total health expenditures	Personal health expenditures	Expenditures for dental services	Dental services as a percent of personal health expenditures
1960	$27.1	$23.9	$2.0	8.4
1965	41.6	35.6	2.8	7.9
1970	74.4	64.9	4.7	7.2
1975	132.9	116.6	8.2	7.1
1980	250.1	219.4	14.4	6.5
1985	422.6	369.7	23.3	6.3
1990	675.0	591.5	34.1	5.8
1995	1,101.9	986.7	46.5	4.7
2000	1,739.8	1,572.1	62.3	4.0

[1] References 44 and 45a.

Table 8.5. *Percentage of national expenditures in billions of dollars for all health and dental services, 1960–2000[1].*

expenditures for dental services were paid by private sources, either out-of-pocket by dental consumers (56 percent) or through private health insurance (34 percent). Less than 4 percent of dental expenditures come from public sources, principally Medicaid.

Out-of-Pocket Payments

The primary source of payment for dental services is out-of-pocket. In 1987, the mean annual out-of-pocket expense for dental services was $165.20 (48). On average, Americans paid almost $50 more out-of-pocket annually for dental services than for ambulatory physician services.

The out-of-pocket cost of dental services can have a significant impact on the poor (that is, those Americans below the Federal poverty level). The poor who sought dental care in 1987 paid an average of $113 per year out-of-pocket, while middle income people paid an average of $164.60 per year out-of-pocket.

Out-of-pocket payments represent a significant source of payment for dental services for two reasons. First, approximately 150 million Americans have no private third-party dental insurance coverage, and there is limited payment for dental services under public programs

Year	All goods and services in urban areas	Hospital services	Physician services	Dental services
1981	90.9	78.1	84.9	86.5
1982	96.5	90.4	92.9	93.1
1983	99.6	100.6	100.1	99.4
1984	103.9	109.0	107.0	107.5
1985	107.6	115.5	113.3	114.2
1986	109.6	122.3	121.5	120.6
1987	113.6	131.1	130.4	128.6
1988	118.3	143.4	139.8	137.5
1989	124.0	158.1	150.1	146.0
1990	130.7	175.4	160.8	155.8
1991	136.2	191.9	170.5	167.4
1992	140.3	208.7	181.2	178.7

[1] Reference 46.

Table 8.6. Consumer Price Index for hospital, physician, and dental services compared with all goods and services in urban areas, United States, 1981–92 (1982–84 = 100)[1].

(48). Second, even for those with dental insurance, the number of covered services may be limited depending on the plan. Copayments and deductibles under some insurance plans may be as high as 50 percent for many dental procedures.

The large proportion of out-of-pocket payments for dental services results in significant amounts of bad debt and free care. In 1987, for example, more than $2 billion of dental services were provided as either bad debt or free care, representing approximately 7 percent of the costs associated with providing dental services (48). Five percent of charges for inpatient hospital services and ambulatory physician services and 1 percent of charges for outpatient prescribed medicines were paid by workers' compensation, private charity, other similar sources, and free care from the provider including bad debt.

Dental Insurance

Approximately 95 million Americans have some form of dental insurance (9). The distribution of dental insurance by age group is shown in Figure 8.7. Most persons who have dental insurance are between 25 and 54 years of age or are the dependents of employed adults with dental insurance. Since dental insurance coverage is usually employment-based, persons who do not work or who work part-time are less likely to be insured.

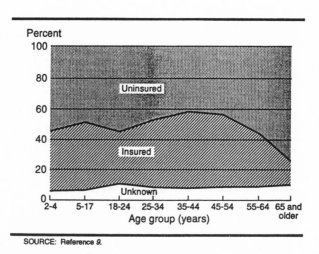

SOURCE: Reference 9.

Figure 8.7. Percentage distribution of persons 2 years and older by private dental insurance status, United States, 1989.

The proportion of dentally insured people decreases in two age groups. Nearly 12 million previously insured young adults lose their dental insurance between the ages of 18 and 24. The percent of people with insurance increases until age 54, when workers begin to retire. By the age 65, only 15 percent have dental insurance, a decrease of more than 33 percent from the 45 to 54 age group.

Whether a person has dental insurance is associated with the annual income level. Approximately 10 percent of people with annual incomes of less than $10,000 have private dental insurance (9). However, almost 60 percent of people with annual incomes of $35,000 or more have private dental insurance. For those below the poverty threshold, only 10.6 percent have dental insurance, while 47.7 percent of those above the poverty level are insured.

Medicaid

In fiscal year 1991, more than $709 million was spent to provide dental services to approximately 5.2 million Medicaid recipients (49). Medicaid recipients receiving dental services represented less than 17 percent of all Medicaid-eligible people, and expenditures for these services represented less than 1 percent of the $77 billion spent on Medicaid in 1991. Expenditures for dental services are the only health service expenditures that have decreased since 1975—by 29.7 percent (45b). Medicaid payments for dental services were principally for children receiving benefits through the Aid to Families with Dependent Children (AFDC) Program (48.6 percent). Yet, only about 20 percent of Medicaid eligible children receive any dental services.

Nationwide in 1991, an average of $136 was spent per recipient for dental services under Medicaid. However, because benefit levels for dental services are determined by each State, there is significant variability in the per capita spending. For example, in 1991, the reported per capita expenditures for dental services ranged from $73 in Pennsylvania, $124 in Georgia, $169 in New York, $223 in California, to $328 in Alaska (49). This considerable variability is due, in part, to differences in covered services, eligibility criteria, and reimbursement levels. In most States, for example, dental services for adults are extremely limited or are not covered.

In 1990, the Office of Technology Assessment (OTA), U.S. Congress, issued a report entitled "Children's Dental Services Under the Medicaid Program" (50). This report included seven States that represent about 45 percent of Medicaid total payments for dental services and about 43 percent of dependent children younger than 21 years enrolled in the program nationwide. The report was prepared in response to a request from the U.S. House of Representatives' Committee on Energy and Commerce and sought to determine whether the dental care programs for Medicaid beneficiaries, particularly children eligible for the Early and Periodic Screening, Diagnosis, and Treatment Program, conform to a minimum level of dental care. The OTA found that:

• There are significant differences among those States surveyed in the dental services offered through their Medicaid programs.

• Each of the States surveyed failed to adequately cover "basic" dental services in its Medicaid program.

• Some dentists believed that their Medicaid patients younger than 18 years did not receive services equal to those provided young non-Medicaid patients.

• A variety of barriers restrict the low-income child's access to dental services under State Medicaid programs (including administrative problems, paperwork associated with claims submission and prior approval, and low reimbursement rates for dental services).

Medicare

With Medicare, payment for routine dental services is prohibited under statute except in very limited circumstances (for example, medically necessary dental care and surgery on the jaw not involving the teeth). As a result, essentially no Federal dollars are expended for dental services under Medicare.

Comparison of source of payment for dental services and ambulatory physician services. As Table 8.7 illustrates, the distribution of sources of payment for dental services differs from that for ambulatory physician services (48). A much larger percentage of dental services than physician services are paid for out-of-pocket. For example, the poor paid 56 percent of the cost of dental care out-of-pocket, compared with only 19 percent out-of-pocket for physicians' ambulatory care. Medicaid paid for only 15 percent of the expenditures for dental services among the poor in 1987, compared with 31 percent for physicians' ambulatory services in the same group. Medicare paid 22 percent of the expenses for physicians' ambulatory services for the poor in 1987, but 0 percent for dental services.

Dental expenditures under other public programs. Dental services and other oral health programs are covered under several other public programs as well. For example, in 1991, approximately $60 million was spent by the Indian Health Service (IHS) to provide dental services to more than 355,000 Native Americans (according to the Dental Branch, IHS, Public Health Service, Rockville, MD, February 1993). Total expenditures for dental services in the IHS are projected to increase to $70 million by the year 2000.

Public expenditures for oral health services at the State and territorial level totaled approximately $55.7 million in 1989 (51). Information collected by the Public Health Foundation shows the growth in dental expenditures from 1984 to 1989 for both dental health and fluoridation programs (see Table 8.8). Oral health comprised less than 1 percent of all public health expenditures in this period. While absolute expenditures for oral health services increased between 1984 and 1989, oral health spending as a percent of total public health expenditures actually declined (51).

Source of payment	Dental services		Ambulatory physician services	
	Poor[2]	U.S. average	Poor[2]	U.S. average
Out-of-pocket	56	56	19	26
Private insurance.......	16	34	10	38
Medicare	0	0	22	14
Medicaid	15	2	31	8
Other public programs..	3	1	12	10
Workers' compensation, private charity, and free from provider including bad debt	10	7	5	5

[1] Reference 48.
[2] Poor are those persons earning less than 100 percent of the Federal poverty level.

Table 8.7. *Sources of payment and percentage for dental and ambulatory physician services, United States, 1987[1].*

87

Fiscal year	States reporting	Public health expenditures	Oral health expenditures	Oral health as a percent of public health expenditures	States without categorical oral health expenditures
1984	43	$5.3	$0.0381	0.72	3
1986	48	6.9	0.0491	0.71	6
1988	50	7.7	0.0531	0.69	8
1989	50	8.95	0.0557	0.62	8
Percent change 1984–89..........		68.87	46.19	...	...

[1] Reference 51.

Table 8.8. Public health and oral health expenditures in billions and percent of oral health to public expenditures, fiscal years 1984, 1986, and 1989[1].

Characteristic	1983	1986	1989
All ages[2]	55.0	57.1	57.2
2–4 years..............	28.4	31.3	32.1
5–17 years	67.0	70.3	69.0
18–34 years	57.0	58.0	56.9
35–54 years	57.4	60.5	61.4
55–64 years	51.3	51.2	54.0
65 years and older	38.6	41.7	43.2
Race:			
White	57.0	59.2	59.3
African American.....	41.8	43.6	44.5
Family income:			
Less than $10,000....	38.8	40.9	40.9
$10,000–$19,999	47.5	47.5	43.4
$20,000–$34,999	61.4	61.0	58.3
$35,000 and more....	74.0	73.5	73.0

[1] Reference 9.
[2] Includes persons of other races and unknown income (not shown separately).

Table 8.9. Percent of persons 2 years and older with dental visits in past year, by selected characteristics, United States, 1983, 1986, and 1989[1].

Use of Dental Services

Since 1983, the proportion of Americans with at least one dental visit per year has increased modestly from 55 percent to 57.3 percent, representing about 135 million persons in 1989 (9). As table 8.9 illustrates, from 1983 to 1989, African Americans and poor and low-income persons were less likely to have had a dental visit in the past year when compared with white Americans or higher income groups.

Use of dental services remains quite variable throughout the population (9). Race and ethnicity, age, and income were significant factors in use of dental services. Those with a dental visit in the past two years were more likely to be white, non-Hispanic, have a higher income, have at least a high school education, and have dental insurance (see Table 8.10). Unfortunately, poor and low-income groups—the same groups that have the highest levels of dental disease—have the lowest utilization rates.

Characteristic	Less than 2 years	2 years or more	Never
Race:			
White	68.6	22.1	4.4
African American	55.5	32.0	5.8
Other	61.3	24.8	6.7
Hispanic origin:			
Non-Hispanic	67.9	22.8	4.1
Hispanic	56.5	27.6	9.7
Mexican American	49.4	31.1	13.1
Other Hispanic	65.5	23.6	5.1
Education level:			
Less than 9 years	39.6	49.0	5.9
9–11 years	49.7	43.8	1.3
12 years	65.2	29.4	0.5
13 years or more	78.7	17.2	0.2
Family income:			
Less than $10,000	53.1	36.4	7.0
$10,000–$19,999	55.7	33.5	6.6
$20,000–$34,999	68.7	23.6	4.6
$35,000 or more	80.3	14.0	2.9
Dental insurance coverage:			
Yes	79.1	15.8	3.3
No	61.5	29.6	6.0

[1] Reference 9.
NOTE: Rows do not sum to 100 percent because "unknowns" are not included in table.

Table 8.10. Interval since last dental visit for percent of persons by selected characteristics, 1989[1].

Among edentulous Americans older than 35, less than 13 percent had a dental visit during the year preceding the interview, and more than 60 percent had not been to a dentist in more than five years.

While dental insurance increased the utilization rate for all groups, differences in utilization among the insured were also found (9). African Americans and persons with lower incomes who had dental insurance had less utilization and fewer visits than similarly covered white Americans (see Table 8.11). Indeed, African American children with dental insurance had fewer visits (1.6 visits per child) than white children without dental insurance (2.0 visits per child) (9).

Characteristic	Visits per person per year	Percent with 1 or more visits in previous year
Race:		
White	2.9	71.6
African American......	1.7	57.6
Family income:		
Less than $10,000.....	2.0	59.4
$10,000–$19,999	2.2	54.8
$20,000–$34,999	2.5	66.2
$35,000 and more.....	3.2	77.3

[1] Reference 9.

Table 8.11. *Age-adjusted dental visits per person per year and percent with dental visit in previous year among persons with dental insurance by selected characteristics, 1989[1].*

Reasons for seeking dental care vary according to the individual. According to a national survey, in 1985-86, nearly three million African Americans (29.7 percent) sought dental care most recently for either a toothache or to have a tooth extracted (13). Less than 13 percent of white Americans sought care for these reasons (see Figure 8.8). There are many explanations for differences in not using dental services. About one-half of those surveyed who had not seen a dentist in the previous year did not perceive they had a dental problem (see Table 8.12) (9), although epidemiologic data would suggest that this perception is incorrect. Cost was the second most common reason offered for not visiting the dentist for persons up to the age of 35 years. Fear of the dentist did not appear to be a major factor in failure to seek care.

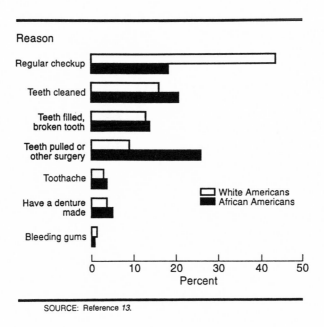

Figure 8.8. Main reason given by employed persons for last visit for dental care by race, United States, 1985.

Characteristic	Fear	Cost	Access problem	No perceived dental problem	No teeth	Not important	Other reasons
Age (years):							
All ages	4.3	13.7	1.7	46.8	14.3	2.3	8.7
2–17	1.3	15.0	1.5	56.8	0.2	1.9	11.9
18–34	5.9	19.1	2.4	52.4	0.7	3.2	9.5
35–64	5.8	12.8	1.5	43.3	17.8	2.2	8.4
65 and older	2.2	4.1	1.1	31.2	49.7	1.1	3.9
Family income:							
Less than $10,000	3.8	19.7	1.7	42.8	22.5	1.4	6.4
$10,000–$19,999	4.0	18.8	1.5	47.0	17.4	1.7	6.5
$20,000–$34,99	4.8	13.7	1.7	51.3	11.5	2.3	11.1
$35,000 or more	5.9	6.8	2.6	52.3	8.1	4.1	14.1
Dental insurance coverage:							
Have dental insurance	6.2	7.2	2.5	53.2	10.1	3.4	15.2
Without dental insurance . . .	4.0	18.5	1.5	48.7	17.2	2.0	7.0
Insurance status unknown . .	1.6	3.9	0.7	23.8	9.3	0.8	2.9

[1] Reference 9.

Table 8.12. *Percent of persons reporting various reasons for no dental visits in past year, according to selected demographic characteristics, United States, 1989.*

Condition	Poor[1]	African American	Hispanic	U.S. average
5–17-year-olds with untreated dental caries	. . .	35.1	37.6	24.0
Any private dental insurance.	7.8	31.9	28.7	44.3
Dental sealants	4.3	4.2	5.1	10.9
At least 1 dental visit in the preceding year	48.8	49.9	47.9	61.7
Average number of dental visits per year.	1.1	1.0	1.6	2.1

[1] Family income under $10,000.

Table 8.13. *Oral health status and use of dental services among U.S. children (percent or number)*

Condition	Poor[1]	African American	Hispanic	U.S. average
18–64-year-olds with untreated dental caries	. . .	50.43	42.86	29.69
Any private dental insurance.	13.3	35.6	31.2	43.9
At least 1 dental visit in the preceding year	43.5	44.9	46.0	58.3
Edentulous	8.5	4.2	2.3	4.8
Average number of dental visits per year.	1.4	1.3	1.5	2.1

[1] < $10,000.

Table 8.14. *Oral health status and use of dental services among U.S. adults 18-64 years of age (percent or number)*

Condition	Poor[1]	African American	Hispanic	U.S. average
Any private dental insurance.........	5.7	11.1	15.6	15.0
At least 1 dental visit in the preceding year..........	25.8	22.5	40.2	43.2
Edentulous	51.1	37.9	[2]24.9	34.1
Average number of dental visits per year..............	1.3	0.6	1.2	2.0

[1] < $10,000.
[2] For ages 65–74 years only.

Table 8.15. *Oral health status and use of dental services among U.S. adults 65 years and older (percent or number).*

Summary

Tables 8.13–8.15 summarize information on the oral health of children, adults, and the elderly and their use of dental services.

Major findings for children (Table 8.13) follow:

- African Americans and other minorities have a higher percentage of untreated disease than the U.S. average.

- Poor children and minorities have less private dental insurance than the average for all children.

- Smaller proportions of minority and poor children have dental sealants.

- Ten percent fewer minority and poor children had a dental visit in the preceding year compared with the U.S. average, although these groups have a higher percent of untreated disease.

- The average number of dental visits per year for poor and minority children is less than the U.S. average.

The findings for adults (Table 8.14) follow:

- The level of untreated dental caries among minorities is greater than the national average.

- Smaller proportions of minorities and poor adults have dental insurance than the national average.

- Smaller proportions of minorities and poor adults had a dental visit in the preceding year.

- The average number of dental visits for poor and minority adults is less than the average for all U.S. adults.

- Almost 9 percent of poor adults are edentulous compared with 4.8 percent of the adult population.

Major findings among U.S. elderly include these observations (Table 8.15):

- Only 15 percent of the elderly have any private dental insurance, and Medicare does not reimburse for routine dental services.

- More than 22 percent of elderly African Americans, and 26 percent of poor elderly had at least one dental visit in the preceding year, about one-half of the national average for all elderly.

- Minority and poor elderly have fewer visits than the U.S. average; elderly African Americans have less than one-half the average number of visits among the elderly.

- More than one-half of the poor elderly had lost all their teeth.

Conclusion

While significant improvements have been made in preventing and controlling dental caries and periodontal diseases during the past two decades, millions of Americans have been left behind, resulting in needless pain, increased cost, decreased health, and loss of self-esteem. Almost all Americans have been affected by oral diseases; however, poor and low-income persons, minorities, and persons with little education are particularly at risk. Oral diseases remain an unnecessary obstacle to better health.

Access to primary and preventive dental care can be difficult, especially for those that cannot afford dental care. Regrettably, Americans for whom the burden of oral disease is greatest often have the most difficulty gaining access to the dental care system. Access to needed services is critical to narrow the disparity in disease between the poor and the middle class and among whites, African Americans, and other minorities. Access to dental care for elderly Americans is particularly difficult, since they often lose their dental benefits at retirement, and Medicare does not pay for dental services. The elderly are at risk of losing a lifetime's worth of investment in oral health.

Regular dental care is important for a number of other oral diseases besides dental caries and periodontal diseases. Oral cancer, which affects primarily adults older than 55, results in significant morbidity and disfigurement associated with treatment, substantial cost, and more than 8,000 deaths annually. The percent of persons with oral cancer who survive five years is 22 percent lower among African Americans than whites. Routine dental examinations are the best strategy to narrow the gap in survival between African Americans and whites, since early detection and treatment are imperative. Yet, African Americans are less likely to have a dental visit than whites.

Dental and oral diseases have a significant impact on general health. For example, dental and oral diseases and treatment associated with these diseases can result in infective endocarditis (which has a 50 percent mortality rate), infections of artificial knee, hip, or shoulder joints, and in complications associated with organ and bone marrow transplantations. Oral complications associated with HIV infection also can have a significant impact on overall health, resulting in loss of appetite, painful mouth sores, hospitalization, and potentially life-threatening fungal infections. Most of these complications among people with HIV-AIDS can be managed by a dentist in an outpatient setting. However, because many people with AIDS cannot afford dental care, access is often compromised. As the number of AIDS cases continues to rise, barriers to obtaining oral health care can only exacerbate the problem.

One of the principal barriers to dental care is cost. More than 150 million Americans have no dental insurance coverage. Public programs pay for less than 3 percent of all dental services, and eligibility for these programs is highly variable. Most States provide only limited dental services for adults, or none at all. In many States, benefits available to children covered by the Medicaid Program do not even include basic dental services. The 30 percent decrease in per capita payments for dental services under Medicaid between 1975 and 1990 stands in stark contrast to all other medical expenditure categories under Medicaid, none of which declined during this period.

For persons who do not have access to physician or other primary health care services, hospital emergency rooms provide a safety net to ensure that at least some level of care, albeit expensive, is available. For oral health problems, however, no such mechanism exists. Few hospitals provide dental services, and those that do offer only emergency services to relieve pain and provide palliative treatment for injuries and infections.

Dental schools and hospital-based postdoctoral dental education programs are a source of care for some of those who cannot afford to pay, but not all people, especially poor people, have the time, resources, or transportation necessary to seek care at dental education institutions. The additional financial burden "free care" places on these schools can be significant.

Community and migrant health centers (CMHCs) may be a source of dental care but are not found in every community. Further, only about one-half of existing CMHCs provide basic dental care services (according to the Bureau of Primary Health Care, Health Resources and Services Administration, Public Health Service, Rockville, MD, February 1993). More importantly, CMHCs do not have the resources to meet this need alone. The unfortunate reality is that people who cannot afford routine dental care and who are not covered by either public programs or private dental insurance do not receive care.

Fiscal crises in many of the States place ever-increasing burdens on the poor. The Center for Budget and Policy Priorities recently found that during each of the last two years, State programs assisting the poor were cut more deeply than at any time since the early 1980s (52). The center reported that during the last two years, reductions in general assistance benefits, a program of last resort for the non-elderly poor who do not quality for AFDC, affected more than half a million recipients. In addition, seven States made cuts in their general medical assistance programs for low-income people who do not qualify for Medicaid. Given that Medicaid beneficiaries eligible for dental services have restricted or no access to dental care currently and that such a substantial proportion of dental services are paid for out-of-pocket, these reductions by the States can only mean less access to dental care for those most at risk for disease.

The current dental care delivery system has not adequately met the oral health needs of all Americans, especially those who are unable to afford dental care, who have no dental insurance, and who are at high risk of dental and oral diseases. Further improvement of the oral and general health of Americans can be accelerated by ensuring improved access to primary preventive and early intervention services for all and the removal of barriers to the care system.

References

1. Kozol, J.: *Savage inequalities: children in America's schools*. Crown Publishers, Inc., New York, 1991, pp. 20-21.

2. *National Institute of Dental Research: Oral health of United States children: the National Survey of Dental Caries in U.S. School Children, 1986-1987*. NIH Publication No. 89-2247, Bethesda, MD, 1989.

3. Newbrun, E.: Effectiveness of water fluoridation. *J Public Health Dent* 49: 279-289, special issue No. 5 (1989).

4. Glass, R. L.: Fluoride dentifrices: the basis for the decline in caries prevalence. *J Soc Med* 79 (supp. 14): 15-17 (1986).

5. Ismail, A. I., et al.: Findings from the dental care supplement of the National Health Interview Survey, 1983. *J Am Dent Assoc* 114: 617-621, May 1987.

6. Clovis, J., and Hargreaves, J. A.: Fluoride intake from beverage consumption. *Community Dent Oral Epidemiol* 16: 11-15, February 1988.

7. Naylor, M. N.: Possible factors underlying the decline in caries prevalence. *J R Soc Med* 78 (supp. 7): 23-25 (1985).

8. *Public Health Service: Healthy people 2000: national health promotion and disease prevention objectives*. DHHS Publication No. (PHS) 91-50212, Washington, D.C., 1990.

9. Bloom, B., Gift, H. C., and Jack, S. S.: Dental services and oral health; United States, 1989. *Vital Health Stat* [10] No. 183. DHHS Publication No. (PHS) 93-1511. National Center for Health Statistics, Hyattsville, MD, 1992.

10. Kuthy, R. A.: Charges for sealants and one-surface, posterior permanent restorations: three years of insurance claims data. *Pediatr Dent* 14: 405-406, November/December 1992.

11. Broderick, E., Mabry, J., Robertson, D., and Thompson, J.: Baby bottle tooth decay in Native American children. *Public Health Rep* 104: 5054, January-February 1989.

12. Kelly, M., and Bruerd, B.: The prevalence of nursing bottle decay among two Native American populations. *J Public Health Dent* 47: 94-97, spring 1987.

13. *National Institute of Dental Research: Oral health of United States adults: the National Survey of Oral Health in U.S. Employed Adults and Seniors: 1985-1986.* NIH Publication No. 87-2868. Bethesda, MD, 1987.

14. Reinhardt, J. W., and Douglass, C. W.: The need for operative dentistry services: projecting the effects of changing disease patterns. *Operative Dentistry* 14: 114-120, summer 1989.

15. Jack, S. S., and Bloom, B.: Use of dental services and dental health: United States, 1986. *Vital Health Stat* [10] No. 165. DHHS Publication No. (PHS) 88-1593. National Center for Health Statistics, Hyattsville, MD, 1988.

16. *American Cancer Society: Cancer facts and figures-1992.* Atlanta, GA, 1992.

17. *Centers for Disease Control and the National Institutes of Health: Cancers of the oral cavity and pharynx: a statistics review monograph*, 1973-1987. Atlanta, GA, 1991.

18. *National Institute of Dental Research: Broadening the scope: long-range research plan for the nineties.* NIH Publication No. 90-1188, Bethesda, MD, 1990.

19. Barone, R., et al.: Prevalence of oral lesions among HIV-infected intravenous drug abusers and other risk groups. *Oral Surg Oral Med Oral Pathol* 69: 169-173, February 1990.

20. Feigal, D.W., et al.: The prevalence of oral lesions in HIV-infected homosexual and bisexual men: three San Francisco epidemiological cohorts. *AIDS* 5: 519-525, May 1991.

21. Barr, C. E., and Marder, M. Z.: *AIDS: a guide for dental practice.* Quintessence Publishing Co., Chicago, 1987, pp. 49.

22. Carranza, J. R., and Fermin, A.: *Glickman's clinical periodontology.* Ed. 7, W. B. Saunders Co., Harcourt Brace, Jarovich. Inc., Philadelphia, PA, 1990, pp. 567-586.

23. Sande, M. A., Kaye, D., and Root, R. K.: *Endocarditis.* Churchill Livingston, New York, 1984, pp. 7-8.

24. Durack, D. T., and Peterson, R. G.: *Changes in the epidemiology of endocarditis.* American Heart Association Monograph, Series 52, 1977, pp. 3-8.

25. Jacobson, J. J., Schweitzer, S., DePorter, D. J., and Lee, J. J.: Chemoprophylaxis of dental patients with prosthetic joints: a simulation model. *J Dent Educ* 52: 599-604, November 1988.

26. Tsevat, J., Durand-Zaleski, I., and Pauker, S. G.: Costeffectiveness of antibiotic prophylaxis for dental procedures in patients with artificial joints. *Am J Public Health* 79: 739-743, June 1989.

27. Shuman, S. K.: A physician's guide to coordinating oral health and primary care. *Geriatrics* 45: 47-51,54,57, August 1990.

28. Wilson, R. L., Martinez-Tirado, J., Whelchel, J., and Lordon, R. E.: Occult dental infection causing fever in renal transplant patients. *Am J Kidney Dis* 2: 354-356. November 1982.

29. Harms, K. A., and Bronny, A. T.: Cardiac transplantation: dental considerations. *J Am Dent Assoc* 112: 677-681, May 1986.

30. Locker, D.: The burden of oral disorders in a population of older adults. *Community Dent Health* 9: 109-124, June 1992.

31. Cushing, A. M., Sheiham, A., and Maizels, J.: Developing socio-dental indicators-the social impact of dental disease. *Community Dent Health* 3: 3-17 (1986).

32. Reisine, S.: Dental health and public policy: the social impact of dental disease. *Am J Public Health* 75: 27-30, January 1985.

33. Bailit, H. L.: The prevalence of dental pain and anxiety: their relationship to quality of life. *NY State Dent J* 53: 27-30, August-September 1987.

34. Locker, D., and Grushka, M.: The impact of dental and facial pain. *J Dent Res* 66: 1414-1417, September 1987.

35. Reisine, S. T.: The impact of dental conditions on social functioning and the quality of life. *Annu Rev Public Health* 9: 1-19 (1988).

36. Sternbach, R. A.: Survey of pain in the United States: the Nuprin Pain Report. *Clin J Pain* 2: 49-53 (1986).

37. Kiyak, H. A., and Mulligan, K.: Studies of the relationship between oral health and psychological well-being. *Gerodontics* 3: 109-112, June 1987.

38. Marbach, J. J., Lennon, M. C., Link, B. G., and Dohrenwend, B. P.: Losing face: sources of stigma as perceived by chronic facial pain patients. *J Behav Med* 13: 583-604, December 1990.

39. Erlandsson, S. I., Rubinstein, B., Axelsson A., and Carlsson, S. G.: Psychological dimensions in patients with disabling tinnitus and craniomandibular disorders. *Br J Audiol* 25: 15-24, February 1991.

40. Schnurr, R. F., Brooke, R. I., and Rollman, G. B.: Psychosocial correlates of temporomandibular joint pain and dysfunction. *Pain* 42: 153-165, August 1990.

41. Keller, D. L.: Reduction of dental emergencies through dental readiness. *Mil Med* 153: 498-501, October 1988.

42. Gift, H. C., Reisine, S. T., and Larach, D. C.: The social impact of dental problems and visits. *Am J Public Health* 82: 1663-1668, December 1992.

43. Adams, P. F., and Benson, V.: Current estimates from the National Health Interview Survey, 1991. *Vital Health Statistics* [10] No. 184. DHHS Publication No. (PHS) 93-1512. National Center for Health Statistics, Hyattsville, MD, 1992.

44. Bruner, S. T., Waldo, D. R., and Mckusick, D. R.: National health expenditures projections through 2030. *Health Care Finance Rev* 14: 1-29, fall 1992.

45. *Committee on Ways and Means, U.S. House of Representatives: Overview of entitlement programs*. Publication No. 052-070-06807-8, U.S. Government Printing Office, Washington, D.C., 1992, (a) pp. 286-291, (b) p. 1666.

46. Bureau of Labor Statistics, U.S. Department of Labor: CPI detailed report. Washington. DC. 1993.

47. *Health Resources and Services Administration: Health personnel in the United States. Eighth report to Congress, 1991*. DHHS Publication No. HRS-P-OD-92-1. Washington, D.C., 1992.

48. Hahn, B., and Lefkowitz, D.: *Annual expenses and sources of payment for health care services. National Medical Expenditure Survey Research Findings* 14. AHCPR Publication No. 93-0007. Agency for Health Care Policy and Research, Rockville, MD, 1992.

49. Health Care Financing Administration, Office of the Actuary: *A statistical report on Medicaid*. Baltimore, MD, 1992.

50. Office of Technology Assessment: *Children's dental ser vices under the Medicaid Program-background paper*. Publication No. OTA-BP-H-78. U.S. Government Printing Office, Washington, D.C., 1990.

51. Lockwood, S.: *Public health and oral health expenditures, FY84-FY89 abstractions*. American Public Health Association, Washington, D.C., 1992, p. 338.

52. States' fiscal crises force cuts in programs for poor. *The Washington Post*, Feb. 10, 1993, p.A2.

Acknowlegement

B. Alex White, DDS, DrPH, of the National Institute of Dental Research, was the editor of this chapter. The report was prepared under the auspices of the Oral Health Coordinating Committee of the Public Health Service and approved in March 1993.

Contributing to the chapter were Jane A. Weintraub, DDS, MPH; Daniel J. Caplan, DDS; M. Cathenne Hollister, RDH, MSPH; Rosemary G. McKaig, RDH, MPH; and Cathenne A. Watkins, DDS, MS; all of the University of North Carolina at Chapel Hill. They provided information on the epidemiology of dental diseases, utilization of dental care, and the impact of oral health status on systemic health and quality of life. Chester W. Douglass, DMD, PhD, and John Da Silva, DMD, MS, Harvard University, provided information on the financing and reimbursement of dental care and on dental insurance.

— by Oral Health Coordinating Committee,
Public Health Service.

Chapter 9

Results of the National Oral Health Survey

The National Institute of Dental Research (NIDR) nationwide survey of oral health in children and adults provides a snapshot of the nation's dental health status. The survey provides the most reliable estimates yet of dental disease in several population subgroups, including children under age 5, adults age 60 and over, and black Americans and Mexican Americans—the two largest minority groups in the U.S.

What emerges from the first three years, or Phase I, of the 1988-94 National Health and Nutrition Examination Survey—called NHANES III—is a more complete picture of the dental treatment needs of children and adults from Mexican American, non-Hispanic black, and non-Hispanic white backgrounds. The NIDR, which is one of the Federal government's National Institutes of Health, sponsored the oral health component of NHANES III in collaboration with the National Center for Health Statistics.

"While there has been remarkable improvement in the nation's dental health over the past couple of decades, the survey findings point to many challenges for the American public and the dental community," said NIDR Director Harold Slavkin, DDS. "For example, it appears that caries in permanent teeth continues to decline among school-aged children, and that's good news, but the other side of the coin is that 45 percent of children and adolescents still suffer from this preventable infectious disease: there is our shared challenge."

Press Release date Released." From NIDR Website, http://www.os.dhhs.gov/cgi-bin/waisgate?W. Contact: NIDR/Jody Dove, (301) 496-4261

Tooth Decay in Children and Adolescents

NHANES III dental examiners found no caries, or tooth decay, in the permanent teeth of 55 percent of children and adolescents aged 5 to 17. Only a couple years earlier, a 1986-87 survey had found that 50 percent of 5-17-year-olds were caries-free in their permanent teeth. The NHANES III survey showed that black children enjoyed the highest caries-free rate in permanent teeth—61 percent, followed by white children at 55 percent and Mexican American children at 51 percent. (Throughout this paper, white and black refer to people of non-Hispanic white and black backgrounds.)

Unfortunately, tooth decay continues to affect millions of U.S. children and adolescents, with the majority experiencing caries by their late teens. Only 33 percent of 12-17-year-olds were caries- free in their permanent teeth. Caries in the permanent teeth was not distributed evenly among children and adolescents, the survey showed. Most of the caries—80 percent—was found in a quarter of the 5-17-year-olds.

The survey showed that most of the caries (80 percent) in the permanent teeth of children and adolescents had been treated, or filled. Although black and white youngsters had about the same amount of caries in their permanent teeth, black children had more than twice as much untreated decay as did white children.

Sixty-two percent of children aged 2-9 had no caries in their primary (baby) teeth, the survey found. While caries rates in primary teeth were similar for girls and boys, they increased with age and differed among race-ethnicity groups.

Among 2-4-year-olds, more white children were caries-free in their primary teeth (87 percent) than either black or Mexican American youngsters (78 percent and 68 percent, respectively). Among 5-9-year-olds, about half of white and black children had no caries in their primary teeth, while only about a third of Mexican American children were caries-free.

Untreated decay in primary teeth was a major problem uncovered by the survey. Nearly half (47 percent) of the caries in the primary teeth of 2-9-year-olds had not been treated. Mexican American children had the highest percentage of untreated decay—62 percent, followed by 59 percent for black children and 41 percent for white children.

NHANES III revealed that use of dental sealants more than doubled since 1986-87, but still remained low. Sealants are plastic films painted onto the chewing surfaces of teeth to protect them from decay. The survey found sealants on the primary teeth of less than 2 percent of children, and the permanent teeth of 19 percent of children and adolescents. Use of sealants on permanent teeth was three times as common in white children (22 percent had sealants) as in black children (8 percent) or Mexican American youngsters (7 percent).

Tooth Decay and Tooth Loss in Adults

Tooth decay is nearly universal among American adults. The survey found that 94 percent of people age 18 and older had either untreated decay or fillings in the crowns of their teeth. On average, American adults had 22 decayed, missing, or filled coronal surfaces (out of 128 possible surfaces).

Women had more caries than men (24 decayed, missing, or filled surfaces, versus 21 in men), but they also had slightly less untreated decay. Whites had approximately twice as much coronal caries (24 surfaces) as did blacks (12 surfaces) and Mexican Americans (14 surfaces); however, blacks and Mexican Americans had more tooth surfaces in need of treatment than did whites. Blacks had an average of 3.4 untreated surfaces, Mexican Americans had 2.8, and whites had 1.5.

When gums recede, tooth roots become exposed and subject to decay. The survey found root caries in 23 percent of adults. On average, adults had only one decayed or filled root surface. Decay of tooth roots was more prevalent in black and Mexican American adults than in whites. Half the root caries found in white adults had been treated, but most of the root caries in black and Mexican American adults was untreated.

The survey also showed that 10 percent of adults are missing all their teeth. The remaining 90 percent have, on average, 23.5 teeth. Almost a third of adults have all 28 teeth. Gender did not play a role in tooth loss, the survey found, but age and race- ethnicity did. Virtually none of the adults aged 18 to 24 were toothless, but 44 percent of those age 75 and older were missing all their teeth. Mexican American adults had an average of four more teeth than did black or white adults.

Removable complete or partial dentures are a fact of life for millions of Americans, the survey showed. About 20 percent of adults aged 18 to 74 wore some type of removable denture, with use more common in women than men and more common in white adults (22 percent) and black adults (21 percent) than in Mexican American adults (9 percent). As expected, denture use increased with age; half of Americans age 55 and older wore a partial or complete denture. A high percentage of denture wearers—60 percent—reported problems with their appliances.

Treatment Needs

Untreated caries is one indicator of dental treatment needs, but it doesn't tell the whole story. The survey looked at a number of dental conditions that might benefit from treatment, including defective fillings, crowns, and bridges; loss of healthy tooth structure as a result of restorations or trauma; recurrent caries (decay that develops around a tooth restoration); and damage to the pulp, or soft tissue at the center of the tooth.

They found that more than 40 percent of adults who had teeth—or almost 62 million Americans—had at least one tooth or tooth space that might benefit from treatment. No differences were found by gender or race, but problems did increase with age.

Periodontal Disease in Adolescents and Adults

Periodontal (gum) problems continue to plague millions of Americans. NHANES III looked at such key indicators of periodontal disease as attachment loss—or loss of bone support for the teeth—and bleeding gums, which indicate inflammation. Overall, women had better periodontal health than did men, and whites had fewer periodontal problems than did blacks or Mexican Americans. The survey found that the prevalence and extent of periodontal attachment loss increased with age. Moderate attachment loss of 3-4 mm was found in 30 percent of 25-34-year-olds, 63 percent of 45-54-year-olds, and 80 percent of people over 65. More severe periodontal destruction—attachment loss of 5 mm or more—was found in 15 percent of those surveyed. Bleeding gums were most prevalent among adolescents; three-fourths of 13-17-year-olds had gums that bled on gentle probing.

Tooth Trauma and Occlusal Problems

NHANES III was the first national survey to look at the prevalence of tooth trauma in children and adults. The survey found that 25 percent of Americans aged 6 to 50 had sustained some sort of injury to the incisors—the eight front teeth. The most common injury was a chipped tooth, and trauma was more common in males than in females.

The survey was the first national survey in 25 years to examine problems with occlusion, or positioning and alignment of the teeth. The results show that one-fourth of children and adults aged 8 to 50 had perfect alignment of the front teeth. A comparison of the survey findings to those of a survey conducted in 1966—70 showed a 20 percent increase in adolescents with a normal overbite.

The survey also revealed that 18 percent of children and adolescents and 20 percent of adults had undergone orthodontic treatment. Both malocclusion and orthodontic treatment were more common in whites than in blacks or Mexican Americans.

Note: Oral health results from Phase I of NHANES III, which was conducted from 1988 to 1991, are reported in the February 1996 Special Issue of the *Journal of Dental Research*. An article on dental caries and sealant use in children based on the NHANES data appears in the March 1996 issue of the *Journal of the American Dental Association*. Data from the second phase of NHANES III, conducted from 1991 to 1994, are not yet available. NHANES III was designed to collect nationally representative data on many aspects of health and nutrition, including oral health.

Abstracts for the papers in the February 1996 Special Issue of the Journal of Dental Research can be found on the Internet under the home page for the International Association for Dental Research (address: http://medhlp.netusa.net/iadr/iadr.htm). From the home page, select "Publications Information," then "Journal of Dental Research." Click on "Special Issue (NHANES)" to get a list of the 10 abstracts, then click on the abstract you wish to view.

Part Two

Teeth

Chapter 10

Toothpaste: Does It Matter Which Product You Pick?

Fights plaque. Controls tartar. Reduces sensitivity. Gone are the days when a toothpaste promised only to prevent cavities. To clean and protect your teeth, what type of toothpaste do you really need?

Why brush?

After you eat, bacteria in your mouth convert food into acids. Tooth decay starts when bacterial acids penetrate and erode minerals on the surfaces of your teeth. These acids form sticky deposits called plaque that cling to the surface of your teeth.

Plaque can decay teeth and cause cavities. Plaque also irritates your gums and other tooth-supporting tissues, which may lead to tooth loss. And plaque is a major cause of bad breath.

Although the mechanical action of brushing your teeth removes some bacteria and plaque, detergents and abrasives in toothpaste enhance cleaning. And since its introduction in 1955, fluoridated toothpaste has greatly improved cavity prevention.

Fluoride protects against decay by reinforcing the tooth surface. If your gums are receding, fluoride's protection is essential because tooth surfaces below your normal gum line are soft and decay easily.

The combination of fluoride in your water supply and fluoridated toothpaste is the best defense against cavities.

©1994. Reprinted from August, 1994 *Mayo Clinic Health Letter*, with permission of Mayo Foundation for Medical Education and Research, Rochester, Minnesota 55905. For subscription information, call 1-800-333-9038.

How do I choose the right toothpaste?

With few exceptions, most toothpastes have enough fluoride to protect your teeth against decay. But a growing awareness of dental health has led to a burgeoning array of specialty products.

According to the September 1992 *Consumer Reports* magazine, at least 10 varieties of toothpaste line drugstore shelves. Here's our analysis of some popular claims:

- **Anti-plaque**. Products claim to remove plaque or kill bacteria that can cause plaque. But all toothpastes remove some plaque if you brush and floss well. Regardless of the product, you can't remove all plaque by brushing alone. Even if you use a plaque-fighting toothpaste, be sure to have regular dental checkups.

- **Tartar control**. When mixed with minerals in saliva, plaque hardens into a white or yellowish deposit called tartar. Anti-tartar pastes can help prevent a buildup of tartar. However, regular brushing and flossing remove plaque, leaving little plaque to harden anyway. No toothpaste can remove tartar— that takes a professional cleaning by your dentist. An anti-tartar paste may increase your teeth's sensitivity to cold. If so, change to a product without tartar control.

- **Baking soda.** Baking soda is a mild abrasive and stain re-mover. But when wet, it loses some of its stain-removing power. Manufacturers may add hydrogen peroxide to help kill bacteria and loosen plaque. However, effective brushing with a fluoride toothpaste serves the same purpose.

- **Desensitizing.** Receding gums can make your teeth more sen-sitive to temperature. Desensitizing pastes contain chemicals that block pain perception in your teeth. Before using these products, though, check with your dentist. Sometimes sensitive teeth may be a sign of a problem that needs treatment, not cover-up.

- **Extra whiteners.** Whitening toothpastes, using ingredients such as peroxide bleach or papaya enzymes, claim to make your teeth look whiter. Smokers' pastes contain strong abrasives to scrape off tobacco, coffee, tea and other stubborn stains.

Both types of products may be harsh on delicate gum tissue, especially if you have receding gums. Before using any type of over-the-counter whitening gel or polishing cream, ask your dentist for advice.

- **Natural.** Most products don't contain artificial ingredients like sweeteners. But be sure the one you buy has fluoride. Without it, natural pastes won't effectively fight decay.

Chapter 11

Plaque:
What It Is and
How to Get Rid of It

People used to think that as you got older you naturally lost your teeth. We now know that's not true. By following easy steps for keeping your teeth and gums healthy—plus seeing your Dentist regularly—you can have your teeth for a lifetime!

Plaque: What Is it?

Plaque is made up of invisible masses of harmful germs that live in the mouth and stick to the teeth. Some types of plaque cause tooth decay, other types of plaque cause gum disease. Red, puffy or bleeding gums can be the first signs of gum disease. If gum disease is not treated, the tissues holding the teeth in place are destroyed and the teeth are eventually lost.

Dental plaque is difficult to see unless it is stained. You can stain plaque by chewing red "disclosing tablets," found at grocery stores and drug stores, or by using a cotton swab to smear green food coloring on your teeth. The red or green color left on the teeth will show you where there is still plaque—and where you have to brush again to remove it.

Stain and examine your teeth regularly to make sure you are removing all plaque. Ask your dentist or dental hygienist if your plaque removal techniques are O.K.

NIH Publication No. 91-324.

How to Fight Plaque

Floss

Use floss to remove germs and food particles between teeth. Rinse. Ease the floss into place gently. Do not 'snap' it into place; this could harm your gums. Another way of removing plaque between teeth is to use a dental pick, a thin plastic or wooden stick. These picks can be purchased at drug stores and grocery stores.

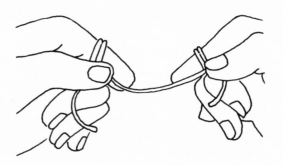

Figure 11.1. *Holding the floss.*

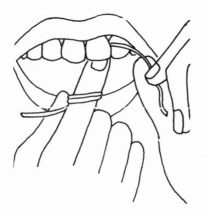

Figure 11.2. *Using floss between the upper teeth.*

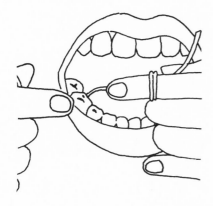

Figure 11.3. Using floss between the lower teeth.

Brush Teeth

Use any tooth brushing method that is comfortable, but do not scrub hard back and forth. Small circular motions and short back and forth motions work well. Rinse. To prevent decay, it's what's on the toothbrush that counts. Use fluoride toothpaste. Fluoride is what protects teeth from decay. Brush the tongue for a fresh feeling! Rinse again.

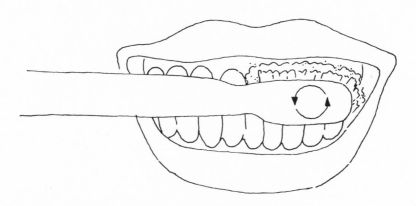

Figure 11.4. Brush using small circular motions.

117

Remember: Food residues, especially sweets, provide nutrients for the germs that cause tooth decay, as well as those that cause gum disease. That's why it is important to remove all food residues, as well as plaque, from teeth. Remove plaque at least once a day twice a day is better! If you only brush and floss once daily, do it before going to bed.

Chapter 12

Dental Amalgam: Filling a Need or Foiling Health?

Amalgam restorations—better known as "silver fillings"—are probably more familiar to millions of Americans than they would like.

Dental amalgam is the most widely used material to fill cavities in decayed teeth, technically known as caries. It has been used for 150 years; only gold has been used longer.

Amalgam is composed of approximately equal parts of liquid mercury and alloy powder containing silver, tin, copper, and sometimes lesser amounts of zinc, palladium or indium.

Despite amalgam's long history of use, some scientists and consumers are concerned that the mercury from amalgam restorations might be harmful. Nearly half of 1,000 adult Americans surveyed by the American Dental Association in 1991 said they believed amalgam could cause health problems.

Besides having the broadest range of use in dental procedures, "amalgam is the most forgiving to place," says William Kohn, D.D.S., National Institute of Dental Research, part of the National Institutes of Health. "It is not as sensitive to moisture [saliva], which can be a problem. With other restorations, the dentist has to be more meticulous or the restoration fails when the filling is placed."

Dental amalgam, which the Food and Drug Administration regulates as a medical device, is used in children and adults alike for:

- stress-bearing areas and small-to-moderate-sized cavities in back teeth, such as molars

FDA Consumer, December 1993.

119

- severe tooth damage

- when finances prohibit use of more expensive alternative filling materials

- as a foundation for cast-metal, metal-ceramic, and ceramic restorations

- when patient cooperation during the procedure or commitment to personal oral hygiene is poor. (Silver is cheaper and easier to place, more resistant to decay than other materials, such as composite [plastic, tooth-colored fillings], and less costly to replace.)

"Dental amalgam is the only material I'm aware of that, when it initially degrades, the restoration improves," says Stephen Corbin, D.D.S., from the National Centers for Disease Control and Prevention. "A byproduct builds up and seals the interface between the tooth and the restoration. There may be drawbacks, but amalgam has allowed people to keep teeth in their mouths."

Amalgam is not used when appearance is important (as in front teeth), in patients allergic to mercury, or for large restorations when use of costlier materials is not prohibitive.

In 1990, nearly half of the more than 200 million tooth fillings performed in the United States involved dental amalgam. This is down 38 percent from 1979.

Dental amalgam use began to decrease in the 1970s, primarily because dental caries among school children and young adults declined and new alternative materials were developed and improved.

Not only has the incidence been reduced, but also the type of dental caries has changed, possibly as a result of fluoride used in toothpaste and topical gels and in water, sealant use, improved oral hygiene practices, and dietary changes.

Corbin says that dentists see fewer caries, which are generally less aggressive once they start, and that today early caries can actually be reversed clinically.

The decision to fill a tooth is complex, whether you are replacing a filling, repairing a damaged tooth, or filling a tooth for the first time. "The decision was simpler in the past. Today there are more choices to make because we see different disease patterns," says Kohn.

Alterative dental restorative materials (composites, glass ionomers, ceramics, and others) are being used more often because cavities are usually smaller and amalgam is therefore not the only choice. Since the alternatives are not as durable as amalgam, the most commonly used alternatives are not used for large fillings or stress-bearing areas. According to Kohn, this is often an inappropriate choice.

Approximately 70 percent of the fillings performed each year are replacements. Most replacements require amalgam or other metallic materials because, as more tooth is drilled away, the new area is larger with each replacement. Some patients do not want the silver showing in their teeth and choose other filling materials that match the natural tooth color.

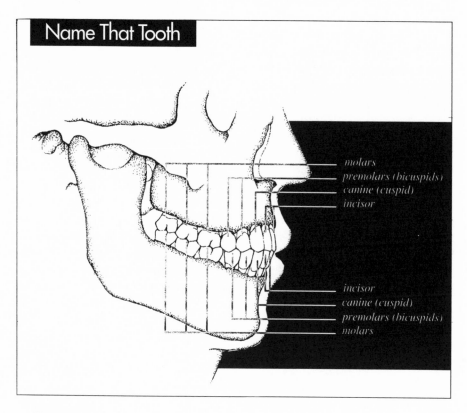

Name That Tooth

molars
premolars (bicuspids)
canine (cuspid)
incisor

incisor
canine (cuspid)
premolars (bicuspids)
molars

Figure 12.1.

Amalgam Risks and Benefits

According to *Dental Amalgam: A Scientific Review and Recommended Public Health Service Strategy for Research, Education and Regulation*, published January 1993 by the Department of Health and Human Services, scientists have shown that dental amalgam emits minute amounts of mercury vapor.

The toxicity of high-dose mercury levels in industrial settings has been established. Although mercury vapor can be absorbed through breathing and eating, research has not shown that low levels of mercury-containing amalgam are harmful except in rare cases of mercury allergies.

A literature review of amalgam research by the U.S. Public Health Service (PHS) found no sound scientific evidence linking amalgam to multiple sclerosis, arthritis, mental disorders, or other diseases, as has been suggested by some critics of amalgam.

The PHS subcommittee, which prepared the amalgam report, reviewed the research of low-dose mercury toxicity. According to the findings, a fraction of the mercury in amalgam is absorbed by the body. People with amalgam fillings have higher concentrations of mercury in their blood, urine, kidneys, and brain than those without amalgam. A small proportion of patients may manifest allergic reactions to these restorations, but, Corbin says, there are only 50 cases of amalgam allergies, reported in the scientific literature.

According to the PHS report, the few human studies done to determine a possible public health risk from amalgam have been flawed or contained too few subjects. If there are long-term effects from the mercury in amalgam, they likely are subtle—slight neurological or behavioral changes—and difficult to detect.

The subcommittee could not conclude with certainty that mercury in amalgam fillings poses a health threat or that removing them is beneficial. Removal itself may, in fact, expose patients to additional mercury absorption since drilling into the amalgam filling releases mercury into the air. Many questions remain unanswered, but for now the PHS report does not recommend either removing or not using amalgam. The report does, however, recommend more research into what the specific health effects of low-level mercury exposure might be, whether these effects can be produced by amalgam, and whether certain population groups, such as women and children, might be particularly sensitive. The report also recommends research on the safety of amalgam alternatives.

Alternatives

No single material can completely replace dental amalgam. Gold and ceramic inlays and crowns can replace amalgam in larger back cavities or in medium-sized cavities on other stress-bearing tooth surfaces. Smaller cavities in premolars and molars can now be restored with resin-based composite materials, glass ionomers, or compacted gold.

Alternatives to dental amalgam are not as durable, however, especially in larger cavities, and can cost significantly more.

"A wholesale conversion to non-amalgam materials would drive up national dental health-care costs by about $12 billion in the first year, a tremendous cost impact," says Robert C. Eccleston, assistant to the director at FDA's Center for Devices and Radiological Health. "The cost would also increase in the years following any across-the-board conversion."

Also, according to the PHS report, it is possible that alternative dental restorative materials could have long-term toxicity problems of their own that have not yet been discovered. Since no definitive data exist to show that mercury in dental amalgam is directly linked to illness, and since amalgam is less expensive, easier to place and more durable than alternatives, dental, amalgam should continue to be used.

Composites

Composites, made from synthetic resins, are used to make attractive restorations in the front teeth. Dentists use a combination of composites and sealants, technically known as preventive resin restorations, to treat small cavities and conserve tooth structure. But the use of composites as substitutes for restorations in stress-bearing areas may be inappropriate because composites can leave a tooth susceptible to recurrent decay.

Pit and Fissure Sealants

In its report, PHS recommends dental sealants to prevent caries. Sealants prevent cavities by sealing with thin plastic coating the natural pits (round holes) and fissures (grooves) in their molars. Pits and fissures in permanent first molars account for 91 percent of the surface cavities in children up to 11 years of age.

"The best restoration that is ever placed cannot be as good as the sound tooth structure that was there in the beginning," Corbin says. "But some of the preventive materials [sealants] actually improve tooth structure."

Glass Ionomers

Glass ionomers, introduced to dentistry in the 1970s, chemically bond to the tooth structure and have the beneficial side effect of releasing fluoride.

Ionomer placement technique requires limited drilling, so the procedure is quick and the result fairly attractive. Because glass ionomers are generally not used in occlusal surfaces (biting surfaces), their use is limited to baby teeth and primarily root surfaces.

Gold Foil

Although not widely used today, gold foil restorations (compacted gold) date back many centuries. These fillings may last 20 years or longer, but are not used for large or very visible areas. Gold foil restorations require more skill and careful attention to detail during placement to prevent harm to the tooth pulp (nerve) and gums. Its high cost also makes gold foil a less popular choice.

Cast Metal and Metal-ceramic

Cast metal and metal-ceramic restorations generally require two or more dental appointments and are typically used for inlays, onlays, crowns, and bridges. Use of metal and metal-ceramic materials depends on the degree of tooth destruction from decay, breakage. or amount of tooth removed by drilling. It is also determined by the number of missing teeth, how important looks are to the patient, and the patient's oral hygiene and financial situation.

These restorations cost approximately eight times more than amalgam and are most often used:

- in teeth involved in the stress from chewing and biting,
- when moderate to severe breakdown of the tooth requires replacement,
- if the patient demands a more pleasing appearance than that produced by amalgam.

Critical Parameters in Evaluating Posterior Restorative Materials	AMALGAM	COMPOSITE	GLASS IONOMER	GOLD FOIL	GOLD ALLOY (CAST)	METAL-CERAMIC CROWNS
Median Longevity Estimate	8 to 12 years	6 to 8 years when used in conservative non-stress bearing situations	No data;[1] 5 years predicted	No data; 10 to 15 years estimated	12 to 18 years	12 to 18 years
Relative Surface Wear	Wears slightly faster than enamel	Excessive wear in stress-bearing situations	Excessive wear in stress-bearing situations	Excessive wear in stress-bearing situations	Wears similar to enamel	Porcelain surface may wear opposing tooth
Resistance to Fracture	Fair to excellent	Poor to excellent	Poor	Fair to good	Excellent	Excellent
Marginal Integrity (leakage)	Fair to excellent Self-sealing through corrosion products	Poor to excellent Polymerization shrinkage can cause poor margins	Poor to excellent	Poor to excellent	Fair to good Depends upon fit and type of luting agent used	Poor to excellent Depends on fit and type of luting agent used
Conservation of Tooth Structure	Good	Excellent	Excellent - if initial restoration, not if replacement	Good	Poor	Poor
Esthetics	Poor	Excellent	Good	Poor	Poor	Excellent
Indications:						
Age range	All ages	All ages	All ages	Adult	Adult	Adult
Occlusal stress	Moderate stress	Low-stress-bearing	Adult - Class V and low-stress primary teeth	Class III and V and crown repair	High-stress areas	High-stress areas
Extent of caries	Incipient to moderate-size cavity	Incipient to moderate-size cavity	Class I and II child incipient to moderate-size cavity	Incipient to moderate-size cavity	Severe tooth destruction	Severe tooth destruction or esthetic considerations
Cost to Patient[2]	1X	1.5X	1.4X	4X	8X + gold	8X

[1] Longevity estimates reflect medians from published studies; however, under different clinical situations many restorations will last longer. For materials which have emerged in the last decade and gold foil, estimates are speculative.

[2] Relative cost to patient, in relation to amalgam (1X). There may also be considerable geographic variation.

Table 12.1.

Cast metal or metal-ceramic restorations are generally not used if:

- there is a danger of exposing the tooth pulp while preparing the tooth for restoration—for example, in patients under 18 whose pulp is higher in the tooth,

- the patient shows evidence of extensive teeth grinding or clenching,

- the patient is known to be allergic to the metals used in casting alloys (gold and certain non-precious casting metals).

Regulation

The PHS report recommends that FDA require restorative material manufacturers to identify the ingredients used in their products, and FDA is considering such an action. Industry disclosure of product ingredients would provide dentists with information necessary to prevent sensitivity reactions in allergic patients.

The PHS findings indicate that it is inappropriate to recommend restrictions on the use of dental amalgam unless more studies show a definite link between amalgam and illness.

"The science simply doesn't justify such an action," FDA's Eccleston points out. "There are several reasons for not restricting amalgam. First, current evidence does not show that exposure to mercury from amalgam restorations poses a serious health risk in humans, except for a very small number of allergic reactions. Second, there is insufficient evidence that alternative materials have fewer potential health effects than amalgam. And, as stated previously, amalgam use is declining."

For a copy of *Dental Amalgam: A Scientific Review and Recommended Public Health Service Strategy for Research, Education and Regulation* from the Department of Health and Human Services, January 1993, write to:

Les Grams HFZ-220 Subcommittee on Risk Management/CCEHRP
5600 Fishers Lane
Rockville, MD 20857

—by Laura Bradbard

Chapter 13

Endodontics:
Once through the Root Canal

Endodontic Treatment

You're probably reading this chapter because your dentist or endodontist has said you need endodontic treatment. If so, you're not alone. More than 14 million teeth receive endodontic treatment each year. By choosing endodontic treatment, you are choosing to keep your natural teeth as a healthy foundation for chewing and biting for years to come.

If you've never had endodontic treatment—also known as a "root canal"—or if it's been many years since your last procedure, you may have questions or outdated expectations.

This chapter answers your questions and explains how today's endodontic treatment saves teeth. If you would like to know more, be sure to talk with your endodontist.

Who performs endodontic treatment?

All dentists, including your general dentist received training in endodontic treatment in dental school. General dentists can perform endodontic procedures along with other dental procedures, but often they refer patients needing endodontic treatment to endodontists.

Endodontists are dentists with special training in endodontic procedures. They do only endodontics in their practices because they are specialists. To become specialists, they complete dental school and an

---

©1996 American Association of Endodontists. Reprinted with permission.

additional two or more years of advanced training in endodontics. They perform routine as well as difficult and very complex endodontic procedures, including endodontic surgery. Endodontists are also experienced at finding the cause of oral and facial pain that has been difficult to diagnose.

"Endo" is the Greek word for "inside" and "odont" is Greek for "tooth." Endodontic treatment treats the inside of the tooth.

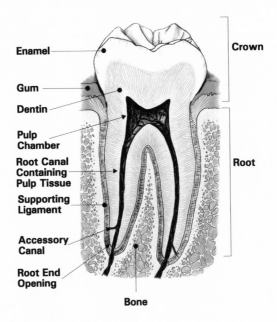

Figure 13.1.

To understand endodontic treatment, it helps to know something about the anatomy of the tooth. Inside the tooth, under the white enamel and a hard layer called the dentin, is a soft tissue called the pulp. The pulp contains blood vessels, nerves, and connective tissue and creates the surrounding hard tissues of the tooth during development.

The pulp extends from the crown of the tooth to the tip of the roots where it connects to the tissues surrounding the root. The pulp is important during a tooth's growth and development. However, once a tooth is fully mature it can survive without the pulp, because the tooth continues to be nourished by the tissues surrounding it.

Why would I need an endodontic procedure?

Endodontic treatment is necessary when the pulp becomes inflamed or infected. The inflammation or infection can have a variety of causes: deep decay, repeated dental procedures on the tooth, or a crack or chip in the tooth. In addition, a blow to a tooth may cause pulp damage even if the tooth has no visible chips or cracks. If pulp inflammation or infection is left untreated, it can cause pain or lead to an abscess.

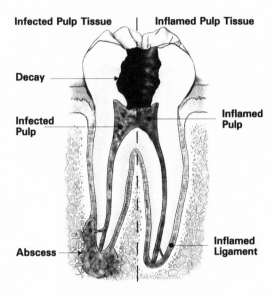

Figure 13.2.

Signs of pulp damage include pain, prolonged sensitivity to heat or cold, discoloration of the tooth, and swelling and tenderness in the nearby gums. Sometimes, there are no symptoms.

How does endodontic treatment save the tooth?

The endodontist removes the inflamed or infected pulp, carefully cleans and shapes the inside of the tooth, then fills and seals the space. Afterwards, you will return to your dentist, who will place a crown or other restoration on the tooth to protect and restore it to full function. After restoration, the tooth continues to function like any other tooth. See below for a step-by-step explanation of the procedure.

Will I feel pain during or after the procedure?

Many endodontic procedures are performed to relieve the pain of toothaches caused by pulp inflammation or infection. With modern techniques and anesthetics, most patients report that they are comfortable during the procedure.

For the first few days after treatment, your tooth may feel sensitive, especially if there was pain or infection before the procedure. This discomfort can be relieved with over-the-counter or prescription medications. Follow your endodontist's instructions carefully.

Your tooth may continue to feel slightly different from your other teeth for some time after your endodontic treatment is completed. However, if you have severe pain or pressure or pain that lasts more than a few days, call your endodontist.

Endodontic Procedure

Endodontic treatment can often be performed in one or two visits and involves the following steps:

1. The endodontist examines and x-rays the tooth, then administers local anesthetic. After the tooth is numb, the endodontist places a small protective sheet called a dental dam over the area to isolate the tooth and keep it clean and free of saliva during the procedure.

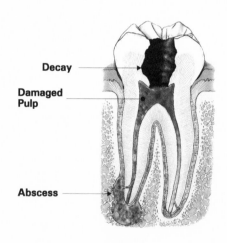

Figure 13.3.

130

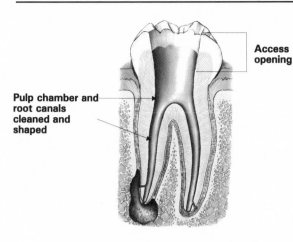

Access opening

Pulp chamber and root canals cleaned and shaped

2. The endodontist makes an opening in the crown of the tooth. Very small instruments are used to clean the pulp from the pulp chamber and root canals and to shape the space for filling.

Figure 13.4.

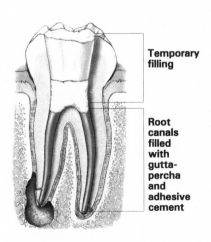

Temporary filling

Root canals filled with gutta-percha and adhesive cement

3. After the space is cleaned and shaped, the endodontist fills the root canals with a biocompatible material, usually a rubber-like material called "gutta-percha." The gutta-percha is placed with an adhesive cement to ensure complete sealing of the root canals. In most cases, a temporary filling is placed to close the opening. The temporary filling will be removed by your dentist before the tooth is restored.

Figure 13.5.

4. After the final visit with your endodontist, you must return to your dentist to have a crown or other restoration placed on the tooth to protect and restore it to full function.

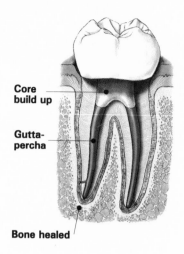

Figure 13.6.

If the tooth lacks sufficient structure to hold the restoration in place, your dentist or endodontist may place a post inside the tooth. Ask your dentist or endodontist for more details about the specific restoration planned for your tooth.

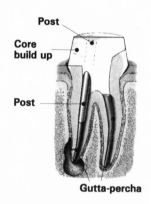

Figure 13.7.

How much will the procedure cost?

The cost varies depending on how severe the problem is and which tooth is affected. Molars are more difficult to treat and usually cost more. Most dental insurance policies provide coverage for endodontic treatment.

Generally, endodontic treatment and restoration of the natural tooth are less expensive than the alternative of having the tooth extracted. An extracted tooth must be replaced with a bridge or implant to restore chewing function and prevent adjacent teeth from shifting. These procedures tend to cost more than endodontic treatment and appropriate restoration.

Will the tooth need any special care or additional treatment?

You should not chew or bite on the treated tooth until you have had it restored by your dentist. The unrestored tooth is susceptible to fracture, so you should see your dentist for a full restoration as soon as possible. Otherwise, you need only practice good oral hygiene, including brushing, flossing, and regular checkups and cleanings.

Most endodontically treated teeth last as long as other natural teeth. In a few cases, a tooth that has undergone endodontic treatment fails to heal or the pain continues. Occasionally, the tooth may become painful or diseased months or even years after successful treatment. Often when this happens, another endodontic procedure can save the tooth.

What causes an endodontically treated tooth to need additional treatment?

New trauma, deep decay, or a loose, cracked or broken filling can cause new infection in your tooth. In some cases, the endodontist may discover very narrow or curved canals that could not be treated during the initial procedure.

Can all teeth be treated endodontically?

Most teeth can be treated. Occasionally, a tooth can't be saved because the root canals are not accessible, the root is severely fractured, the tooth doesn't have adequate bone support, or the tooth cannot be restored. However, advances in endodontics are making it possible to save teeth that even a few years ago would have been lost. And, when endodontic treatment is not effective, endodontic surgery may be able to save the tooth.

What is endodontic surgery?

The most common endodontic surgical procedure is called an apicoectomy or root-end resection. When inflammation or infection

133

persists in the bony area around the end of your tooth after endodontic treatment, your endodontist may perform an apicoectomy. In this procedure, the endodontist opens the gum tissue near the tooth to expose the underlying bone, and the infected tissue is removed. The very end of the root is also removed, and a small filling may be placed to seal the root canal. Local anesthetics make the procedure comfortable, and most patients return to their normal activities the next day.

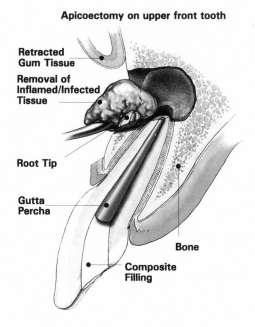

Apicoectomy on upper front tooth

Retracted Gum Tissue

Removal of Inflamed/Infected Tissue

Root Tip

Gutta Percha

Bone

Composite Filling

Figure 13.8.

What are the alternatives to endodontic treatment?

When the pulp of a tooth is damaged, the only alternative to endodontic treatment is extraction of the tooth. To restore chewing function and to prevent adjacent teeth from shifting, the extracted tooth must be replaced with an implant or bridge. This requires surgery or dental procedures on adjacent healthy teeth and can be far more costly and time-consuming than endodontic treatment and restoration of the natural tooth.

No matter how effective modern tooth replacements are—and they can be very effective—nothing is as good as a natural tooth.

For More Information

If you would like further information about endodontic treatment, your endodontist will be happy to talk with you, or you may write to the American Association of Endodontists.

American Association of Endodontists
211 East Chicago Avenue,
Suite 1100
Chicago, Illinois 60611
(312) 266-7255

Chapter 14

Get the Picture on X-Rays

X-rays are important and necessary in dentistry. But many people have questions about the safety of dental x-rays. This chapter should help answer some of those questions.

What Are X-Rays?

X-rays are a form of energy similar to light, microwaves and radio-waves. All of these radiations are electromagnetic; that is, they are electrical and magnetic energy moving together in waves. X-rays can penetrate many kinds of materials including living tissue. This, and their ability to expose photographic film, accounts for their usefulness in medicine and dentistry.

How Do X-Rays Work?

When x-rays pass through your mouth during a dental x-ray examination, more x-rays are absorbed by the denser body parts, like teeth and bone, than by the soft tissues, like the cheek and gums. This creates the picture on the x-ray film, or "radiograph." Structures like teeth appear lighter because fewer x-rays get through to the film. Other areas, including cavities, appear darker because more x-rays get through to the film. The contrast between light and dark allows the dentist to detect small cavities on hidden surfaces of the teeth. It is also possible to detect early signs of cysts, abscesses, infections, impacted teeth and even some kinds of tumors.

FDA 80-8111.

What Are the Different Types of Dental X-Ray Examinations?

We will discuss only a few of the more common dental x-ray exams here. If you have questions about other types of exams, discuss them with your dentist.

The dentist uses the "bitewing" exam to see the tops, or crowns of the teeth, to detect decay between teeth, and to check the condition of the supporting bone. Bitewing exams usually consist of two to four x-ray films, and may be taken during regular checkups.

When the dentist needs information on all the teeth, their roots and supporting bone, a "full mouth series" (usually 16 or more x-ray films) may be taken. When you first see a dentist, a full mouth series may be ordered as a record of your dental condition on your first visit. The dentist also may take a full mouth series periodically to check your dental condition over time.

Another type of examination, called a "panoramic," shows all the teeth and surrounding bone on one large film. A special x-ray machine is needed for this procedure. This type of x-ray is useful in examining the growth and development of children's teeth and jaws and in evaluating the overall condition of the jaws in people who have no remaining teeth or have a suspected fracture or abnormality in the jaw.

A special x-ray examination that is used in orthodontic dentistry is called a "cephalometric" x-ray. This shows a side view of the head, so that the dentist can see the relationship between the teeth and the skull. Since orthodontic treatment can take many years to complete, the dentist needs to see the changes caused by growth of the patient as well as the development of any conditions that might interfere with treatment.

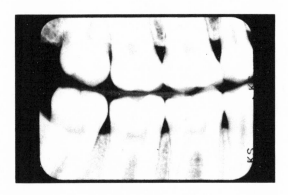

Figure 14.1. *Bitewing Examination*

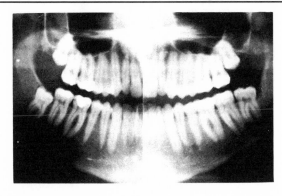

Figure 14.2. Panoramic Examination

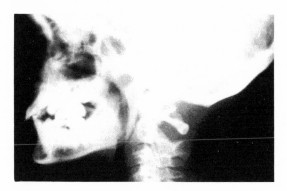

Figure 14.3. Cephalometric Examination

Are Dental X-Ray Examinations Safe?

It depends on what you mean by "safe." It's never "absolutely safe" to have an x-ray. But, it's certainly "safe enough" to have a dental x-ray if it is needed. Here's why:

Large amounts of x radiation—far greater than those used in dentistry—have been shown to increase the risk of getting cancer; to affect the unborn child when directed to the abdomen of a pregnant woman; and, to cause genetic damage that can be passed on to future generations when directed to the reproductive organs. Less is known about the effects from small amounts of radiation such as used in dental x-rays. Many scientists believe that small amounts of radiation may carry the same kind of risks, but that the chance of any harm occurring is much smaller.

139

How Does this Apply to Dental X-Rays?

In a dental x-ray examination, a small amount of radiation is directed for a fraction of a second to the mouth. In most of these exams, the x-ray beam does not go near the reproductive organs or, in the case of a pregnant woman, near the unborn child. So the possibility of genetic damage or of harm to an unborn child from most dental x-rays is practically nonexistent.

As to cancer, the increased risk, if any, to an individual from a dental x-ray exam, or from many such exams over a lifetime, is very small. But, even such small risks should not be taken unless the x-ray is needed for proper dental care.

In trying to explain the safety of a dental x-ray, some people have compared it to spending a day in the sun. This comparison can be confusing. Sunlight contains ultraviolet radiation, not x radiation. Ultraviolet is not as energetic nor as penetrating as x-rays, so its effects are different. Unlike x-rays, the ultraviolet radiation from a "day in the sun" cannot expose the internal tissues of the body. In this sense, there is no valid comparison.

A comparison between dental x-rays and the natural radiation to which we are all exposed makes a little more sense because they both involve very small amounts of similar radiation. This natural radiation, called "background radiation," comes from naturally occurring radioactivity in the soil, building materials, food, water, and even our bodies.

In addition, we are continually exposed to background radiation called "cosmic radiation" that filters through the earth's atmosphere from outer space. Background radiation continuously exposes the whole body, while a dental x-ray limits direct exposure to a small part of the body for a fraction of a second. And unlike background radiation, which provides no benefit to the person exposed, dental x-rays do provide a benefit by helping the dentist to determine your dental health.

So neither of these comparisons are particularly useful. The decision to perform a dental x-ray examination should be based on its benefit to the patient, not on these kinds of "safety comparisons."

Are Lead Shields Needed During X-Ray Exams?

A lead apron is most useful when the reproductive organs or the uterus of a pregnant woman might be in or near the direct x-ray beam. This rarely occurs in dental x-ray examinations, although it is possible during certain procedures.

During any x-ray exam, a very small amount of radiation is scattered about the room and to other parts of the patient's body, including the reproductive organs. A lead apron would block some of this "scatter radiation." But the amount of "scatter" in dentistry is extremely small because the x-ray beam is kept narrow by a device in the machine called a "collimator." Thus, lead aprons are generally not needed for most dental exams. Nevertheless, many patients and dentists find the use of a lead apron reassuring. Some see it as an indication of the dentist's concern about radiation protection.

A special type of lead shield that is placed around the patient's neck, like a collar, may be used during examinations that could expose the thyroid gland to the direct x-ray beam. The thyroid is particularly sensitive to radiation. Thyroid shielding may be used during panoramic, cephalometric, and other examinations in which the middle of the neck is in or near the beam.

How Often Should I Have Dental X-Ray Examinations?

There is no simple answer to this question. The American Dental Association recommends that the dentist "use professional judgment to determine the frequency and extent of each radiographic examination." Each patient's dental condition and needs must be assessed individually. For example, someone who frequently gets cavities or has serious gum disease may need x-rays more frequently than someone with a history of good dental health. Certainly, x-rays should not be taken before the dentist has examined your teeth to determine whether or not x-rays are needed. Feel free to ask your dentist about the need for dental x-rays in your case.

Is Equipment Checked for Safety?

Both Federal and State agencies try to ensure that x-ray equipment in the dental office is working properly. The Bureau of Radiological Health of the Food and Drug Administration requires that all x-ray equipment manufactured since 1974 meet a rigorous radiation safety standard. The standard requires several safety features to be built into the machine so that patient receives minimum radiation. State health departments inspect x-ray equipment in dental offices regardless of the manufacture date. Since each State has its own particular radiation protection program, you may want to ask your dentist about the program in your State. While regulation of x-ray equipment provides some measure of radiation protection, the personnel who order and conduct the x-ray exams play the most important role in keeping dental radiation exposure as low as possible. This is why FDA, State health departments, and professional dental organizations work together on educational efforts on radiation protection.

You Also Have a Role in Dental X-Ray Protection

X-rays can give needed, even lifesaving information. But, like most things, they carry some small risk. That's why x-rays should be taken only when there's a medical need; that is, when they will help determine the diagnosis and treatment. Doctors may suggest an x-ray simply because they are unaware of similar x-rays taken elsewhere. Keep this record and show it when an x-ray is suggested. Another x-ray may not be needed. And even if a new exam is needed, the earlier x-ray may help in the diagnosis.

By communicating with your dentist, you can help avoid unnecessary x-ray risks and costs:

- Ask your dentist why an x-ray is needed. If your doctor orders an x-ray, ask how it will help with the diagnosis.

- Don't decide on your own that you need an x-ray. Don't pressure your dentist into taking x-rays if he or she explains that x-rays are not required for your dental care.

- When you change dentists, ask if your x-ray films can be sent to your new dentist. Sometimes your dentist may be able to use previous x-rays instead of taking new ones. Tell your doctor about any similar x-ray examination you have had.

- Keep an X-Ray Record Card of your dental x-rays if you see different dentists at the same time. This way you have a record of your dental x-rays with you and can help the dentist determine if another x-ray is really needed.

- Ask if gonad shielding can be used (for yourself and for your children) during x-ray exams near the sex organs.

- Tell your doctor if you think you're pregnant before having an x-ray examination of the abdomen.

For More Information

U.S. Department of Health and Human Services
Public Health Service
Food and Drug Administration
Bureau of Radiological Health (HFX-28)
Rockville, Maryland 20857

This information was provided in cooperation with the American Dental Association.

Chapter 15

The Story of Fluoridation

It started as an observation, that soon took the shape of an idea. It ended, five decades later, as a scientific revolution that shot dentistry into the forefront of preventive medicine. This is the story of how dental science discovered—and ultimately proved to the world—that fluoride, a mineral found in rocks and soil, prevents tooth decay.

Although dental caries remains a public health worry, it is no longer the unbridled problem it once was, thanks to fluoride. Today's children have only half as much decay in their teeth as their counterparts did just 40 years ago, when fluoride was first introduced as a preventive measure.

As NIDR Director Dr. Harald Löe says, "Whether it is squeezed from a tube, swished in the mouth as a rinse, or swallowed as an additive in public water supplies, fluoride is the most important discovery that dental research has made—or may ever make—for preventing tooth decay."

A Mysterious Disorder

Fluoride research had its beginnings in 1901, when a young dental school graduate named Frederick McKay left the East Coast to open a dental practice in Colorado Springs, Colorado. When he arrived, McKay was astounded to find scores of Colorado Springs natives with grotesque brown stains on their teeth. So severe could these permanent stains be, in fact, sometimes entire teeth were splotched the color of chocolate candy.

NIH Publication No. 88-1868. National Institute of Dental Research, 1988. *NIDR at 40.*

145

McKay searched in vain for information on this bizarre disorder. He found no mention of the brown-stained teeth in any of the dental literature of the day. Local residents blamed the problem on any number of strange factors, such as eating too much pork, consuming inferior milk, and drinking calcium-rich water.

Thus, McKay took up the gauntlet and initiated research into the disorder himself. His first epidemiological investigations were scuttled by a lack of interest among most area dentists. But McKay persevered and ultimately interested local practitioners in the problem, which was known as Colorado Brown Stain.

A Fruitful Collaboration

McKay's first big break came in 1909, when renowned dental researcher Dr. G.V. Black agreed to come to Colorado Springs and collaborate with him on the mysterious ailment. Black, who had previously scoffed that it was impossible such a disorder could go unreported in the dental literature, was lured West shortly after the Colorado Springs Dental Society conducted a study showing that almost 90 percent of the city's locally born children had signs of the brown stains.

When Black arrived in the city, he too was shocked by the prevalence of Colorado Brown Stain in the mouths of native-born residents. He would write later: "...I spent considerable time walking on the streets, noticing the children in their play, attracting their attention and talking with them about their games, etc., for the purpose of studying the general effect of the deformity. I found it prominent in every group of children. One does not have to search for it, for it is continually forcing itself on the attention of the stranger by its persistent prominence. This is much more than a deformity of childhood. If it were only that, it would be of less consequence, but it is a deformity for life."

Black investigated fluorosis for six years, until his death in 1915. During that period, he and McKay made two crucial discoveries. First, they showed that mottled enamel (as Black referred to the condition) resulted from developmental imperfections in children's teeth. This finding meant that city residents whose permanent teeth had calcified without developing the stains did not risk having their teeth turn brown; young children waiting for their secondary set of teeth to erupt, however, were at high risk. Second, they found that teeth afflicted by Colorado Brown Stain were surprisingly and inexplicably resistant to decay.

The two researchers were still a long way from determining the cause of Colorado Brown Stain, but McKay had a theory tucked away in the back of his head. Maybe there was, as some local residents suggested, an ingredient in the water supply that mottled the teeth? Black was skeptical; McKay, though, was intrigued by this theory's prospects.

The water-causation theory got a gigantic boost in 1923. That year, McKay trekked across the Rocky Mountains to Oakley, Idaho to meet with parents who had noticed peculiar brown stains on their children's teeth. The parents told McKay that the stains began appearing shortly after Oakley constructed a communal water pipeline to a warm spring five miles away. McKay analyzed the water, but found nothing suspicious in it. Nonetheless, he advised town leaders to abandon the pipeline altogether and use another nearby spring as a water source.

McKay's advice did the trick. Within a few years, the younger children of Oakley were sprouting healthy secondary teeth without any mottling. McKay now had his confirmation, but he still had no idea what could be wrong with the water in Oakley, Colorado Springs, and other afflicted areas.

The answer came when McKay and Dr. Grover Kempf of the United States Public Health Service (PHS) travelled to Bauxite, Arkansas—a company town owned by the Aluminum Company of America—to investigate reports of the familiar brown stains. The two discovered something very interesting: namely, the mottled enamel disorder was prevalent among the children of Bauxite, but nonexistent in another town only five miles away. Again, McKay analyzed the Bauxite water supply. Again, the analysis provided no clues.

But the researchers' work was not done in vain. McKay and Kempf published a report on their findings that reached the desk of ALCOA's chief chemist, H. V. Churchill, at company headquarters in Pennsylvania. Churchill, who had spent the past few years refuting claims that aluminum cookware was poisonous, worried that this report might provide fresh fodder for ALCOA's detractors. Thus, he decided to conduct his own test of the water in Bauxite—but this time using photospectrographic analysis, a more sophisticated technology than that used by McKay.

Churchill asked an assistant to assay the Bauxite water sample. After several days, the assistant reported a surprising piece of news: the town's water had high levels of fluoride. Churchill was incredulous. "Whoever heard of fluorides in water," he bellowed at his assistant. "You have contaminated the sample. Rush another specimen."

Shortly thereafter, a new specimen arrived in the laboratory. Churchill's assistant conducted another assay on the Bauxite water. The result? Photospectrographic analysis, again, showed that the town's water had high levels of fluoride tainting it. This second and selfsame finding prompted Churchill to sit down at his typewriter in January 1931, and compose a five-page letter to McKay on this new revelation. In the letter, he advised McKay to collect water samples from other towns "where the peculiar dental trouble has been experienced . . . We trust that we have awakened your interest in this subject and that we may cooperate in an attempt to discover what part 'fluorine' may play in the matter."

McKay collected the samples. And, within months, he had the answer and denouement to his 30-year quest: high levels of water-borne fluoride indeed caused the discoloration of tooth enamel.

New Questions Emerge

Hence, from the curious findings of Churchill's lab assistant, the mystery of the brown stained teeth was cracked. But one mystery often ripples into many others. And shortly after this discovery, PHS scientists started investigating a slew of new and provocative questions about water-borne fluoride. With these PHS investigations, research on fluoride and its effects on tooth enamel began in earnest.

The architect of these first fluoride studies was Dr. H. Trendley Dean, head of the Dental Hygiene Unit at the National Institutes of Health (NIH). Dean began investigating the epidemiology of fluorosis in 1931. One of his primary research concerns was determining how high fluoride levels could be in drinking water before fluorosis occurred.

To determine this, Dean enlisted the help of Dr. Elias Elvove, a senior chemist at the NIH. Dean gave Elvove the hardscrabble task of developing a more accurate method to measure fluoride levels in drinking water. Elvove labored long and hard in his laboratory, and within two years he reported back to Dean with success. He had developed a state-of-the-art method to measure fluoride levels in water with an accuracy of 0.1 parts per million (ppm).

With this new method in tow, Dean and his staff set out across the country to compare fluoride levels in drinking water. By 1936, he and his staff had made a critical discovery. Namely, fluoride levels of up to 1.0 ppm in drinking water did not cause mottled enamel; if the fluoride exceeded this level, however, fluorosis began to occur.

Proof That Fluoride Prevents Caries

This finding sent Dean's thoughts spiralling in a new direction. He recalled from reading McKay's and Black's studies on fluorosis that mottled tooth enamel is unusually resistant to decay. Dean wondered whether adding fluoride to drinking water at physically and cosmetically safe levels would help fight tooth decay. This hypothesis, Dean told his colleagues, would need to be tested.

In 1944, Dean got his wish. That year, the City Commission of Grand Rapids, Michigan—after numerous discussions with researchers from the PHS, the Michigan Department of Health, and other public health organizations—voted to add fluoride to its public water supply the following year. In 1945, Grand Rapids became the first city in the world to fluoridate its drinking water.

The Grand Rapids water fluoridation study was originally sponsored by the U.S. Surgeon General, but was taken over by the NIDR shortly after the Institute's inception in 1948.

During the 15-year project, researchers monitored the rate of tooth decay among Grand Rapids' almost 30,000 school children.

After just 11 years, Dean—who was now director of the NIDR—announced an amazing finding. The caries rate among Grand Rapids children born after fluoride was added to the water supply dropped more than 60 percent. This finding, considering the thousands of participants in the study, amounted to a giant scientific breakthrough that promised to revolutionize dental care, making tooth decay for the first time in history a preventable disease for most people.

A Lasting Achievement

Almost 30 years after the conclusion of the Grand Rapids fluoridation study, fluoride continues to be dental science's main weapon in the battle against tooth decay. Today, just about every toothpaste on the market contains fluoride as its active ingredient; water fluoridation projects currently benefit over 200 million Americans, and 13 million school children now participate in school-based fluoride mouthrinse programs.

As the figures indicate, McKay, Dean, and the others helped to transform dentistry into a prevention-oriented profession. Their drive, in the face of overwhelming adversity, is no less than a remarkable feat of science—an achievement ranking with the other great preventive health measures of our century.

Chapter 16

Fluoride: Cavity Fighter on Tap

A decade ago, the National Institutes of Health called it "the leading chronic disease of childhood." An editorial published in the *Journal of the American Medical Association* just a few years before that, in 1975, went further, terming it "the most common disease of mankind."

The scourge referred to, dental caries (non-dentists call it tooth decay), is a malady that may well be on its way out, thanks mostly to fluoride, a remedy supplied by nature in some parts of our nation and applied by human ingenuity in others. It's now a major ingredient in 95 percent of the toothpaste we purchase. It's also an ingredient in the community water supplies serving most of our citizens.

Interest in the role of fluoride arose when it was observed that people in some parts of the country had a surprisingly low incidence of tooth decay. The areas, it turned out, were those in which fluorides occur naturally in the drinking water.

By the mid-1950s, the results of decade-long controlled studies of water supply fluoridation had established beyond a doubt both the effectiveness and the safety of fluoridation in reducing tooth decay. The practice was—and continues to be—endorsed by the American Medical Association, the American Dental Association, the U.S. Public Health Service (PHS), and the National Research Council.

Exceeding Expectations

Every 10 years, PHS (of which FDA is a part) determines national health objectives for the decade ahead. In setting dental health goals

FDA Consumer, January 1992.

in 1980, PHS declared that by 1990, the proportion of 9-year-olds who had never had cavities in their permanent teeth should rise to 40 percent.

At the time, 40 percent seemed a sensible expectation (the most recent data then available showed that in the mid-1970s, the figure was under 30 percent). Yet, even then a new survey was under way, and it soon became clear that at the time the goal was set, it had already been not only achieved, but surpassed.

In 1982, the National Institute of Dental Research released the results of its 1979-80 survey, based on a sampling of 40,000 children nationwide, showing that more than half of the 9-year-olds (51 percent) were decay-free. In fall of 1988, PHS announced that, according to preliminary results from a 1986-87 survey, over 65 percent of American 9-year-olds had never had decay in their permanent teeth, and the trend continues.

Cavity-Fighter on Tap: How Fluoride Helps

There are three requirements for the creation of cavities: teeth, which are extremely susceptible to attack by certain acids; bacteria—notably *Streptococcus mutans*—that produce those acids; and food on which the bacteria can feed. Carbohydrates, especially sucrose (ordinary sugar), make fine fare for *S. mutans* and kin.

No vaccine against caries-causing bacteria is in sight. Nor has anyone found a way to enforce immediate after-meals tooth-brushing to remove the bacteria-nourishing nutrients. Enter fluoride, which structurally bolsters the teeth's resistance to acid invasion. If babies receive fluoride from the start (even when still in the womb), while their teeth are still developing, and continue to do so all through formation of both their baby teeth and the permanent set, stronger teeth will erupt, teeth that are more resistant to attack by decay-causing bacteria.

To achieve resistance, children growing up in an area where the water is neither naturally nor artificially fluoridated may need to receive supplements.

Only fluoride taken internally, whether in drinking water or dietary supplements, can strengthen babies' and children's developing teeth to resist decay. Once the teeth have erupted, they're beyond help from ingested fluoride.

For both children and adults, fluoride applied to the surface of the teeth can nonetheless add protection, at least to the outer layer of enamel, and it has unquestionably also played a role in reducing decay. The most familiar form, of course, is fluoride-containing toothpaste, introduced in the early 1960s. Fluoride rinses are also available, as are applications by dental professionals. All these products are regulated by FDA. They are considered effective adjuncts to ingested fluoride—and they are the only useful sources of tooth—strengthening fluoride for teenagers and adults.

Fluoride Risks

There is one proven adverse effect of fluoride on the teeth: too much fluoride can cause a condition called dental fluorosis. In its mildest form, this condition causes small, white, virtually invisible opaque areas on teeth. In its most severe form, it causes a distinct brownish mottling. However, dental fluorosis doesn't result from artificial fluoridation alone, because the levels are kept low enough to avoid this effect.

Over the years, many studies of dental fluorosis patterns have established optimal levels for fluoride in drinking water-levels that will provide protection against decay but will cause no, or negligible fluorosis. Fluoride levels are stated in parts per million (ppm) concentrations. About 1 ppm is ideal. Less than 0.7 ppm isn't adequate to protect developing teeth; more than about 1.5 to 2.0 ppm can lead to mild fluorosis. Artificial fluoridation of water uses an optimum standard set by the Environmental Protection Agency of 0.7 to 1.2 ppm, depending on locality (a lower amount is needed in warmer parts of the country, where people drink more water).

Dental fluorosis affects only the teeth. In its mildest form, it isn't at all apparent to the untrained eye and can be detected only by an experienced dentist or specially trained technician. Somewhat greater discoloration does become a cosmetic problem, a condition that an individual may feel mars his or her appearance even though it's not truly harmful. Severe fluorosis poses a threat to health, since the discoloration may be accompanied by actual pitting of dental enamel-rendering affected teeth possibly more, rather than less, susceptible to decay. As with the benefits of fluoride, once permanent teeth have erupted, there is no longer any threat of dental fluorosis.

A study reported in the *Journal of the American Dental Association* in 1983 by a team from the National Institute of Dental Research clearly described the impact of excess fluoride. Seven Illinois communities where water consumption was likely to be similar were compared; their natural fluoride concentrations ranged from an optimal 1.06 ppm up to an excessive 4.07 ppm. Experienced clinicians examined the teeth of youngsters aged 8 to 16. Where the fluoride level was optimal, the examiners could find no fluorosis in 86 percent and detected only mild signs in another 12 percent; severe fluorosis was found in 0.6 percent. At two to three times optimal levels, severe cases were found in 5 to 8 percent. At the highest level, the figure jumped to a disturbing 23 percent—almost a quarter of the youngsters examined.

EPA is the federal authority responsible for ensuring that naturally occurring fluoride levels meet safety standards. Above the concentration that protects against tooth decay, fluoride is considered a contaminant, and the states must report local levels to EPA.

As Edward V. Ohanian, Ph.D., of the human and environmental criteria division in EPA's Office of Water explains, the agency has established two "maximum contaminant levels (MCLs)" for fluoride, 2 ppm and 4 ppm. The first MCL is considered the point above which cosmetic effects, in the form of a degree of dental fluorosis, can occur and is intended to ensure public awareness of that possibility. Although EPA cannot compel the states to hold fluorides to this level, the 4-ppm MCL is legally enforceable, since it is based on the possibility of adverse health effects above that level. Local authorities may be ordered to defluoridate the water if levels exceed that figure.

In accordance with the Safe Drinking Water Act, EPA periodically re-examines its standards and is currently reviewing information that has become available since 1985. A report is expected by late 1992 or 1993.

Fluoride Supplements

To be sure that teeth incorporate decay-fighting fluoride during structural development, infants and children need to receive fluoride on a regular basis. Whether or not supplements are needed, and how much, depends on both the local water supply and sources in a child's diet.

Fluoride supplements, which are regulated by FDA as drugs, may take the form of drops or, for older youngsters, chewable tablets. They are available both alone and in combination with vitamins.

The daily requirement rule of thumb suggested by the American Dental Association and the American Academy of Pediatrics is 0.25 milligrams per day up to age two, 0.5 mg for ages two and three, and 1.0 mg after age three and until the teen years. Children who consume tap water with a fluoride concentration of less than 0.3 parts per million (ppm) need full supplementation. At water supply levels between 0.3 and 0.7 ppm, only half the need is met; if the water supply provides 0.5 ppm, for example, an average 5-year-old should receive 0.5 milligrams of supplemental fluoride per day. Breast-fed infants are exceptions to the rule, since breast milk contains almost no fluoride (nor do ready-to-drink formulas).

Further, doctors need to consider both the local water supply and the baby's diet as a whole in calculating needs and prescribing supplements, points out Katherine Karlsrud, M.D., a clinical instructor in pediatrics at Cornell University Medical College.

The process can be complicated for physicians in some "mixed" geographical areas. Karlsrud practices in New York City, which offers what she pronounces a "perfect" fluoride level—but she also cares for children from surrounding counties where the level is zero.

"Each baby's need," she says, "has to be individually figured out. If a baby in Manhattan, for example, is being partly breast-fed, but half that baby's diet consists of formula reconstituted with tap water, half the child's need for fluoride is being met." That would not be true, though, for an infant in nearby Suffolk County, on Long Island, where the citizenry at this writing continues to reject health officials' recommendation that the water supply be fluoridated.

In areas where the drinking water provides protective fluorides, over 0.7 ppm, breast-fed babies who have been weaned need no further supplementation.

Tips for Parents

While parents should be sure that their children are getting fluoride's protection for their teeth, they should also be aware of what FDA's Ronald Coene calls the "total body burden of fluoride" and be sure their children aren't ingesting unneeded amounts. (Only ingested fluoride, not topical application, has been associated with dental fluorosis or any other systemic effect.)

Some guidelines on various fluoride sources:

- **Drinking Water:** Find out from local health officials the fluoride concentration in your community's water supply. If it's below protective levels, see that your children receive supplements until their teen years. If the level's just right and a physician or dentist prescribes supplements, question him or her about it (exceptions would be breast-feeding babies who drink very little or no water). If the level is naturally too high, contact your local EPA office.

Some promoters of bottled water, which some families choose for drinking instead of tap water, claim their products come from springs of remarkable purity. According to Neil Sass, Ph.D., a science policy advisor in FDA's Center for Food Safety and Applied Nutrition, "Perhaps 50 percent of bottled waters are taken from municipal water supplies, which may or may not be fluoridated. Some are put right into the bottles; others are filtered. In many cases, any fluoride content may be removed before bottling."

One researcher who checked out a number of popular bottled water brands reported in the *New England Journal of Medicine* in 1989 that, except for three imported carbonated brands, none had fluoride levels above 0.25 parts per million; of those three, two fell short of the cavity-fighting range and one exceeded it (the fluoride level of the sample tested was 1.9 ppm).

- **Fluoride Supplements:** If they're needed, be sure the doses are appropriate, taking into consideration, for example, such factors as an infant's varied diet.

- **Toothpaste:** The fluoride concentration in toothpaste is high, and toothpaste is meant to be applied to the surface of the teeth, not swallowed. According to Assistant Secretary for Health James O. Mason, M.D., if the average 2-year-old brushing twice a day swallows the toothpaste, it could add 0.5 milligrams per day to the child's fluoride intake—full supplement dosage for a child of this age. He suggests that children be carefully taught never to swallow toothpaste and to use only a pea-sized amount on the brush.

- **Rinses:** FDA has concluded that these nonprescription products can indeed boost the anti-cavity effect of fluoride toothpaste. They are best used after brushing but should not be used by children under six unless recommended by a dentist. (Nor should they be used by anyone who may be apt to swallow some of the product.)

- **Dental-Office Application:** This is the most concentrated topical form of fluoride, and can be quite helpful in preventing cavities in children and adults alike. The likelihood of harm from proper application is virtually nil, says Jack Klatell, D.D.S., chairman of the department of dentistry at Mount Sinai School of Medicine: "The application is usually in the form of a paste or gel inside a mouth guard, which is placed in the mouth and left in contact with the teeth for a period of time and then removed."

A Community Decision

Along with caries reduction, PHS set another dental health objective a decade ago—that by 1990, at least 95 percent of the population using community water systems would be drawing optimally fluoridated water from their taps. But by 1985, that figure was only 62 percent, and growth in community water fluoridation had slowed to 1 to 2 percent a year. Why are so many fluoride-deficient water supplies still unfluoridated?

There is no national law requiring fluoridation, and the question must be decided locally. Although most Americans are aware that many substances are routinely added to our water to ensure that it's safe and drinkable, there are still some apprehensions about the addition of chemicals that don't occur naturally. And some misunderstandings have arisen.

Four Ill-Fated Rats

The most recent misunderstanding occurred in the spring of 1990, with the news of an experimental animal study. Some abbreviated reports of the study were interpreted as confirming a "weak link" between fluoride and cancer. However, a more detailed look at the study results shows this was not the case. In the study by PHS's National Toxicology Program, four male rats given very high doses of fluoride developed osteosarcoma, a rare form of bone cancer.

They were among 50 rats and mice of both sexes given the highest doses of fluoride they could tolerate in their drinking water for two years. One rat that developed cancer received fluoride at a level of 45 ppm; the other three received it at a level of 79 ppm. There were no cancers found in female rats, or in mice of either sex, at these fluoride levels; nor were cancers found in any animals at lower levels.

Despite the weakness of the association, the Department of Health and Human Services assembled a panel to review all current and past research relating to fluoride safety. The group, the Ad Hoc Subcommittee on Fluoride of the Committee to Coordinate Environmental Health and Related Programs, included scientists from more than a dozen federal agencies and was chaired by former FDA Commissioner Frank E. Young, M.D., Ph.D.

The subcommittee's report, released in February 1991 after months of examining the evidence, concluded there was no cause for alarm and no reason to link fluoridation of water with any human disorder or disease, including osteosarcoma or other malignancies. And a study published in the April 1991 issue of the *American Journal of Public*

Health, comparing the incidence of osteosarcomas in fluoridated and unfluoridated areas of New York state, found no difference in the rates.

The PHS report did observe that there are multiple sources of fluoride and commented that, "in accordance with prudent health practice of using no more than the amount necessary to achieve a desired effect, health professionals and the public should avoid excessive and inappropriate fluoride exposure."

Clearly, the levels of fluoride added to water supplies do not represent a public health hazard. But the risk of adverse effects, specifically of fluorosis in young teeth, is real if infants and children ingest appreciably more fluoride than they need for decay prevention.

Ronald F. Coene, an engineer and water supply specialist at FDA's National Center for Toxicological Research, who served as executive secretary of the special subcommittee, points out that, "it is possible for a child to get too much fluoride. That can happen when more than maximum allowable levels occur naturally in drinking water, or from swallowing toothpaste. It can also result from unneeded dietary supplements. Sometimes, dentists recommend fluoride tablets when the local water supply is fluoridated. Too much fluoride can cause fluorosis. That was the concern of the committee when it comes to overexposure—fluorosis, not cancer."

—by Dodi Schultz

Dodi Schultz is a freelance writer in New York City and a contributing editor of *Parents* magazine.

Chapter 17

Community Water Fluoridation

What Is Community Water Fluoridation?

Community water fluoridation is the process of adjusting the fluoride content that occurs naturally in a community's water to the best level for preventing tooth decay.

A key word in this definition is "adjusting" because all drinking water supplies contain some fluoride naturally. Fluorine is the 13th most abundant element in nature. It is present in small and varying amounts in all soils, plants, animals and water supplies and, therefore, all diets contain fluoride. There is no such thing as a fluoride-free water supply. A community that fluoridates its water is simply modifying the amount of fluoride already found naturally in the water to a level that is best for the dental health of its residents. Thus adjusted water fluoridation means that the appropriate amount of fluoride is being maintained in the community's water supply.

Getting the right amount of ingested fluoride is important to prevent tooth decay. However, where water fluoride levels occurs in nature at too high a level or dietary fluoride supplements or fluoride toothpaste are misused, discoloration of the teeth (dental fluorosis) also can occur. Thus, water plant operators continuously monitor the fluoride content of drinking water in communities that fluoridate.

Research has shown that the most favorable concentration for community water fluoridation in the United States varies from 0.7 parts-per-million (ppm) in hot climates to 1.2 ppm in cold climates. For

---

Centers for Disease Control, October 1992.

moderate climates, one part fluoride in one million parts of water (1 ppm) is recommended. (One ppm is the same as 1 mg/L.) This amount is extremely small. To appreciate how small, think of it compared with other units of measurement.

One ppm is equivalent to:

- 1 inch in 16 miles
- 1 minute in 2 years
- 1¢ in $10,000

What Are the Benefits of Community Water Fluoridation?

Hundreds of studies carried out in the United States and many other countries during the past half century prove that community water fluoridation prevents tooth decay. At a time when the only fluoride available was that found naturally in drinking water, studies showed that children who grew up in fluoridated communities experienced about 50 to 60 percent less decay than those in non-fluoridated ones. Because fluoride was so successful in preventing decay, it later was incorporated into many oral health products, such as toothpastes and mouthrinses. Most people in non-fluoridated communities now receive some protection against cavities from fluoride contained in these toothpastes and mouthrinses and in foods and beverages processed in fluoridated communities. This is why recent measures of dental decay prevention from community water fluoridation in the United States have been smaller, generally in the 20 to 40 percent range. This remains a substantial reduction in disease.

Do Adults Benefit from Drinking Fluoridated Water?

It has been a popular misconception that fluoridation helps only children. Adults as well as children benefit from drinking fluoridated water throughout their lives. Several studies show that people in their sixties who have lived all of their lives in areas with sufficient fluoride in the drinking water have much less tooth loss and tooth decay than do adults in non-fluoridated communities. Because more people are living longer and keeping more of their natural teeth, and older persons often experience receding gums and exposed roots, the problem of decay on the root surfaces of teeth is increasing. Recent studies have shown that adults who live in communities with optimal levels of fluoride in the water supply have much less root-surface decay than do adults of the same ages in low-fluoride communities.

In areas where other fluoride methods have not been widely available, studies of community water fluoridation historically have shown reductions in tooth decay of approximately 60 percent. With use of other fluoride products such as fluoride containing toothpaste, rinses and gels, currently widespread in most areas of the United States, the measurable benefits from water fluoridation now are:

- 20 to 40 percent less dental decay in persons of all ages,
- more children free of dental decay,
- many fewer extracted permanent first molars ("6-year molars") in children,
- lower dental bills for repairing decayed teeth, and
- less need for procedures that require anesthesia and drilling.

Why Is Community Water Fluoridation an Ideal Public Health Method?

Community water fluoridation is effective, safe, inexpensive, and practical. The average cost of fluoridation is about 50 cents per person a year. This is one of the best bargains in health today. Studies in the United States, Canada and New Zealand have shown that the annual costs of children's dental care decrease after community fluoridation has been in operation for several years.

The entire community benefits from community water fluoridation, regardless of a person's age, income, level of education, or access to dental care services. Everyone automatically benefits when they drink fluoridated water and consume foods and beverages prepared with it.

Is Community Water Fluoridation Safe?

The safety of community water fluoridation has been studied more thoroughly than any other public health measure during the past 45 years, with results of hundreds of clinical, animal and laboratory studies supporting its safety. One reason for the large amount of this research is that opponents of fluoridation have made so many inappropriate claims of harm, including assertions that water fluoridation causes heart disease, cancer, Down's syndrome, premature aging and even acquired immune-deficiency syndrome (AIDS). Much additional research has been conducted which refutes these unsupported claims. Each study has reaffirmed the safety of fluoridation.

Who Supports and Who Opposes Community Water Fluoridation?

Community water fluoridation has the unqualified approval of every major health organization in the United States and many other countries as well. The American Dental Association and the U.S. Public Health Service have endorsed community water fluoridation since 1950, and the American Medical Association, since 1951. In 1958, the World Health Organization recognized it as a practical and effective public health measure and has repeated its support at successive World Assemblies. The U.S. Department of Health and Human Services recently reaffirmed its support.

The Consumers Union has published excellent review articles in support of fluoridation. Other organizations have adopted policies in support of fluoridation, including The American Academy of Pediatrics, American Cancer Society, American Heart Association, American Public Health Association and International Association for Dental Research. Based on an extensive review of 50 years of experience with fluoridation, the American Association of Public Health Dentistry in 1992 reaffirmed its unqualified support of fluoridation.

Efforts to begin community water fluoridation, however, have frequently been hampered because of organized opposition to fluoridation. Frequently, these opponents also take issue with such basic health practices as the pasteurization of milk and immunization against infectious diseases. These groups try to attract support by appealing to popular generic issues, such as individual rights, freedom of choice, anti-pollution, natural diets and substances in the environment that lead to cancer.

In many areas, proposals to fluoridate the water have become political issues, decided by public referenda or by elected officials who sometimes lack specific knowledge about the benefits and safety of fluoridation or fail to seek expert advice on health matters. During these campaigns, opponents often resort to scare tactics and spread false, irrelevant and misleading information. As a result of such misinformation, doubts raised in voters' minds may lead them to rejection of fluoridation.

What Is the Status of Community Water Fluoridation?

More than half of the U.S. population (about 135 million persons) live in communities served by fluoridated water supplies (0.7 ppm or more). This includes about 10 million people who live in communities with sufficient naturally occurring fluoride in their drinking water. About 30 million Americans cannot benefit from fluoridation because they live in areas, largely rural, that lack community water supplies.

Currently, 42 of the 50 largest cities in the U.S. fluoridate their drinking water supplies. Several of them, including San Francisco, Baltimore, Pittsburgh and Washington, D.C., have had fluoridated water for about 40 years. However, eight of the nation's 50 largest cities, including Los Angeles, San Diego, San Antonio and Honolulu, still have not fluoridated their water supplies and, consequently, are not providing the known dental benefits of fluoridation to their residents.

Community water fluoridation has not been adopted as widely by smaller U.S. cities and towns. The reasons are usually economic or political, or sometimes simply reflect a lack of perceived need.

As of December 31, 1989, the International Dental Federation (FDI) reported that its member countries estimated that about 275 million persons living in 24 of those countries drank fluoridated water that was adjusted properly. The estimates showed that another 300 million persons in the world drank water with naturally occurring, appropriate amounts of fluoride.

The Republic of Ireland passed legislation requiring national fluoridation in the early 1960s. The municipal water supplies in Hong Kong and Singapore have been fluoridated for many years.

Is the Drinking Water in Your Community Fluoridated?

Surveys have shown that many Americans do not know if their community has fluoridated water, even in those cities that have been fluoridated for many years. There are several ways to learn if your community maintains adequate levels of fluoride in its drinking water. A telephone call or letter to the utility that provides water for your community is probably the easiest way. You also can ask physicians, dentists, and pharmacists in your community, or check with your local, county or state health department.

In summary, community water fluoridation is the most efficient way to prevent tooth decay. The following key facts about fluoridation summarize why this is so.

- Fluoridation is the least expensive and most effective way to reduce tooth decay.
- Fluoridation is safe.
- Fluoridation benefits children and adults.

- Fluoridation provides benefits that continue for a lifetime when consumption of fluoridated water continues.
- Fluoridation reduces the need for and cost of dental treatment.
- Fluoridation is the surest way for everyone in the community to benefit.
- Fluoridation benefits everyone when they drink fluoridated water and consume foods and beverages prepared with it.

The American Association of Public Health Dentistry urges you to support the adoption or continuation of community water fluoridation for your community. Find out if your community water is fluoridated. If it isn't, ask your political leaders and local health officials why not. You have a right to the improved oral health that results from living in a fluoridated community!

For additional information, contact:

American Association of Public Health Dentistry
10619 Jousting Lane
Richmond, VA 23235-3838
(804) 272-8344

American Dental Association Council on Community Health,
Hospital, Institutional and Medical Affairs
211 E. Chicago Avenue
Chicago, IL 60611
(800) 621-8099 Ext. 2862

Centers for Disease Control
Division of Oral Health
Mailstop F10
1600 Clifton Road
Atlanta, GA 30333
(404) 488-4450

Chapter 18

Tips on Rinsing and the Benefits of Fluoride

Used daily, fluoride dental rinses provide excellent protection against cavities along with brushing, flossing and drinking fluoridated water. Rinsing is one of the fastest and easiest ways to keep your teeth, and your children's teeth, healthy and strong.

There's proof.

Independent clinical studies show that children who use a daily non-prescription fluoride rinse reduce cavities up to 40 percent. That's over and above the protection they receive from regular brushing with a fluoride toothpaste and drinking fluoridated water. For this reason, dental professionals recommend that people over the age of six use a fluoridated rinse daily.

Fluoride rinses can be especially helpful for adults with receding gums. The fact is, a fluoride rinse aids in the replacement of lost minerals and the overall strengthening of teeth.

When gums recede, they expose the area of your teeth that's not protected by hard enamel. This area becomes especially susceptible to cavities. A fluoride rinse is shown to reduce root cavities significantly over brushing with a fluoride toothpaste alone.

If you live in an area with fluoridated drinking water or brush with fluoridated toothpaste, you may think a fluoride rinse is overdoing it. It has been shown, however, that fluoride rinses actually provide supplemental benefits.

Johnson & Johnson. One of four Oral Care "Tips" booklets. To collect the full series, see your dental professional or call 1-800-526-3967 (8 a.m. to 6 p.m. EST). Reprinted with acknowledgement.

Drinking water, for instance, is called systemic fluoride, which is swallowed and works from the inside out. On the other hand, fluoride rinses and toothpaste are called topical fluorides, which work from the outside in. Together, these three provide maximum cavity protection.

- **Mouthwashes:** Most antiseptic mouthwashes provide only a temporary reduction of the amount of bacteria in the mouth and freshen your breath.

- **Fluoride rinses:** A fluoride rinsed used daily, provides a different effect than mouthwash. Though both are capable of freshening your breath, fluoride rinses have a therapeutic effect in that they actually strengthen your teeth and make them more resistant to cavities.

- **Dental fluoride treatments:** A dental fluoride treatment, applied in the dentist's office, provides your teeth with a concentrated dose of fluoride. However, for optimal benefit, teeth need to be strengthened with fluoride on a daily basis, in conjunction with professional treatments.

1. For best results, rinse every day, especially before bedtime. This way, the fluoride will have a chance to work longer.

2. Squeeze 10 ml into the dosage meter, then into a cup.

3. Swish the rinse around in your mouth for about 60 seconds. Do not swallow. Then, spit out.

4. Do not eat or drink anything for at least 30 minutes after rinsing. This will give the fluoride rinse enough time to provide its full protection.

Rinsing Away Cavities Has Never Been So Refreshing

- **Visit your dentist regularly.** Regular visits are the best way to detect gum disease and tooth decay in their early stages when they're easiest to treat.

- **Follow a healthy diet.** Eat a balanced diet containing foods from the five major food groups. Dental professionals recommend limiting snacks between meals.

- **Brush twice a day.** The morning and before bed are good times to brush.

- **Use a high quality, ADA Accepted soft bristle toothbrush:** one that's comfortable in your hand as well as in your mouth. And remember to replace your brush every three months, or sooner if the bristles are worn.

- **Use an ADA Accepted fluoride toothpaste.** Adults should use a small amount. Children should use a pea-sized dab.

- **Clean in between your teeth every day.** Brushing alone doesn't reach everywhere. Proper flossing or the use of interdental cleaners like STIM-U-DENT® Plaque Removers are important to clean areas that toothbrushes can't reach.

- **Use a fluoride rinse daily.** This goes for both kids over age six and adults. Regular use of a fluoride rinse is shown to reduce root cavities up to 71 percent and children's cavities up to 40 percent over brushing with a fluoride toothpaste alone.

- **Consult your dentist.** For questions, concerns or advice on oral care, always consult your dentist.

Chapter 19

Healthy Start:
Fluoride Drops or Tablets for
Children in Child Care and
Preschool Settings

Settings such as preschool and child care centers offer exciting opportunities to help children get a healthy start in life. One way is to foster healthy teeth; there are procedures available that will assure improved oral health by reducing tooth decay.

The best way to prevent tooth decay is to adjust the amount of fluoride in a community's drinking water. When fluoridated water is used from birth, tooth decay is reduced by as much as 65 percent. However, one-sixth of all Americans cannot have fluoridated water because they live in areas without central water supplies. Unfortunately, an additional one-third of the U.S. population is not receiving this benefit because their communities have not yet adopted water fluoridation.

For children who live in fluoride-deficient areas, taking a fluoride supplement each day is an effective alternative method for prevention of tooth decay. Physicians or dentists can prescribe the correct amount of fluoride drops for infants and fluoride tablets for older children. Fluoride drops may be placed directly into the infant's mouth with a dropper or they may be added to juice or other liquid consumed by the infant. The tablets are chewed or dissolved in the mouth and the resulting solution swished between the teeth for one minute before swallowing. Used in this manner, fluoride tablets benefit the teeth already present in the mouth (topical benefits), as well as the teeth that are still developing in the jaws (systemic benefits). The greatest effectiveness occurs if fluoride supplements are taken each day from

NIH Publication. National Institute of Dental Research Fact Sheet.

infancy through the teen years. Daily use of fluoride supplements at home is recommended for highly motivated families who have dentists or physicians to prescribe them. Conscientious daily use of fluoride supplements from birth can provide protection against tooth decay equivalent to that provided by optimally fluoridated drinking water.

Another way is to give children, with parental permission, a fluoride tablet each day in preschool and child care settings. Research studies have demonstrated that school programs can reduce tooth decay by about 35 percent. For best results, the procedure should be started as early as possible in preschool and child care settings and be continued until at least the eighth grade and preferably through the teen years.

The daily use of fluoride drops or tablets in preschool and school settings is desirable because:

- The procedure effectively reduces tooth decay by providing systemic as well as topical benefits to teeth.
- It is safe and is inexpensive.
- There are no paper products used, eliminating waste disposal problems.
- Little time is required—approximately three minutes per day for an average group of children.
- The procedure is easy for preschool or child care children to learn and to do.
- After minimal training, teachers, aides or volunteers can effectively supervise the procedure.

A fluoride tablet program in a preschool or child care setting provides an excellent opportunity to help young children get a healthy start and ensure good dental health.

A healthy smile is a beautiful sight. Help your children keep a healthy, beautiful smile. For more information on how to initiate a fluoride tablet program in your preschool program, contact your local or state health department or:

Science Transfer and Research Analysis Branch
National Institute of Dental Research
Westwood Building, Room 522
5333 Westbard Avenue
Bethesda, Maryland 20892

Chapter 20

Dental Sealants: Sealing out Decay

Imagine being able to protect your children's teeth from decay instead of both of you having to undergo the stress and discomfort often associated with getting teeth filled. Imagine that such protection is available now from your regular dentist.

Sound too good to be true? Well, the good news is that your children's teeth most at risk of cavities can be protected by a sealing process that is safe, effective, and relatively inexpensive. Moreover, today's sealants are long-lasting, easily applied, and can virtually eliminate the kinds of cavities kids get most often.

The bad news, however, is that sealants have been underused. Many in the general public have not known they are available, and health insurers and other third-party payers often have not reimbursed for them. Fortunately, though, more dentists are beginning to encourage patients to use sealants. People are also becoming aware of them through public education programs, and more insurers are beginning to include sealant coverage in their dental policies.

"We have the means today to prevent most tooth decay" says Preston Littleton Jr., D.D.S., deputy director of the National Institute of Dental Research (NIDR) in Bethesda, Md. "We'd like to see dental sealants adopted on a much broader scale than they have been so far."

Dental sealants were conceived in the 1950s, developed in the 1960s, and brought into general use in the early 1970s. They are mixtures of the same bisphenol and methacrylate chemicals used in most white dental fillings. The sealants, which are applied as a liquid, may be clear or tinted.

FDA Consumer, November 1989.

Sealants' protective qualities derive from the barrier they form on the chewing surfaces of molars and premolars. A thin, plastic coating seals the teeth surfaces, preventing food particles from becoming trapped in pits and fissures where individual toothbrush bristles often cannot reach.

Pits and fissures occur naturally on the chewing surfaces of molars and premolars. Shaped like deep river valleys or rock crevices, they increase the surface area available for grinding food before it is swallowed. Those of concern are the particularly deep and narrow ones at the bottom of larger, more rounded crevices.

Smooth-surface teeth (incisors and canines) do not require sealants because they lack the surface irregularities of molars and premolars. For the former, fluorides and regular brushing remain the best preventive dentistry. But not even topical fluorides can completely stop pit and fissure cavities.

Dental sealants are best applied when permanent molars erupt, usually at ages 6 to 8 and 12, although they can be used effectively later too, according to Louis Ripa, D.D.S., professor and chairman of children's dentistry at the State University of New York's School of Dental Medicine at Stony Brook.

Children are more likely than adults to get cavities, Ripa explains, because they typically eat more sweets than adults usually do. Also, newly erupted molars are more susceptible to and develop decay faster than other teeth. In fact, more than 80 percent of cavities today occur on the chewing surfaces of molars and premolars, Ripa says.

Benefiting from Sealants

How many children could use sealants? NIDR surveys have found a nationwide decline of 36 percent in dental cavities among school-age children. While in 1979-80, the per child average was 4.8 decayed, missing or filled teeth, by 1986-87, this had decreased to 3.1. Nevertheless, Ripa says, nearly all children would benefit from sealants.

The reason: While 97 percent of 5-year-olds have no decay in their permanent teeth, the percentage falls to 15 percent by age 17, according to John Bogert, D.D.S., executive director of the American Academy of Pediatric Dentistry (AAPD), who agrees with Ripa that the overwhelming majority of school-age children should get sealants.

Michael Roberts, D.D.S., NIDR deputy clinical director says, "Dentists cannot absolutely predict who will get cavities and who will not. If I guess wrong, the child will get decay. If I have to err, I would rather err on the side of preventing decay, and sealants can't hurt."

In Ripa's opinion, however, not all teeth require sealing, nor do all children need to have their teeth sealed. If the pits and fissures are not deep and narrow and if they do not catch the hooked tip of the dentist's metal explorer, he says, perhaps they should be left unsealed.

"It calls for the dentist's best professional judgment," Ripa explains. "The profession may one day agree that all teeth should be sealed," he says, "but that is not the current consensus among dentists."

"It's individually determined on a patient-by-patient and tooth-by-tooth basis," adds AAPD's Bogert.

Roberts also urges sealing the primary molars of children under five. "Baby molars stay in the mouth from age 2 or 3 until 12, when they are replaced," he says. "These teeth are very susceptible to decay." Roberts concedes that getting young children to cooperate long enough to apply sealants is difficult; Thus, he says, sealants probably will continue to be used primarily on older children. At the other end of the age scale, most dentists and dental groups recommend sealing teeth only through age 17. But, Ripa says, given the increasing number of cavities dentists see in older teens and young adults, perhaps they would benefit from sealants, too. By the mid-20s, though, most people have had most of the cavities sealants are designed to prevent.

Before sealants are applied, the teeth to be sealed are first cleaned, then etched using a mild, 30 to 50 percent phosphoric acid solution. The acid creates many small; microscopic pores in the teeth. The liquid sealant flows into the pores, aided by a small brush, and becomes bonded to the teeth. If left unsealed after etching, by the way, the pores would remineralize and naturally fill in.

Sealing Process

Applying sealants causes no pain, Bogert says. Patients might experience an unpleasant taste, but would feel nothing except their teeth being cleaned, the brush applicator, and maybe a little liquid. Afterwards, patients might feel the sealant when they bite down, especially at first, but after a few days it would feel like any other tooth surface.

"The beauty of sealants is they are non-invasive, require no drilling or anesthetic, and do not interfere with normal chewing," Bogert says.

Moreover, the process of applying them is quick, typically taking 7 to 10 minutes a tooth, and relatively inexpensive. While the price varies from city to city and from dentist to dentist, sealants usually cost from $7 to $26 for a single tooth. That is about half the cost of filling a single cavity.

Additionally, Bogert says, if the teeth remain sealed, "you probably will never need a filling" for the surfaces of sealed teeth. Sealants are virtually 100 percent effective in preventing pit and fissure cavities, he adds, noting: "Sealants are the most effective preventive tool dentists have except for fluorides. Together, they can virtually eliminate cavities."

Indeed, Ripa says, numerous scientific studies have found that dental sealants can reduce cavities up to 99 percent for the two years after being applied, up to 85 percent after three years, and up to 62 percent after four. How much protection occurs depends on whether a chemical activator is used to harden the sealant, the skill of the dentist (or, in some states, hygienist) applying them, and whether the sealants are replaced if they begin to deteriorate.

The key, he adds, is good etching, keeping the tooth enamel contamination-free and, most important, maintaining a completely dry tooth until the sealant has hardened.

Sealants may eventually wear down with chewing, and the bond between them and teeth can break down in the mouth's moist environment. But while early sealants usually lasted no more than a year or so, most now remain good for four years, and many last much longer, Bogert says. Still, they should be checked periodically and replaced when necessary.

In addition to being beneficial, sealants are also among the safest of dental materials, according to Robert McCune, D.D.S., associate dean of the Washington University School of Dental Medicine in St. Louis. They are made of chemically inert materials, and there have been no known cases of illness or injury caused by their use. "Once they harden, sealants are just a piece of plastic stuck on a tooth," McCune says.

FDA regulates dental sealants as medical devices under the Food, Drug, and Cosmetic Act. The agency has found no side effects or safety problems with their use either, says Gregory Singleton, D.D.S., the dental officer in FDA's office of device evaluation.

Previously, though, many dentists worried that any bacteria or an early, undetected cavity sealed into a tooth would continue to decay under the sealant. Studies have shown, however, that any decay inadvertently sealed into a tooth will get no worse than it was before sealing, Ripa says. That's because the cavity-causing bacteria would be sealed off from their food source, thus halting the cavity's progress. If the sealant is dislodged later, the cavity might develop further or the tooth might become susceptible to decay again, but no more so than had the sealant never been applied.

Unfortunately, sealant use among American children is low. A 1986-87 nationwide survey sponsored by NIDR found only 7.6 percent of almost 40,000 school children examined had one or more teeth sealed. "We were surprised by the findings," NIDR's Littleton says.

The findings were especially unexpected given the acceptance sealants have received from almost every dental and public health group. The American Dental Association first approved a commercial sealant in 1972 and then accepted sealants in general in 1976. A 1983 National Institutes of Health (NIH) consensus conference called sealants a "safe" and "highly effective means" of preventing cavities. And former Surgeon General C. Everett Koop declared: "The greater use of sealants would lead to an improvement in the public's health, as well as reduce the future need for dental care."

If sealants are safe, beneficial, cheap and widely approved, why have so few children had their teeth sealed? There are no good answers, say numerous dental officials and observers, but there are a number of possible explanations.

Bogert says that while they are no longer new, sealants have been heavily promoted only since the 1983 NIH consensus conference. He adds that some dentists, remembering the low lifetimes and poor reliability of early sealants, are reluctant to try the new ones.

Another reason: Relatively few health insurance plans cover dental sealants. Many dentists are reluctant to advise parents to have their children's teeth sealed if the parents' insurance will not reimburse the cost, Bogert says. The American Academy of Pediatric Dentistry and other groups are urging insurers to offer sealant coverage. To some extent most now do, Bogert says, but only about one in five of their policies contain the coverage.

Increase Seen

Still, some signs indicate sealant use may be going up. The number of dentists applying sealants rose, according to published surveys, from 38 percent in 1978 to 52 percent in 1984. More recently, 85 percent of 1,330 Michigan dentists responding to a 1988 University of Michigan mail survey said they use sealants. But only 22 percent of them said they applied sealants to more than 20 percent of their patients' teeth.

At the same time, Janet Brunelle, an NIDR statistician and co-director of the 1986-87 survey, reports that slightly more 8-, 9- and 10-year-olds (about 11 percent) had at least one tooth sealed than did younger (6.5 percent at age 7) or older (5.5 percent at 17) children.

Brunelle says that is "a good sign" sealant use may be increasing because in years ahead more older children will have sealed teeth and more younger ones will get sealants as they get older.

Meanwhile, several state health departments—assisted by the National Institute of Dental Research, U.S. Centers for Disease Control, American Dental Association, and others—have launched programs to promote more widespread use of sealants. Perhaps the most far-reaching is in Ohio, where a statewide poll conducted earlier this year found only 15 percent of those surveyed had heard of sealants and could correctly state their purpose.

Together with the state dental society, the Ohio Department of Health began a pilot program in Cincinnati in February 1989 that features public service announcements on television and radio, billboard ads, brochures and posters, letters to dentists, and news media and academic journal articles. The Ohio Department of Health has also promoted the distribution of videos on sealants developed by the Columbus (Ohio) health department.

Earlier, the Ohio Department of Health awarded grants to local health departments in eight cities to increase the number of disadvantaged children who get sealants. Under the grants, dentists examine second and sixth-graders in public schools who have returned signed consent forms. Those who need sealants get them on the spot from hygienists. Some 10,000 to 12,000 children a year now receive sealants through this program, up from 2,000 in 1984, when it started.

"We are trying to make more people aware of sealants, to get them to ask their dentists about sealants, and, through school-based programs, to reach those kids who are unlikely to get dental care in a private office," says Mark Siegal, D.D.S., chief dental officer in the Ohio Department of Health. Similar programs are under way in Massachusetts, Utah, and other states.

It is just such programs that give NIDR's Littleton hope that sealant use is rising. "I think the momentum is rolling in the right direction" he says. "We are doing a better job of getting our message across. I'm optimistic that we can at least double the number of kids with sealed teeth in the next decade."

Stony Brook's Ripa agrees. He says dentistry is a profession committed to prevention, pointing to long-standing support of using fluorides in drinking water, toothpaste and mouthwashes to help prevent cavities. "If some dentists are looking for something to do," Ripa says, "sealants are it."

—by Jeffrey P. Cohn

Jeffrey P. Cohn is a freelance writer in Washington, D.C.

Questions and Answers about Dental Sealants

NIH Publication No. 94-489. Reprinted November 1994.

What are dental sealants?

Sealants are thin, plastic coatings painted on the chewing surfaces of the back teeth.

Sealants are put on in dentists' offices, clinics, and sometimes in schools. Getting sealants put on is simple and painless.

Sealants are painted on as a liquid and quickly harden to form a shield over the tooth.

Sealants are clear or tinted. Tinted sealants are easier to see.

Why get sealants?

By covering the chewing surfaces of the molars, sealants keep out the germs and food that cause decay.

What causes decay?

Germs in the mouth change the sugar in food to acid. The acid can eat a cavity in the tooth. The decay has to be cleaned out by drilling and then the tooth has to be filled.

Of course a healthy tooth is the best tooth. So it is important to prevent decay. That's why sealants are so important.

Why do back teeth decay so easily?

The chewing surfaces of back teeth are rough and uneven because they have small pits and grooves. Food and germs can get stuck in the pits and stay there a long time because toothbrush bristles cannot brush them away.

Who should get sealants?

Children should get sealants on their permanent molars as soon as the teeth come in—before decay attacks the teeth.

The first permanent molars—called "6-year molars"—come in between the ages of 5 and 7.

The second permanent molars—"12-year molars"—come in when a child is between 11 and 14 years old.

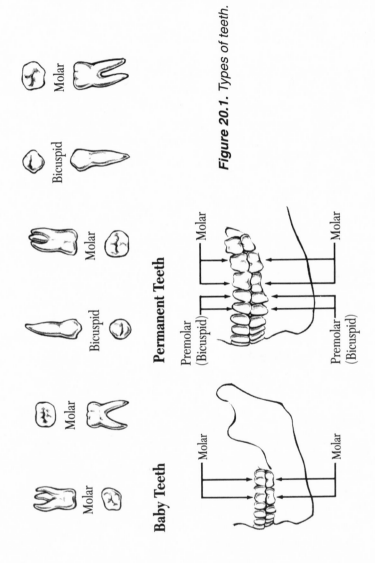

Figure 20.1. Types of teeth.

The other teeth with pits and grooves—called "premolars" or "bicuspids"—right in front of the molars, also may need to be sealed.

Teenagers and young adults without decay or fillings in their molars also may get sealants.

Should sealants also be put on baby teeth?

Your dentist might think it is a good idea, especially if your child's baby teeth have deep pits and grooves.

Baby teeth play an important role in holding the correct spacing for permanent teeth—so it is important to keep baby teeth healthy so they don't fall out early.

How much do sealants cost?

Sealing one tooth usually costs less than filling one tooth.

Having sealants put on healthy teeth now will save you money in the long run by avoiding fillings, crowns, or caps used to fix decayed teeth.

But the most important reason for getting sealants is to avoid tooth decay. Healthy teeth can last a lifetime.

Does insurance pay for sealants?

Many insurance companies pay for sealants. Check with your company for details.

How long do sealants last?

Sealants can last up to 10 years. But they need to be checked at regular dental check-ups to make sure they are not chipped or worn away. The dentist can repair sealants by adding more sealant material.

What if a small cavity is accidentally covered by a sealant?

The decay will not spread because it is sealed off from its food and germ supply.

Are sealants new?

No, sealants are not new. They have been around for about 25 years. Research by NIDR and others led to the development of sealants in the early 1960s.

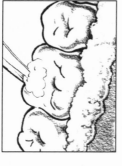

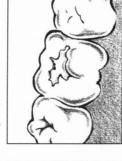

A solution is put on the tooth surface that makes the tooth a little rough. (It is easier for the sealant to stick to a slightly rough tooth.)

The sealant in place

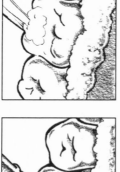

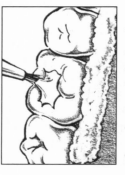

The tooth is dried, and cotton or other material is put around the tooth so it stays dry.

The sealant is applied in liquid form and hardens in a few seconds.

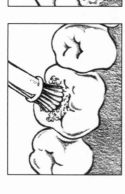

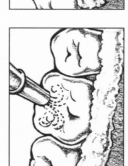

The tooth is cleaned.

The tooth is rinsed and dried. Then new cotton is put around the tooth so it stays dry.

Figure 20.2. *How are sealants put on?*

But many people still do not know what sealants are. In fact, fewer than 20 percent of children in the United States have sealants.

Besides sealants, are there other ways to prevent tooth decay?

Yes. The best way you can help prevent tooth decay is to brush with a fluoride toothpaste and drink fluoridated water (water is fluoridated in about half the cities and towns of the United States). If your water is not fluoridated or if your teeth need more fluoride to stay healthy, your dentist can prescribe it in the form of a gel, mouthrinse or tablet.

If you have a baby or a young child that needs fluoride and do not have fluoride in your water, your physician (pediatrician) or dentist can prescribe fluoride drops or tablets.

Fluoride is the best defense against tooth decay.

How does fluoride help?

- makes teeth more resistant to decay
- repairs tiny areas of decay before they become big cavities
- makes germs in the mouth less able to cause decay

Fluoride helps the smooth surfaces of the teeth the most. It is less effective on the chewing surfaces of the back teeth (molars).

Regular brushing—with fluoride toothpaste—and flossing also help prevent tooth decay. Sealants and fluoride together can prevent almost all tooth decay.

For more information about sealants call your dentist, state or local dental society, or health department. Sometimes sealants are put on at school; check with your school or local health department to see if there is such a program in your area.

For more information, write to:

National Institute of Dental Research
P.O. Box 54793
Washington, D.C. 20032

Part Three

Gum Disease

Chapter 21

What You Need to Know about Periodontal Disease

How you say it: Periodontal (per ee oh don tal) Diseases

The word "periodontal" comes from the two Greek words that mean "around the tooth."

What are periodontal diseases?

Infections of the gum and bone that hold the teeth in place. They are commonly called gum diseases.

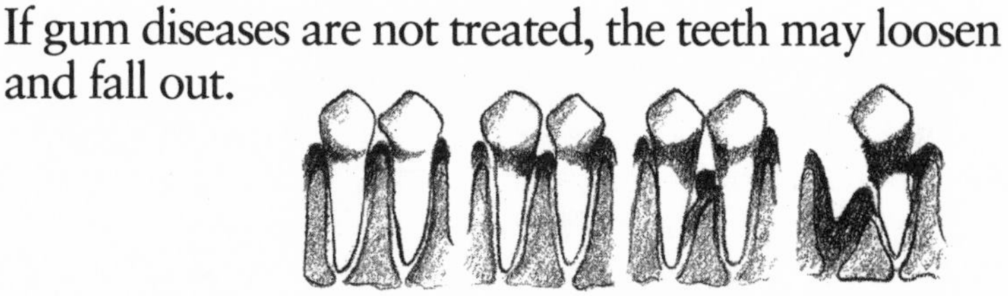

If gum diseases are not treated, the teeth may loosen and fall out.

Figure 21.1. *If gum diseases are not treated, the teeth may loosen and fall out.*

NIH Publication No. 94-1142.

What causes these diseases?

Dental plaque—a sticky mass of harmful germs. Dental scientists have found that about a half dozen of the nearly 300 germs found in the mouth can cause gum diseases.

Can I prevent gum diseases?

Yes. You can prevent them by removing dental plaque.

- Brush your teeth twice a day
- Floss your teeth once a day
- Have your teeth cleaned professionally at least once a year
- Also once a year: have a check-up by the dentist to make sure any signs of gum diseases are caught early.

How can I tell if I'm removing all the plaque?

Dental plaque is hard to see unless it's stained. You can stain plaque by chewing red "disclosing tablets," found at grocery stores and drug stores, or by using a cotton swab to smear green food coloring on your teeth. The red or green color left on the teeth will show you where there is still plaque—and where you have to brush again to remove it. Ask your dentist or dental hygienist if your plaque removal techniques are okay. If plaque is not removed, you may develop gingivitis, a condition that can be the first step toward the breakdown of your gums and bone that hold teeth in place.

Poor Oral Hygiene→Plaque Build-Up→
Gingivitis→Periodontitis→Possible Tooth Loss

Gingivitis is an infection of the gums. As a result of the infection, the gums become red, inflamed and can bleed during brushing.

It is a mild form of gum disease that does not include any loss of the bone and tissue that hold teeth in place. Gingivitis can usually be reversed with regular brushing and flossing.

Gingivitis is the first sign that something is wrong with your gums. If it is not treated it can progress to a more destructive type of gum disease called periodontitis.

Periodontitis is an infection of the tissues that help anchor the teeth. The infection can lead to loss of the bone that holds the tooth in its socket and might lead to tooth loss.

Since periodontitis affects more than just the gums, it is not controllable with regular brushing and flossing. Periodontitis must be treated by a dentist or periodontist (a dentist who specializes in treating gum diseases).

In its early stages, periodontitis usually does not have obvious symptoms. Pain, loosening of teeth, and abscess do not occur until the disease is very advanced. So it's important to visit the dentist on a regular basis so he or she can check for early signs of gum diseases. If gum diseases are not treated, the teeth may loosen and fall out.

Will my dentist refer me to a periodontist?

Your dentist might refer you to a periodontist if you have an advanced case of a gum disease, or if you have a milder form that is not responding to regular treatment.

Who gets gum diseases?

People usually don't show signs of advanced gum diseases until they are in their 30s or 40s. But it is not uncommon for teenagers to have gingivitis, the early stage of gum disease. The most common types of gum diseases develop as a result of neglect—poor brushing and no flossing.

Special Cases

Teenagers can develop a very severe form of gum disease called juvenile periodontitis. Scientists think this rare but aggressive type of gum disease might be inherited. Pregnancy, diabetes and other medical conditions also may trigger gum diseases. Smoking can make you prone to gum diseases. In fact, one study showed that smokers are five times more likely than nonsmokers to have gum diseases.

Diagnosis

Three ways a dentist can tell if you have periodontitis:

- By looking at the gums to see if they are red, swollen, and inflamed and by checking for tartar-hardened plaque—beneath the gumline. The dentist also will check for gum recession.

- By using an instrument called a probe to see if the gums bleed when they are probed and by checking for and measuring the periodontal pockets—spaces that form when unhealthy gums pull away from teeth. Usually, there is a space of 1-3 mm between healthy gums and teeth. Deeper pockets may signal advanced disease.

- By taking mouth x-rays to check for any loss of the bone that helps anchor teeth, another sign of periodontitis.

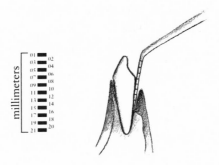

Figure 21.2. *The dentist uses the probe to measure the periodontal pocket. Most people find probing only mildly uncomfortable.*

Treatment

How are gum diseases treated?

By controlling the infection.

- the dentist or hygienist removes the plaque that contains harmful germs

How?

By scaling and root planing. These are deep-cleaning procedures that get rid of the plaque.

Scaling means scraping off the tartar from above and beneath the gumline. Planing the tooth root until it is smooth gets rid of rough spots where germs gather and allows the gums to heal closer to the teeth.

- Your dentist might also prescribe a special anti-germ mouthrinse containing a chemical called chlorhexidine. These are the only mouthrinses approved for treating periodontitis.

- Sometimes, the dentist will prescribe an antibiotic that will help kill the germs that are causing periodontitis. After the dentist scales and planes your teeth, you must brush and floss at home to keep the plaque from returning. You also will have to have a checkup with the dentist to see if the treatment has helped. Scaling and planing may need to be repeated every three to four months.

What About Gum Surgery?

Surgery might be necessary if:

1. scaling and planing do not bring the gum disease under control, or

2. the gum disease is very advanced and includes bone loss around the teeth.

Flap Surgery

A local anesthetic is given so the patient will not feel any pain or discomfort. Flap surgery involves lifting back the gums, removing the tartar, and then sewing the gums back in place.

Can baking soda help periodontitis?

Although baking soda and most toothpastes can be used to remove dental plaque, there is no evidence that they can stop or reverse tissue and bone loss caused by periodontitis.

I've heard a lot about lasers recently. How do they work and can they be used to treat periodontal diseases?

Simply put, a surgical laser works by emitting a concentrated beam of light strong enough to cut through tissue. Lasers can be used on soft tissue for certain surgical procedures related to the treatment of periodontal diseases. At this time, though, the Food and Drug Administration has not approved lasers for use on hard tissue—teeth and bone.

Research is under way to see if lasers can be used on teeth and bone.

Diagnosis: On the Horizon

1. Computer-linked probes. A computer attached to the probe regulates the probing pressure so it is always the same. The computer also can compare the results of the current test to the previous one, since it stores measurements from each reading.

189

2. Temperature probe. Detects temperature of the periodontal pockets to 1/100th of a degree centigrade. The hotter the site, the more likely there is gum disease.

3. New X-ray technology:

    - **Taking x-rays.** Taking x-rays with an instrument similar to that found in a home video camera uses much less radiation than does the standard x-ray.

    - **Reading x-rays.** The computer can compare two x-rays and highlight even the smallest changes in bone surrounding the teeth. Using the computer allows dentists to see details that would not be visible on a regular x-ray.

4. Determining which germ is causing the infection. Knowing what type of bacterium is causing the infection could help determine the best treatment. Some bacteria can be removed by scraping plaque off the teeth, a process known as scaling. Others are harder to get rid of and may require an antibiotic—a medicine that can kill germs.

5. Quick test for identifying active gum disease. The dentist takes a sample of fluid leaked from the gums that is found at the base of the teeth. It is analyzed for substances associated with active tissue and bone destruction.

Treatment: On the Horizon

1. **Slow-release antibiotics** placed directly into the periodontal pockets. Tiny fibers or gels containing antibiotics are put into the pockets next to the tooth root where the medication seeps onto the affected area.

2. **Barrier membranes.** During flap surgery, the dentist inserts these small, mesh-like pieces of fabric between the gum flap and the affected teeth. The mesh helps the soft tissue and bone grow back in place. A second surgery is needed to remove the mesh. The newest mesh will be able to break down and be absorbed by the body, eliminating the need for the second surgical procedure.

3. **High-powered ultrasonic cleaning.** A cleaning instrument that uses high-frequency sound waves is useful in breaking up tartar and removing plaque.

4. **Chemically modified antibiotics.** These drugs lack the antibiotic property but have the ability to inhibit tissue destruction. They should help stop gum disease and should be safe for long-term use, without causing bacterial resistance.

5. **Low-Dose antibiotics.** Researchers have found that low doses of doxycycline can slow the destruction of tissue and bone. At low doses, the drug doesn't seem to encourage the development of antibiotic-resistant germs.

6. **NSAIDs—Non-Steroidal Anti-Inflammatory Drugs.** These aspirin-like medicines have been shown to slow bone loss in patients with periodontitis. Researchers are testing these medications.

Chapter 22

Brushing up on Gum Disease

Getting your teeth pulled because of a sore arm may sound far-fetched. But it has happened more than once, says Saul Schluger, D.D.S., professor emeritus at the University of Washington's school of dentistry in Seattle.

Schluger has been involved in the treatment and study of gum, or periodontal, disease for more than 50 years, and he recalls that the patients in these cases were professional baseball players who had the ill luck to have developed their dental (and arm) problems when the "focal infection" theory of periodontal disease was in vogue earlier this century.

The theory held that periodontal disease always worsened, could only be stopped by pulling teeth, and that it could spread—not only from one area of the gums to another, but to other parts of the body. In the case of an affected ballplayer with a sore arm, explains Schluger, it was considered possible that migrating infection from the gums might be the cause of the sore arm. To prevent further problems it was sometimes thought best to simply pull the player's teeth.

For ordinary people, a more common scenario was the wholesale pulling of teeth at the first sign of gum disease. The reaction, says Schluger, was "almost Pavlovian. If you had gum disease, you had your teeth out. It was the cause of a lot of dentures."

FDA Consumer, May 1990.

Old Beliefs, New Data

Though the focal infection era is now behind us, its legacy remains. Many older people are toothless and wearing dentures for reasons now considered unnecessary. And many fears and beliefs formed during that period continue to hold sway.

For instance, periodontal disease is commonly said to be responsible for 70 percent of the teeth lost after childhood. But, according to Brian Burt, Ph.D., a dental epidemiologist in the School of Public Health at the University of Michigan, this oft-repeated statement is based largely on a single study conducted in the early 1950s. A more recent study published in the January 1987 *Journal of the American Dental Association* found that dental decay was the most common disease-related reason for adult tooth extractions in the late 1970s and early 1980s; only 9 percent were necessitated by periodontal disease.

Clearly, much has changed. So what is the threat of periodontal disease today? And what can be done about it?

What Is Periodontal Disease?

In the broadest sense, periodontal disease can be considered any form of ill health affecting the periodontium, the tissues that surround and support the teeth. These include the gums (or gingiva), the bone of the tooth socket, and the periodontal ligament, a thin layer of connective tissue that holds the tooth in its socket and acts as a cushion between tooth and bone.

Inflammation or infection of the gums is called gingivitis, that of the bone, periodontitis. These conditions can arise for a variety of reasons. A severe deficiency of vitamin C can lead to scurvy and result in bleeding, spongy gums, and eventual tooth loss. And at least one periodontal disease—the uncommon but highly destructive juvenile periodontitis—is thought to have a strong genetic basis. But as the terms periodontal disease, gingivitis, and periodontitis are most commonly used, they refer to disease that is caused by the buildup of dental plaque.

Plaque is a combination of bacteria and sticky bacterial products that forms on the teeth within hours of cleaning. Its source is the natural bacteria in the mouth, of which more than 300 different species have been identified. In small amounts and when newly formed, plaque is invisible and relatively harmless. But when left to accumulate, it increases in volume (in large amounts, plaque can be seen as a soft whitish deposit), and the proportion of harmful species in the plaque grows.

Separating Gingivitis . . .

The role played by plaque in the development of gingivitis was demonstrated in the early 1960s. Dental researchers had people stop brushing their teeth and let the plaque in their mouths build up. Within two to three weeks, signs of inflammation appeared (redness, swelling, and an increased tendency to bleed) and when brushing resumed, the inflammation went away.

Gingivitis is fairly common. Just about everybody, says Burt, has it in some degree. A recent nationwide survey by the National Institute of Dental Research, for example, found that 40 to 50 percent of the adults studied had at least one spot on their gums with inflammation that was prone to bleeding.

At one time gingivitis and periodontitis were thought to be different phases of the same disease, meaning that the sort of inflammation detected in this study would lead inevitably to periodontitis if left untreated. Yet, dental researchers no longer believe this to be true. In the April 1988 Dental Clinics of North America, National Institute of Dental Research director Harald Löe, D.D.S., describes an ongoing study, then in its 15th year, of Sri Lankan tea workers who practice no oral hygiene. All have gingivitis, but not all have periodontitis.

This and other studies with similar results have led dental researchers to two conclusions. One, says dental epidemiologist Ronald J. Hunt, of the College of Dentistry at the University of Iowa, is that "gingivitis is not a particularly serious disease." The other is that "gingivitis and periodontitis are different disease entities."

. . . From Periodontitis

Some people with gingivitis do, nonetheless, develop periodontitis. The plaque that causes gingivitis is located at or above the gum line and is referred to as supragingival plaque. With time, areas of supragingival plaque can become covered by swollen gum tissue or otherwise spread below the gum line (where it is called subgingival plaque), and in this airless environment the harmful bacteria within the plaque proliferate. These bacteria can injure tissues through the direct secretion of toxins. But they cause the greatest damage by stimulating a chronic inflammatory response in which the body in essence turns on itself, and the periodontal ligament and bone of the tooth socket are broken down and destroyed. This is similar to what happens in rheumatoid arthritis and, like rheumatoid arthritis, periodontitis is now considered primarily an inflammatory disease.

The bone destruction from periodontitis can be fairly even, resulting in receding gum lines. But more often it causes deep crevices between an individual tooth and its socket. These crevices are called periodontal pockets, and just as it once was thought that gingivitis inexorably progressed to periodontitis, so it was once believed that shallow periodontal pockets inevitably deepened, eventually becoming deep enough to jeopardize the socket's support of the adjacent tooth.

Recently, however, dental researchers have collected substantial evidence to support a theory called the burst hypothesis. This theory states that periodontal bone loss is not a steady process but results instead from periodic flare ups of infection and inflammatory response inside the pocket. Writing in a 1988 issue of the *Journal of Clinical Periodontology*, researchers from the British Medical Research Council say this theory helps explain epidemiologic and clinical findings that many, if not most, periodontal pockets are not actively diseased. Rather, they are remnants of past infections that the body has overcome. Further, not all periodontal pockets inevitably deepen; some apparently partially heal and get shallower.

What triggers a destructive "burst" inside a periodontal pocket (or, for that matter, the transition from gingivitis to periodontitis) is unknown. But, as described by these British researchers, such events are most likely the result of unfavorable fluctuations in the balance between the type, quantity and location of bacteria in a person's mouth, the ability to resist bacterial infection, and the unique characteristics of an individual's inflammatory response.

Good News-Bad News

It's estimated that only 30 percent of the U.S. population cleans their teeth adequately using only a toothbrush, floss, and toothpaste.

All this has something of a good news-bad news flavor to it. The good news is that most of us have less to fear than we may have been led to believe. Periodontal disease is often described as almost universal, a disease that can or will affect almost everyone and that can have "devastating" results. But most such statements are based on studies that are not only old (dating from the 1950s and early 1960s) but that also combine gingivitis and periodontitis under the single heading "periodontal disease."

More recent studies suggest that only about 10 percent of adults have periodontitis severe enough to possibly cause tooth loss. The percentage is lower in younger people and higher in older people. Even among these people, says epidemiologist Burt, it is unusual to have more than a few affected teeth. In one 1985 study of nearly 55,000 Italians, among those who had what are considered deep periodontal pockets the average number of affected teeth was fewer than one.

The "bad" news generated by all this new research into the causes and natural history of the periodontal diseases (as gingivitis and periodontitis are now referred to collectively) is that while most of us may be at lower risk than previously thought, it is still impossible to say who is at high or low risk individually. It can't be predicted who with gingivitis will develop periodontitis or who with shallow periodontal pockets will go on to develop deep pockets and possibly lose teeth.

Researchers are, however, working rapidly on methods to make such predictions. These techniques will involve tests of immune function and the types of bacteria in a person's mouth. Once available, they are expected to dramatically change current approaches to the treatment of periodontitis.

Today, periodontitis is treated either by surgically eliminating periodontal pockets or by cleaning affected tooth roots in a process known as scaling and planing. The current trend is toward the latter, and the ability to predict who is susceptible to worsening disease could accelerate the move in this direction. By one estimate, such predictions could make 90 percent of "pocket elimination" surgeries unnecessary.

Fighting Plaque

As yet, however, dentists can't make such predictions. And because both gingivitis and periodontitis are caused by the buildup of plaque, one dental maxim is as true now as ever: If you want to keep your teeth you have to keep them clean.

Only a dentist can diagnose and treat periodontitis. And only a dentist can remove the subgingival plaque responsible for periodontitis and its worsening. Nonetheless, according to Sebastian Ciancio, D.D.S., professor and chairman of the Department of Periodontology at the School of Dental Medicine, State University of New York at Buffalo, controlling the buildup of plaque above the gum line helps control both the quantity and harmful nature of plaque below the gum line. He says an ideal plaque control program involves periodic professional examinations and cleanings, "so you can start out with a clean mouth," coupled with good cleaning at home.

The most effective method of plaque control at home is brushing and flossing. According to dental experts, most people don't brush their teeth properly and frequently miss some areas of their mouths, so it is a good idea to get instructions in effective brushing from a dentist or dental hygienist. One way to help determine how well you are brushing is through the use of disclosing agents (available over-the-counter), which make plaque easier to see.

As for toothbrush selection, studies show that soft bristles are better than hard at removing plaque. Toothbrushes are also less effective when splayed or matted and for this reason should be replaced at the first signs of wear. These considerations aside, virtually any toothbrush can be effective if properly used, and a choice can usually be made based on personal preference or a dentist's advice.

There is a large and growing selection of dental flosses on the market today. According to the August 1989 *Consumer Reports*, which evaluated "anti-plaque" products, waxed and unwaxed floss are equally effective. Flosses do vary in strength and resistance to shredding, but as long as it doesn't break, the kind of floss you choose is less important than how well you use it—and whether you use it at all. Surveys show that fewer than 20 percent of Americans floss their teeth daily.

Though flossing is the only effective way to clean between the teeth, toothpastes can help in the removal of plaque from more accessible tooth surfaces. This is not because they have special "anti-plaque" ingredients, but because they contain abrasives and detergents that aid in the mechanical removal of plaque that occurs during tooth brushing. This is the source of the "anti-plaque" statements made on some toothpaste labels.

Several toothpastes are also now being marketed for preventing the buildup of "tartar." Tartar, which is plaque that has calcified and hardened on the teeth, was once thought to contribute to or even cause periodontal disease by physically irritating the periodontal tissues. It is now considered far less important, however, and, according to the January 1988 *Journal of the American Dental Association*, tartar control toothpastes have a "cosmetic benefit" only. They have no effect on gingivitis or periodontitis.

Theoretically, a toothbrush, floss, and toothpaste are all you need to control supragingival plaque. Yet estimates are that only 30 percent of the U.S. population cleans their teeth adequately using these mechanical means alone. For this reason, dental researchers have been searching recently for additional ways to help people control plaque. In particular, this search has focused on mouthwashes.

There have been differences of opinion over the anti-plaque claims made for various mouthwashes. But regardless of how effective a mouthwash might be, Ciancio points out that not everyone needs such products. "People who don't have periodontal problems don't need an anti-plaque mouthwash," he says. "If you are having problems, for instance, gums that bleed when you brush see your dentist. If an anti-plaque mouthwash is recommended, what I advise is using the product for three to six weeks to see what a clean mouth feels like. Then stop and see if you can maintain that feeling with mechanical means alone. If not, resume the mouthwash for another few weeks, then try again to maintain a clean mouth mechanically."

This kind of conscientious effort at good plaque control holds great promise. When combined with researchers' rapidly growing knowledge about the causes of periodontal disease and how it can best be treated, the future offers a realistic prospect, says NIDR's director Löe, that "no one need ever lose a tooth to periodontal disease."

Anti-Plaque Mouthwashes

The use of mouthwashes in the quest for a healthy mouth has a long history. According to Irwin Mandel, D.D.S., professor of dentistry at Columbia University's School of Dental and Oral Surgery, an ancient Chinese text contains the first known recommendation for the use of a mouthwash in the treatment of gum disease: Rinse the mouth with urine.

In the intervening 5,000 years, urine (which from a healthy person is sterile) has been used as a mouthwash in cultures around the world. By lowering the acidity of the mouth it may, says Mandel, help reduce the formation of cavities. But against the periodontal diseases it's unlikely to have an effect.

The modern era of mouthwashes might be said to have begun in 1920. It was then that Listerine, which had already been sold for more than 40 years as a general antiseptic, was first marketed as a remedy for bad breath. A new advertising campaign for the product introduced the American public to the term "halitosis" and its social undesirability. The pitch was so successful it is now considered a classic.

Such promotional activities no doubt contributed to what Mandel describes as a longstanding "disdain" of mouthwashes by members of the dental and scientific communities. This view was further reinforced by a widely held assumption that any effect mouthwashes had against oral bacteria was only temporary. In the early 1980s, however, studies began to appear suggesting that some mouthwashes might indeed reduce supragingival plaque and plaque-related gingivitis. There is no evidence that mouthwashes can affect subgingival plaque or periodontitis.

A prescription product (trade name Peridex) containing the anti-microbial chlorhexidine was approved by FDA in 1986 based on studies showing that it reduced gingivitis by up to 41 percent. Chlorhexidine mouthwashes have long been used in Europe, and an article that year in *The Journal of Periodontal Research* called chlorhexidine "the most effective and most thoroughly tested anti-plaque and anti-gingivitis agent known today."

Shortly after Peridex was approved for marketing, the American Dental Association awarded it its "Seal of Acceptance"—the first ever granted a mouthwash by the ADA. This seal (which can have considerable marketing value and is probably most familiar as a result of its being displayed on many brands of toothpaste) indicated that Peridex had met a series of guidelines established by the ADA for evaluating products making anti-plaque, anti-gingivitis claims.

In 1987 the ADA awarded its second (and so far only other) Seal of Acceptance to a mouthwash for use in the reduction of plaque and gingivitis. This seal went to Listerine, and its manufacturer has since used the ADA seal in promoting the product as a plaque-fighter. FDA, however, has not yet approved Listerine for this use; In fact, FDA has sent letters to the makers of Listerine and several other over-the-counter (OTC) products making anti-plaque claims stating that in its opinion the products are being marketed in violation of the Federal Food, Drug, and Cosmetic Act and are "at risk of regulatory action."

The basis for these letters is that no ingredient for use in an OTC drug product has yet been recognized as safe and effective for the prevention or reduction of plaque or gingivitis in FDA's ongoing evaluation of OTC drug products. FDA therefore considers as unproven claims that a product's ingredients have such effects.

In part, the reason for this stance (and for the difference between the actions of FDA and those of the ADA with respect to Listerine) has to do with timing. Data concerning the claims of the OTC anti-plaque, anti-gingivitis products were not available until after FDA's review of OTC dental products was well under way. Such data have since been submitted and in the case of Listerine, says Jeanne Rippere, a microbiologist in FDA's over-the-counter drug evaluation division, the information is probably much the same as that presented to the American Dental Association and on which the awarding of its Seal of Acceptance was based. In a continuation of its ongoing OTC drug review, FDA plans to have a panel of non-government experts evaluate ingredients that might be used in OTC drug products making anti-plaque and anti-gingivitis claims. Steps are being taken to facilitate this process, and it may begin within the next year.

What about Baking Soda?

In the late 1970s and early 1980s an oral hygiene program known as the Keyes Technique was widely promoted in the United States. Aimed at combatting plaque-related periodontal diseases, the program included not only such conventional advice as frequent professional cleanings, but also the recommendation that patients apply to their gums and brush their teeth with a mixture of salt, hydrogen peroxide, and baking soda.

Laboratory studies showing these agents had some effectiveness against harmful bacteria were the principal basis for this recommendation But critics pointed out that what worked in the laboratory didn't always work in the mouth. A study by the technique's proponents showed some effectiveness in humans. However, it lacked a control group, so it was impossible to say how the technique compared to more traditional methods of oral hygiene. Furthermore, the subjects in this study had been liberally treated with antibiotics, so it wasn't known if the benefits they had experienced were actually due to the baking soda brushing regimen.

To resolve these issues, dental researchers at the University of Minnesota, led by Larry Wolff, Ph.D., D.D.S., conducted a four-year study involving 171 adults with moderate periodontitis. The study's design enabled the researchers to compare the effectiveness of a baking soda, salt, and hydrogen peroxide mixture with that of ordinary toothpaste. The results, published in the January 1989 *Journal of the American Dental Association*, showed that while the baking soda mixture did help in the maintenance of oral health it was no more effective than ordinary toothpaste.

Wolff and his colleagues also found that, compared to the patients using ordinary toothpaste, those using the baking soda regimen were three times as likely to stop following their oral hygiene program because it was inconvenient. Overall, they said, there was no evidence that a baking soda brushing regimen "will contribute more toward periodontal health than use of a commercial toothpaste, a toothbrush, and dental floss."

Steven Shepherd, M.P.H.

Steven Shepherd is a medical writer in San Diego.

Chapter 23

Vaccine Slows Gum Disease

Researchers at the University of Washington have shown for the first time that immunization can slow the progression of periodontal disease in monkeys. The study, conducted at NCRR's Regional Primate Research Center in Seattle, Washington, and supported by the National Institute of Dental Research, indicates that one day it may be possible to develop a human vaccine to prevent periodontitis, the major cause of tooth loss among older Americans.

"We know enough already to say that a human periodontitis vaccine seems feasible, but it may be a decade before we see full-fledged clinical trials of such a vaccine," says Dr. Roy C. Page, director of the Research Center in Oral Biology at the University of Washington School of Dentistry, Seattle.

Periodontitis is a common infectious disease in which the tissues and bones surrounding and supporting the teeth are destroyed by invading bacteria. Treatment to restore tooth support can be costly and time-consuming. One of the primary culprits in periodontal disease is the gram-negative bacterium *Porphyromonas gingivalis*. The University of Washington researchers, working with scientists at the University of Texas in San Antonio and the Bristol Myers Squibb Pharmaceutical Research Institute in Seattle, have developed a vaccine containing killed *P. gingivalis*. The vaccine was tested in long-tailed macaque monkeys (*Macacafascicularis*).

NCRR Reporter, May 1994.

Twenty monkeys were enrolled in the study. They had pre-existing *P. gingivalis* infection. Ten randomly chosen monkeys received the vaccine and 10 received placebo inoculations at the start of the study and again at 3, 6, and 16 weeks. At the time of the final injection, the investigators wrapped silk thread beneath the gum line of eight teeth in each of the monkeys to induce bacterial buildup and periodontal disease.

Examination of the animals' gums at intervals after the silk thread was placed showed that the amount of *P. gingivalis* and gum inflammation increased significantly in both groups of animals, indicating that the vaccine was not effective in clearing *P. gingivalis* from the gum tissue. However, dental X rays and bone density measurements taken 30 and 36 weeks after the inoculations showed that the non-vaccinated monkeys had lost twice as much tooth-supporting bone as had the vaccinated animals.

Although the vaccine elicited relatively large amounts of antibody against *P. gingivalis*, the antibody response did not appear to be long-lasting. Antibody titers peaked after the third injection (at week 6), decreasing by 50 percent by week 12. The titer increased again following the fourth injection (at week 16), but dropped by more than half by week 36.

In spite of the dissipating antibody response, vaccination protected the monkeys against a challenge with the bacteria. In a test conducted at week 36, Dr. Page and his colleagues applied live *P. gingivalis* bacteria directly to the gum lines of six monkeys—three vaccinated and three non-vaccinated animals. Eight weeks later, the vaccinated animals appeared to be completely resistant to this bacterial onslaught, while the control animals showed rapid and dramatic bone loss.

"It appears that immunization may in fact block bacterially induced bone loss," says Dr. Page. "Over the next five years we're going to study why the vaccine works, how it works, and whether we will be able to produce a vaccine that effectively reduces the level of bacteria in the gum tissue."

—by Maureen Curran

Chapter 24

Lasers in Dentistry: Only for Gum Disease, for Now

Lasers are now part of our lives in many ways. They are in our computer printers and compact disc players, they record prices at the supermarket check-out, they light up rock concerts, and they guide weapons and measure distances between planets. Lasers have also revolutionized many surgical procedures, minimizing bleeding, swelling, scarring, and pain. And now they're beginning to blaze a new trail in dentistry.

The potential benefits of laser use in dentistry include procedures done on soft tissues of the mouth. Because laser techniques cause less pain than traditional methods, they are also likely to reduce the fear that many people have of the dentist. At the very least, lasers in some dental applications would eliminate the noise of the instruments that to some patients are nearly as disturbing as the physical discomfort.

However, it may be quite a while before you can have your cavities drilled or root canals cleaned with a painless flash of a laser. "FDA has cleared for marketing certain lasers for soft tissue use, such as gingivectomies [removing excess gum tissue], but not for hard tissues," says Gregory Singleton, D.D.S., senior dental officer in the Center for Devices and Radiological Health at FDA. The hard tissues include tooth and root, while soft tissues of the mouth refer to the gums, the ligaments and fibers that bind tooth to socket, and the tissue supporting the tongue.

So far, lasers seem to be living up to their promise in the latter area. "For soft tissue surgery, lots of patients report less postoperative

FDA Consumer, January 1995.

pain. There are sealed off nerve endings, so recovery is less painful," says Marilyn Miller, D.M.D., co-director of the Princeton Dental Resource Center in Princeton, NJ. But she adds that healing may be slightly slower, because the laser also seals off blood vessels, which would bring in clotting factors to help heal cut tissues.

Laser Basics

Since the mid-1960s, lasers have proven to be powerful surgical tools. The word "laser" is an acronym for "light amplification by stimulated emission of radiation," which means that the intense and narrow beam of light is of one wavelength. Ordinary "white" sunlight, in contrast, is a continuum of light of many wavelengths, corresponding to the colors of the visible spectrum plus the infrared (heat) and ultraviolet wavelengths that sandwich them. Sunlight passing through a prism separates into its component colors; a laser light remains a single color.

A medical laser device includes a source of electricity, mirrors to direct the beam, a crystal or gas that is stimulated to emit the light, and tubing to deliver the light energy. The nature of the material through which the light passes determines the specific properties of the laser, and therefore what it can do in the human body. Instrument design is tailored to specific uses. Many dental lasers, for example, include long narrow tubing so that the dentist can use it in the narrow confines of a person's mouth.

Types of Dental Lasers

FDA has cleared four types of lasers for dental use: carbon dioxide, Nd:YAG, argon, and holmium:YAG.

A carbon dioxide (CO_2) laser uses CO_2 gas. Watery tissue absorbs this type of laser energy, which doesn't penetrate very deeply, but vaporizes surface cells. A CO_2 laser leaves a residue of carbon, called char. If a dentist leaves char in place, it serves as a biological dressing, maintaining sterility.

Because the beam from a CO_2 laser is invisible, a second laser beam, based on the elements helium and neon, adds a red beam, so the dentist can see the laser energy.

A CO_2 laser is used in gingivectomies, biopsies, and removal of benign and malignant lesions. A CO_2 laser is particularly good for a frenectomy. "The frenum (the tissue under the tongue) is tight in some people, and it can be quickly loosened up with laser treatment," says

Michael Yessik, president of Incisive Technologies, a laser manufacturer in San Carlos, CA.

For lesions extending into tissue deeper than the 0.1 millimeter that the CO_2 laser penetrates, a neodymium:yttrium-aluminum-garnet (commonly called an Nd:YAG) laser is appropriate. As with the CO_2 laser, an accompanying red beam makes the energy visible. A jet of cool water or air limits possible heat damage that can result when a super-heated gas, called a plasma, forms on the tissue surface as it is being treated. An Nd:YAG laser can harm thin tissue, such as the gum in the lower front of the mouth. The CO_2 and Nd:YAG lasers are used in some of the same procedures that remove soft tissue.

The argon laser is based on gas of the element argon, and emits a bluish-green light. It is cleared for marketing for a different application, curing composite resins. These tooth-colored materials are used in reconstructing chipped teeth, filling cavities in visible areas of the mouth, or sealing teeth to protect them from decay. The dentist paints on the composite, and then focuses a narrow beam of light to harden, or cure, it. The intense light alters the physical properties of the composite, linking its small molecules into longer ones, which adds great strength. Robert Pick, D.D.S., clinical associate professor at Northwestern University Dental School, writes that he thinks the argon laser will soon become the standard method for curing dental composite resins, replacing ultraviolet light.

Another device used on soft tissues is the holmium:YAG laser. Oral and maxillofacial surgeons have used it experimentally to surgically remove the damaged disc separating the condyle of the mandible from the base of the skull. The disc can be damaged due to trauma or chronic inflammatory diseases such as osteoarthritis that can cause symptoms commonly known as temporomandibular joint (TMJ) syndrome. (An oral and maxillofacial surgeon is a dentist specializing in correcting abnormalities of the jaws and face with surgical procedures.) TMJ syndrome can cause facial pain, headaches, pain in front of the ear, noise when the jaw opens, ear congestion, dizziness, ringing in the ears, difficulty swallowing, nervousness, insomnia, difficulty chewing, sensitive teeth, numb fingertips, and backache.

Choosing the Best Laser

The challenge to dentists is finding the best laser type and strength for a particular application. Lasers can vary in chemical basis (CO_2, Nd:YAG, holmium:YAG, argon, and others), wavelength of emitted light, power, whether it is applied continuously or in short pulses, and whether the laser is applied directly (a contact laser) or through a tip of some sort (non-contact).

The effect of a particular laser must be evaluated for each type of dental tissue: such as enamel, dentin, pulp, bone, and gingiva. Light can have one of four fates when it hits a tissue; it may be absorbed, reflected, scattered within the tissue, or transmitted. This is important, because light energy that is transmitted or scattered may harm surrounding tissue. Reflected laser light dissipates so quickly that it does no damage.

Whether or not anesthesia is needed for soft tissue dental laser procedures depends on the duration of the treatment and the amount of tissue removed. CO_2 laser procedures may require local anesthesia, but Nd:YAG treatment usually does not.

"About 70 to 80 percent of procedures using dental lasers are done without anesthesia. It depends on the power level needed to perform the procedure," says Yessik.

Safety Measures

Several precautions to dental staff and patient must accompany laser use. Everyone in the room must wear protective glasses—dark green tinted for argon and YAG lasers, and clear for CO_2 lasers. Wet gauze pads are placed in the patient's mouth surrounding the treated area. Reflective surfaces, such as instruments and mirrors, are covered so that stray light beams cannot ricochet around the room.

It is very important that all anesthetic gases be removed from the room. They are explosive, and could be ignited by a laser beam. The dentist must also suction off vaporized soft tissue, and the smoke, or laser "plume," emitted during procedures. The plume can carry viruses. This is one reason that some dentists do not like to use a laser to remove herpes lesions in the mouth. Treatment with a CO_2 laser provides rapid pain relief and speeds healing.

Zapping Away Cavities—Not Yet

If you dream of having a cavity treated with a painless, soundless zap of a laser, you will have to wait awhile. Although lasers have great potential for one day replacing the drill, there is still too much danger of their damaging the pulp under the enamel, according to Gerard Kugel, D.M.D., assistant clinical professor of restorative dentistry at Tufts University School of Dental Medicine in Boston. The problem is the amount of heat generated in hard tissue treatment.

"It may take a different intensity or type of laser energy to remove debris from soft tissue than to remove the hard calculus or plaque from a tooth's root," says Dennis Mangan, Ph.D., director of the Periodontal Research Program at the National Institute of Dental Research in Bethesda, MD. (A periodontist specializes in diseases of the gums and supporting structures of the teeth.) Also, a laser could not produce the uneven edges carved intentionally with a drill so that dental amalgam or other filling materials can be retained properly. Lasers could not be used to repair existing fillings either, because they would vaporize the amalgam component mercury, which would make it highly toxic.

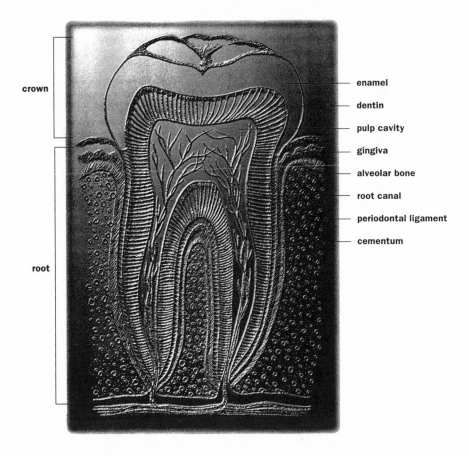

Figure 24.1. Anatomy of a Tooth

But dental researchers are actively investigating the safety and efficacy of lasers for hard tissue applications on freshly extracted human teeth and in animal and human trials.

Researchers at the University of California at San Francisco School of Dentistry carried out one human study using a pulsed Nd:YAG laser at relatively low power. They used the laser on 163 cavities in 97 people at three private dental clinics in 1987 and 1988. At follow-up three years later that included 35 participants, the areas where the laser had removed decay had all remineralized well, with no complications.

Still, much more study is needed before the dentist's drill becomes a thing of the past. "The FDA feels there is not enough support for use of lasers on hard tissues, and dental organizations, such as the American Dental Association, do not support non-FDA-approved laser procedures," says Miller.

A Look Ahead

Despite the slow evolution of lasers in dentistry, researchers say the day will indeed come when a variety of lasers play a more prominent role in maintaining a healthy mouth. "And it won't be just one laser that will do all dental procedures. Researchers envision a laser unit in which you can switch on or off different types of lasers depending upon the procedure," says Miller.

"It's an exciting technology, and patients are really intrigued at the idea of a laser. The lay press exaggerated, saying now we can throw away dentists' drills. But research is showing that we will be able to do that—eventually," she says. "But we haven't yet found the right laser."

Some Current Dental Laser Procedures

Replacing conventional soft tissue dental surgery with lasers often eliminates the need for sutures and anesthesia. Today lasers can:

- Remove excess gum tissue, which can develop as a side effect of taking certain drugs, poor oral hygiene, or orthodontia, in a procedure called gingivectomy.

- Expose dental implants, replacement tooth roots made of steel or titanium surgically embedded in the jawbone, which can become covered with too much soft tissue. A CO_2 laser can quickly expose the implant for the dentist to work on.

- Relieve the pain of aphthous ulcers, mouth sores. Both CO_2 and Nd:YAG lasers can relieve the pain instantly, used on low power, without an anesthetic.

- Remove excess tissue under the tongue in less than two minutes, in a procedure called frenectomy.

- Biopsy or sample tissue from a lesion to see whether it is cancerous. A laser biopsy does not require suturing and heals well. This is particularly useful on the tongue, where bleeding can be profuse.

- Remove soft tissue in the mouth to even out wrinkles that form when a person smiles.

- Hasten clotting of bleeding caused by other procedures.

Ricki Lewis, Ph.D.

Ricki Lewis is a freelance science writer in Scotia, N.Y., and author of college biology texts.

A Laser for Gum Disease

FDA Consumer, September 1990.

U.S. dentists have access to the world's first YAG laser designed for general dentistry, following FDA's permission in May 1990 for the American Dental Laser to be marketed to treat gum disease.

In clinical trials at the University of California in San Francisco and in countries where the device is already approved, treatments in which the laser was used as a scalpel to cut soft tissue such as the gingiva and gums led to substantial reduction in bleeding and in use of anesthesia.

The laser pulses its energy in short bursts through a flexible fiber optic (an ultra-thin tube that carries a light). This design overcomes problems of destructive heat levels and inability to reach the recesses of the mouth, which confronted earlier laser inventors.

Sunrise Technologies Incorporated of Sunnyvale, CA., developed and manufactures the instrument for American Dental Laser Incorporated, Birmingham, MI., which owns the patents and markets it.

The firms said they expect to expand the indications for the American Dental Laser to introduce new methods of treatment to dentistry and to make current procedures easier, faster, and less invasive.

Chapter 25

Women and Gum Disease

As a woman, you know that your health needs are unique. You know that brushing and flossing daily, diet, exercise and regular visits to your physician and dentist are all important to help you stay in shape. You also know that at specific times in your life, you need to take extra care of yourself. Times when you mature and change for example, puberty or menopause, and times when you have special health needs, such as menstruation and pregnancy. Did you know that your oral health needs change at these times, too?

During these particular times, your body experiences hormonal changes. These changes can affect many of the tissues in your body, including your gums. Your gums can become sensitive, and at times react strongly to the hormonal fluctuations. This may make you more susceptible to gum disease.

What Is Gum Disease?

Gum disease, or periodontal disease, is caused by the bacteria and toxins in dental plaque, a sticky colorless film that constantly forms on the teeth. Gum disease affects the gums and supporting structures of the teeth. The earliest stage of gum disease, gingivitis, usually causes the gum tissue to swell, turn red and bleed easily. There is usually little to no pain at this time. Sometimes swelling and bleeding can be seen only by the dentist.

If left untreated, gum disease can progress to a more serious stage where the bone and tissue surrounding the teeth are damaged or destroyed. If still not treated, teeth eventually become loose and may be lost.

Without diligent home oral care, including brushing and flossing, and regular trips to the dentist, you put yourself at risk for gum disease. In addition, as mentioned before, hormonal changes at certain stages in life can be a contributing factor in your chances of getting some kinds of gum disease or can make an existing gum problem worse.

The following will give you an idea of some of the symptoms you might experience with your oral health during puberty, menstruation, pregnancy and menopause and help to answer some of the questions you might have.

Puberty

During puberty, an increased level of sex hormones, such as progesterone and possibly estrogen, in a young woman's maturing system causes increased blood circulation to the gums. This, in turn, may cause an increase in the gums' sensitivity which leads to a greater susceptibility or reaction to any irritation including food particles, plaque bacteria and calculus (or tartar).

The gums react to local irritants and swell. Since the cause of this swelling is due to local irritants, these must be removed by a dental professional. Afterwards, careful oral home care (including brushing and flossing) is necessary, or the swelling will return. If not treated, the bone and tissue surrounding, the teeth can be damaged.

As a young woman progresses through puberty, the tendency for her gums to swell so much in response to a small amount of irritants will lessen. However, it is important that she remember to brush and floss daily and seek regular professional dental care.

Menstruation

Gingivitis (red, swollen, tender or bleeding gums) can be much more prevalent during menstruation. Again, this is due to an increased amount of progesterone in your system before your period begins, accompanied by plaque accumulation.

Occasionally, some women experience sores or bleeding in the mouth three or four days before their period begins. Another rare occurrence for some women is gingivitis during menstruation, which is marked by reappearing gingival (gum) bleeding, a bright red swelling of the gums between the teeth and sores on the tongue and the inside of the cheek.

Menstruation gingivitis usually occurs right before a woman's period and clears up once her period has started. As always, good home oral hygiene, including brushing and flossing, is important to maintain oral health, especially during these hormonal fluctuations.

Pregnancy

There used to be an old wives' tale that said "A tooth lost for every child." While it may seem far-fetched, it actually was based loosely in fact. Your teeth and gums are affected by your pregnancy, just as other tissues in your body.

Most commonly, women experience increased gingivitis beginning in the second or third month that increases in severity through the eighth month and begins to decrease in the ninth month. This condition, called **pregnancy gingivitis** is marked by an increased amount of swelling, bleeding and redness in the gum tissue in response to a very small amount of plaque or calculus. This again is caused by an increased level of progesterone in the system.

If your gums are in good health before you get pregnant, you are less likely to have any problems. Pregnancy gingivitis usually affects areas of previous inflammation, not healthy gum tissue. If you experienced some swelling and bleeding of your gums before pregnancy, you might be at an increased risk for pregnancy gingivitis.

Just like any other type of gingivitis, if left untreated, pregnancy gingivitis can have damaging effects on the gums and bone surrounding your teeth, resulting in tissue (bone and gum) loss.

As there will be a great increase of estrogen and progesterone in your system throughout your pregnancy, you may experience more gingival problems at this time. Because your oral tissues are more sensitive due to increased progesterone, they will react strongly to any local irritant present.

In order to reduce gingival problems, it is important to seek a professional cleaning to remove irritants and keep up a diligent daily home oral care routine, including brushing and flossing. Now more than ever, regular examinations by your dentist are very important. If your dental checkup is due, don't skip it. In fact, you might benefit from more frequent professional cleanings during your second trimester or early third trimester. Remember, if tenderness, bleeding or gum swelling occurs at any time during your pregnancy, notify your dentist as soon as possible.

Occasionally, the inflamed gum tissue will form a large lump. These growths, called **pregnancy tumors**, usually appear by the third month of pregnancy, but may occur at any time during the course of pregnancy.

A pregnancy tumor is a large swelling of gum tissue and is not cancerous in any way. It is an extreme inflammatory response to any local irritation (including food particles, plaque or calculus) that may be present.

A pregnancy tumor usually looks like a large lump on the gum tissue with many deep red pin-point markings on it. The tumor is usually painless; however, it can become painful if it interferes with your bite or if debris collects beneath it.

If a pregnancy tumor forms, it may be treated by professional removal of all local irritants and diligent home oral care. Any further treatment or removal would need to be discussed with your dentist and your obstetrician.

Pregnancy gingivitis and pregnancy tumors usually diminish following pregnancy, but they do not go away completely. If you experience any gum problems during your pregnancy, it is important, upon completion of your pregnancy, to have your entire mouth examined and your periodontal health evaluated. Any treatment you might need can be determined at this time.

Oral Contraceptives

If you are taking any oral contraceptives (birth control pills), you may be susceptible to those same oral health conditions that affect pregnant women. As the hormones in oral contraceptives will increase the levels of progesterone in your system, any local irritants (food, plaque, etc.) may cause your gums to turn red, bleed and swell.

There are many medications {for example, antibiotics} that can lessen the effect of an oral contraceptive, so it is important for you to tell your dentist or physician you are taking oral contraceptives before he or she prescribes anything for you.

Menopause

For the most part, any oral problem you have while you are in menopause probably is not directly related to the changes going on in your body. If you are taking estrogen supplements during this time, these should have little to no effect on your oral health. However, progesterone supplements may increase your gums' response to local irritants, causing the gums to bleed, turn red and swell.

On rare occasions, a woman may experience a condition called **menopausal gingivostomatitis**. This condition is marked by gums that are dry and shiny, bleed easily and that range in color from abnormally pale to deep red.

Other symptoms include a dry, burning sensation in the mouth, abnormal taste sensations (especially salty, peppery or sour), extreme sensitivity to hot or cold foods or drinks, and finally, difficulty removing any partial bridges or dentures.

If you are diagnosed with menopausal gingivostomatitis, your dentist or periodontist can help you manage your condition with special medications.

Part Four

The Oral Cavity, Including the Tongue, Lips, and Throat

Chapter 26

Dry Mouth (Xerostomia)

Do you feel the need to moisten your mouth frequently? Does your mouth feel dry at mealtime? Do you have less saliva than you once did? Do you have difficulty swallowing? Do you have trouble eating dry foods such as crackers or toast?

If you answer "yes" to these questions, you may be one of the many people who suffer from dry mouth, or xerostomia (pronounced "zero-stoh'-me-a").

Although xerostomia is not a disease in itself, it is a symptom of certain diseases. Dry mouth also is a common side effect of some medications and medical treatments. Most cases of dry mouth are caused by failure of the salivary glands to function properly. But in some people, the sensation of a dry mouth occurs even though their salivary glands are normal.

Dry mouth is a significant health problem because it can affect nutrition and psychological well-being, while also contributing to tooth decay and other mouth infections. Dry mouth also may signal more serious problems in the body. If you have a dry mouth, you should be seen by a dentist or physician to determine the cause of the symptom.

Why Is Saliva Important?

Saliva has many important functions in the body. Each person needs adequate amounts of healthy saliva to:

NIH Publication No. 91-3174.

221

- Limit the growth of bacteria that cause tooth decay and other oral infections,
- Preserve teeth by bathing them with protective minerals that allow early cavities to remineralize and heal,
- Lubricate the soft tissues lining the mouth to keep them pliable and make speaking and chewing easier,
- Dissolve foods and allow us to experience their sweet, sour, salty, and bitter tastes,
- Assist digestion by providing enzymes that break down food,
- Lubricate food so it can be swallowed easily, and
- Cleanse the teeth and mouth of food particles.

What Causes Dry Mouth?

Changes in salivary gland function, such as dry mouth can be brought on by:

Medications. Over 400 commonly used drugs can cause the sensation of dry mouth. The main culprits are the antihypertensives (for high blood pressure) and anti-depressants. Both are prescribed for millions of Americans. Painkillers, tranquilizers, diuretics, and over-the-counter antihistamines can also decrease saliva.

Cancer treatment. Radiation therapy can permanently damage salivary glands if they are in the field of radiation. Chemotherapy can change the composition of saliva, creating a sensation of dry mouth.

Diseases. Sjögren's syndrome is an autoimmune disorder whose symptoms include dry mouth and dry eyes. Some Sjögren's patients also have a connective tissue disorder, most commonly rheumatoid arthritis or systemic lupus erythematosus.

Other Conditions. Bone marrow transplants, endocrine disorders, nutritional deficiencies, anxiety, mental stress, and depression can cause a dry mouth.

Dry mouth can also be due to changes not related to salivary glands, such as:

Nerve damage. Trauma to the head and neck area from surgery or wounds can damage the nerves that supply sensation to the mouth. While the salivary glands may be left intact, they cannot function normally without the nerves that signal them to produce saliva.

Altered perception. Conditions like Alzheimer's disease or stroke may change the ability to perceive oral sensations.

Does Aging Cause Dry Mouth?

Until recently dry mouth was regarded as a normal part of aging. Researchers now know that healthy older adults do not produce less saliva. When older people do experience dry mouth, it is because they suffer from diseases that cause the condition or they take medications that produce dry mouth as a side effect.

What Happens When You Have Dry Mouth?

Dry mouth caused by malfunctioning salivary glands is associated with changes in saliva. The flow of saliva can decrease, or the composition of saliva can change.

Patients with dry mouth have varying degrees of discomfort. Some people feel a dry or burning sensation in their mouths. A dry mouth may affect their ability to chew, taste, swallow, and speak. Changes in saliva also can affect oral and dental health. Severe cases of dry mouth can result in cracking of the lips, slits at the corners of the mouth, changes in the surface of the tongue, rampant tooth decay, ulceration of the mouth's linings, and infection.

Is Relief Available?

Although there is no single way to treat dry mouth, there are a number of steps you can follow to keep teeth in good health and relieve the sense of dryness. These suggestions will not correct the underlying cause of xerostomia, but may help you feel more comfortable.

To Preserve Your Teeth:

- Brush your teeth at least twice a day.
- Use dental floss daily.
- Use a toothpaste that contains fluoride. Ask your dentist about using a topical fluoride.
- Avoid sticky, sugary foods or brush immediately after eating them.
- See your dentist at least three times a year for cleanings and early treatment of cavities.
- Ask your dentist if you should use a remineralizing solution or prescription-strength fluoride.

To Relieve Dryness and Preserve the Soft Tissues:

- Take frequent sips of water or drinks without sugar. Pause often while speaking to sip some liquid. Avoid caffeine-containing coffee, tea, and soft drinks.

- Drink frequently while eating. This will make chewing and swallowing easier and may increase the taste of food.

- Keep a gloss of water by your bed for dryness during the night or upon awakening.

- Chew sugarless gum. The chewing may produce more saliva.

- Eat sugarless mints or hard sugarless candies, but let them dissolve in your mouth. Cinnamon and mint are often most effective.

- Place a small piece of lemon rind or a cherry pit in your mouth. The sucking action helps stimulate saliva.

- Avoid tobacco and alcohol.

- Avoid spicy, salty, and highly acidic foods that may irritate the mouth.

- Ask your dentist about using artificial salivas to help lubricate the mouth.

- Use a humidifier, particularly at night.

What Is Being Done about Dry Mouth?

At the National Institute of Dental Research (NIDR), one of the National Institutes of Health in Bethesda, MD, scientists study the causes of dry mouth and possible treatments for this condition. In 1983, they opened a Dry Mouth Clinic to evaluate, diagnose, and treat patients with salivary gland dysfunction.

Researchers at the NIDR Dry Mouth Clinic have developed better methods of diagnosing salivary gland dysfunction. A complete evaluation of a patient with dry mouth includes measurement of both "stimulated" salivary flow— found when a person actively chews, sips, or tastes sour substances—and "unstimulated" flow—found when a person is at rest or sleeping. Researchers also analyze saliva composition and look at other aspects of saliva secretion to distinguish between salivary gland dysfunction and other causes of dry mouth.

The investigators are now testing a drug (pilocarpine) to treat dry mouth in patients with minimally functioning salivary glands. Their studies show that pilocarpine can stimulate saliva production and relieve a patient's sense of oral dryness without causing untoward side effects. The increased output of saliva might also help prevent tooth decay, ulcerations, and infections. Further studies are needed, however, before the drug will be available to the public. NIDR investigators are also looking into other possible treatments for dry mouth. Several research studies focus on the cause of Sjögren's syndrome and treatment for the dry mouth associated with this condition.

Patient Volunteers

The NIDR Dry Mouth Clinic seeks patients with dry mouth caused by head and neck radiation therapy and Sjögren's syndrome. A number of research studies are underway to examine the causes of salivary dysfunction in these patients, the long-term consequences of salivary changes, and new methods of treatment.

For further information about the NIDR Dry Mouth Clinic, write to:

Dr. Philip C. Fox
The Dry Mouth Clinic
National Institute of Dental Research
Building 10, Room 1N-113
National Institutes of Health
Bethesda, MD 20892

As many as two million Americans may suffer from Sjögren's syndrome. Two voluntary organizations have chapters in major cities around the country that offer support for these patients.

For further information, contact:

Sjögren's Syndrome Foundation, Inc.
382 Main Street
Port Washington, NY 11050

National Sjögren's Syndrome Association
3201 West Evans Drive
Phoenix, Arizona 85023

Questions and Answers about Dry Mouth

Reprinted from September 1993 *Mayo Clinic Health Letter* with permission from Mayo Foundation for Medical Education and Research, Rochester, Minnesota 55905. For subscription information, call 1-800-333-9038.

Our son has "dry mouth" from the lithium he takes for manic depression. Since starting the drug, he's had thousands of dollars worth of dental bills. What can we do?

When saliva is lacking, which is a common side-effect of lithium, tooth decay often results. The first line of defense against cavities is meticulous flossing and brushing with a fluoride toothpaste. Fluoride mouth rinses can help, too. Your dentist also can make a fluoride carrier—similar to an athletic mouth guard—for your son's upper and lower teeth. Fill the carriers with fluoride twice a day and fit them over the teeth for three to five minutes. That should help protect your son's teeth from decay. To make a dry mouth moist and more comfortable, ask your dentist about saliva substitutes. Chewing gum or sucking on hard candy sometimes can stimulate saliva, too. But make sure it's sugarless. Sugar accelerates tooth decay. Finally, ask your doctor whether your son can tolerate a lower dose of lithium.

Chapter 27

Sjögren's Syndrome: Making a Desert of the Body

Good advice from singer Johnny Ray in his old hit song "Cry." But what if you can't cry—physically can't produce tears? This is what happens to some people who have severe Sjögren's syndrome.

Sjögren's syndrome, a surprisingly common, though often undiagnosed or misdiagnosed disorder, robs the body of moisture essential to the smooth functioning of most organs. Named for Henrick Sjögren (pronounced show-gren), a Swedish ophthalmologist, who first described the condition in 1933, the syndrome is marked by dry eyes, dry mouth, and often a connective tissue disease, such as rheumatoid arthritis or systemic lupus erythematosus.

Primary Sjögren's, or "sicca complex," as it is also called, affects about half of all Sjögren's patients and is characterized by dry eyes or dry mouth alone. When associated with a connective tissue disease, the syndrome is called secondary Sjögren's.

As many as two million people in this country may suffer from Sjögren's syndrome. Although men and women of any age can develop Sjögren's, women, mostly middle aged, outnumber men nine to one.

Sjögren's syndrome is an autoimmune disease. That is, the body's immune system has turned traitor, attacking instead of protecting the body. Lymphocytes, white blood cells that normally fight infection, infiltrate the tissues and attack normal structures.

In Sjögren's syndrome, the moisture-producing glands, such as the lacrimal (tear) and salivary glands and glands in the vaginal area, are destroyed by the invading lymphocytes. The skin, respiratory and

FDA Consumer, February 1989.

gastrointestinal tracts, sweat glands, liver, kidneys, lungs, and thyroid glands may also be affected.

What triggers these events is unknown, but a widely held theory is that the culprit is a virus. Heredity may play a role, but some other factors are necessary for a person to develop Sjögren's.

The onset of Sjögren's syndrome is gradual, beginning when the patient is between 40 and 60. In its early stages it is difficult to diagnose, and many patients go from doctor to doctor before the problem is recognized. A constant and depressing symptom that plagues most patients is an overwhelming fatigue and feeling of malaise. As the disease progresses, the symptoms may come and go, or they may remain stable or get worse.

"I look healthy, but I don't feel it as I pull myself out of bed in the morning, stiff and sore, eyes burning and feeling gritty, my mouth so dry I can't swallow, and my nose dry and crusty," says one patient.

Primary Sjögren's is usually the more severe form of the syndrome. The chance that a patient with primary Sjögren's will later develop a connective tissue disease is slim. The reverse is more likely: About 30 percent of people with rheumatoid arthritis develop secondary Sjögren's.

Sjögren's syndrome is "life altering" rather than "life threatening." However, lack of treatment or improper treatment of dry eyes can lead to blindness. Some Sjögren's patients develop lymphoma, cancer of the lymph glands, although this is unusual.

While there is no cure for Sjögren's syndrome, relief for its major symptoms is available.

Dry Eyes

The symptoms of dry eye—or keratoconjunctivitis sicca— include dryness, itching, and a gritty feeling, as if there were something in the eye. There may be eye pain, fatigue, redness, and light sensitivity. The lids may become inflamed. In severe cases, cells from the eye surface mix with mucus to form painful sticky threads, or filaments, on the eye. Eventually, most patients lose the ability to produce tears. They can still feel emotions, but they can't cry. Low humidity in air-conditioned buildings or a windy or dry climate can aggravate symptoms. (Where the humidity is high, patients may not even be aware they have the disorder.)

Diagnosing Sjögren's syndrome is sometimes difficult because dry eyes can be associated with other medical conditions such as an eye infection or vitamin A deficiency, and from use of some common medications, including decongestants, antihistamines, some tranquilizers, antidepressants, and heart and blood pressure medicines.

The mainstay of treatment for most dry eyes is artificial tears, which help lubricate the eye and prevent infection. Artificial tears must be used regularly, as directed by the doctor, not just when there is a feeling of dryness or grittiness. Available without prescription under a variety of trade names (Clerz, Lyteers, Lacril, Tearisol, Tears Plus, Hypotears), these products contain such ingredients as cellulose derivatives, dextran, polyethylene glycol, and polyvinyl alcohol.

In March 1988, the Food and Drug Administration published a standard for over-the-counter ophthalmic drug products, identifying 13 ingredients considered safe and effective for relieving dry eyes. The agency's conclusions, based on recommendations by an advisory panel of experts, are part of FDA's ongoing review of all over-the-counter drugs.

Artificial tears may differ in their viscosity (resistance to flow), their ability to stay in the eye, and in the preservatives used to prevent bacterial contamination. The thicker and longer-lasting drops can be applied less often, but may cause some blurring of vision and leave a residue on the eyelashes.

The preservatives in artificial tears may cause allergic reactions and actually aggravate dry eye in some people. Artificial tears without preservatives are also available over the counter. Two products— Relief and Refresh—come in single-dose form. A third, Unisol, does not and must be discarded after 24 hours.

Another form of relief for dry eyes is the prescription drug Lacrisert, a small pellet about the size of a grain of rice, which contains a reservoir of lubricating material. Placed between the lower eyelid and the eyeball, the pellet releases the lubricant for 6 to 12 hours. Vision may blur, and artificial tears may still be needed occasionally.

Lubrication ointments can be used in severe cases of dry eyes, but they cause significant blurring of vision. Bedtime is a good time to use such ointments. Ten ingredients were listed as safe and effective as eye lubricants in FDA's standard.

Certain drugs called mucolytics help get rid of excessive mucus that often troubles dry eye patients.

Although dry eye victims usually cannot tolerate contact lenses, in some cases a low-water-content soft lens is used as a bandage, preventing evaporation of the tear film between the lens and the eye. Artificial tears still must be used, however.

If these measures don't help, the tiny canals at the inner corner of the eyelids, which drain excess moisture from the eyes, can be temporarily or permanently blocked. This procedure, called punctal occlusion, helps keep any natural or artificial tears in the eye for a longer time.

Wearing watertight swimming goggles, wrap-around sun glasses, or special shielding on regular glasses can help reduce moisture loss and protect the eyes from the elements. Room humidifiers are also beneficial. Car vents and fans should be turned away from the patient's face.

Dry Mouth

Dry mouth, or xerostomia, is sometimes the first symptom of Sjögren's. It is caused by a lack of saliva normally produced by three major glands on each side of the face and carried via ducts to the mouth. Any or all of these glands and ducts may be involved in Sjögren's syndrome.

Saliva protects the teeth from cavity-causing bacteria, provides minerals that keep teeth hard and enzymes that aid digestion, and moistens food so that it can be swallowed. Dry mouth victims often find it difficult to chew and swallow and even to talk. Food sticks to the teeth and the inside of the mouth. There also may be a burning sensation in the mouth and throat. The voice may become hoarse and weak. Cracks develop on the tongue and lips, particularly at the corners of the mouth.

There may be persistent swelling of the salivary glands in front of the ears and under the jaw, resembling a case of the mumps. The senses of smell and taste may also diminish.

Lack of saliva can lead to dental problems, including rampant cavities and swollen gums, often resulting in tooth loss. Wearing dentures may become difficult. Candida (yeast) infections are frequent in patients with dry mouths.

Again, Sjögren's is not the only cause of dry mouth. It can be a side effect of well over 300 drugs, including antihistamines, anti-inflammatories and diuretics, and of chemotherapy, bone marrow transplantation, and radiation treatment to the head and neck. It can accompany anemia, diabetes, stress, depression, and other conditions.

Dry mouth patients are advised to drink a lot of water—particularly when eating—and to avoid dry foods, spices, alcohol and tobacco. Chewing sugarless gum or sucking on sugarless hard candy helps stimulate the production of saliva. (To further help prevent cavities, Sjögren's patients should avoid highly sugared foods such as candy and gum, breath mints, cough drops, and beverages with sugar.) Foods

230

cut into small pieces and moistened with sauces and gravies are easier to swallow.

Artificial salivas in spray form are available over the counter to help moisten the mouth. They contain ingredients such as potassium phosphate, magnesium, calcium and sodium, or sodium carboxymethyl cellulose.

Last July, FDA approved the Salitron System, a medical device that can stimulate saliva production from the glands.

Good dental hygiene is essential for the dry mouth victim, who must brush and floss more often than others. Use of a "Water-Pik" also helps keep teeth clean. At least three visits a year to the dentist are a must. Fluoride treatment and oral remineralizing solutions can replace minerals normally provided by saliva.

Connective Tissue Diseases

The major symptoms of the connective tissue diseases associated with Sjögren's include joint pain, primarily in the fingers, wrists and knees; joint swelling and stiffness, especially in the morning; pain and color change in the fingertips or toes in low temperatures; and a distinctive rash on the face.

Secondary Sjögren's usually develops after the patient has had a connective tissue disease for many months or years. Because the symptoms are less severe that those of primary Sjögren's, the disease may even go unnoticed by a patient with severe arthritis. Early diagnosis is important, however, since delaying treatment can result in complications.

Treatment of the underlying arthritic disease is the same, regardless of whether the patient also has dry eye or dry mouth symptoms. In the case of rheumatoid arthritis, drugs such as aspirin, fenoprofen, ibuprofen, indomethacin, sulindac, or gold compounds may be prescribed. Care must be taken, however, since some arthritis medications, such as the gold compounds and penicillamine, can cause dry eyes.

Other Sjögren's Symptoms

Nasal dryness and symptoms of sinusitis, the result of the decreased functioning of the moisture-producing glands in the nose and mouth, can be treated with saline sprays (such as Ocean, Solinex, Ayr) and humidifiers at night. Nasal irrigation (washing out the nose) with normal saline often proves helpful, as well.

Dry skin and lips can be soothed with creams and lotions, which are best applied after a shower or bath while the skin is still moist.

Antifungal creams are useful in healing cracking at the angles of the cheek due to Candida infection.

Vaginal dryness, which can cause intercourse to be painful, can be reduced with K-Y jelly, Surgilube, or other sterile lubricants.

Antidepressant drugs are sometimes used to help regulate sleep patterns and treat fatigue. Care must be taken to use products that do not have a drying side effect.

In general, a balanced program of rest and mild exercise can help the Sjögren's patient. It is important for patients to pace their daily activities to avoid fatigue. When symptoms flare up, more rest may be needed. Whenever possible, sources of irritation—such as extremely cold or dry climates and exposure to wind, smoke and hot air—should be avoided.

To cover all the bases, Sjögren's patients should be under the medical supervision of several physicians: an ophthalmologist for eye care, a dentist for mouth care, and, for those with a connective tissue disease, a rheumatologist.

Research

Research into Sjögren's syndrome is under way in the United States and abroad on several fronts. Since 1983 the Dry Mouth Clinic of the National Institute of Dental Research in Bethesda, MD., has been screening dry mouth patients to determine how their Sjögren's began. Bromhexine, a cough medicine ingredient, is being tested for its ability to increase salivary and tear gland function. Other experiments include using the patient's own blood serum to create artificial tears, and a recently completed study suggests that pilocarpine, a drug used to treat glaucoma, can stimulate saliva production.

While there is still no cure for Sjögren's syndrome, today's research holds hope that those who suffer from this moisture-robbing condition can at least find some relief.

Support for Sjögren's Victims

Sjögren's is sometimes called "the lonely disease" because so little seems to be known about it.

Although Sjögren's syndrome was recognized more than 50 years ago, it was not until 1983 that a self-help group for victims of this disease was organized, thanks to the efforts of Elaine Harris, a Great Neck, NY, housewife who suffers from the syndrome.

Frustrated by the lack of information to help her cope with this baffling disease, Harris decided to do something on her own. With the cooperation of her doctors at the Long Island (N.Y.) Jewish Medical Center and the Arthritis Foundation of New York, the first meeting of the fledgling group was held in December 1983, attended by 14 patients and 11 family members. They called themselves "The Moisture Seekers."

The organization was incorporated in the summer of 1985 as the Sjögren's Syndrome Foundation, Inc., and now has 59 contact persons in 29 states and the District of Columbia. Twenty-four groups hold regular meetings in which they hear talks by medical experts and share experiences. In addition, chapters have been started in Canada, England, Japan and Holland. Membership has reached 2,500 and is growing.

The purpose of the foundation, according to Harris, its founder and president, is to educate patients, families, the public, and health professionals on Sjögren's syndrome. This is done through chapter meetings, a newsletter (The Moisture Seekers), an annual symposium held in the New York area, and exhibits at medical meetings. Another service is a telephone "hot line" to provide instant information for those who suffer from Sjögren's.

The *Sjögren's Syndrome Handbook*, a booklet for laymen published by the foundation, includes tips from patients on how to cope.

For further information, write the

Sjögren's Syndrome Foundation
29 Gateway Drive
Great Neck, N.Y. 11021
(516) 487-2243

—by Annabel Hecht

Annabel Hecht is a free-lance writer in Silver Spring, MD, specializing in health reporting.

Chapter 28

Salivary Electrostimulation in Sjögren's Syndrome

Introduction: What Is Sjögren's Syndrome?

Sjögren's syndrome is a chronic inflammatory and autoimmune disease in which the salivary and lacrimal glands undergo progressive destruction by lymphocytes and plasma cells resulting in decreased production of tears and saliva. Sjögren's syndrome is seen predominantly in middle-aged and elderly women. Females are involved 10 times more commonly than males. Secondary effects of xerostomia include impairment in the normal movement of lips and tongue, thereby hampering speech, mastication, and swallowing. Additional signs include oral soreness, adherence of food to buccal surfaces, fissuring of the tongue, an altered sense of taste, and a marked increase in dental caries and infection. Soreness and redness of the mucosa are usually the result of candidal infection, which is found in approximately 70 percent of the Sjögren's syndrome patients.

Complaints resulting from dryness of the mouth are varied and often describe the difficulties encountered in trying to eat dry foods without sufficient lubrication. Many subjects require frequent ingestion of liquids. They may resort to carrying water bottles or hard candy.

The parotid gland enlarges in many patients secondary to cellular infiltration and ductal obstruction. Usually asymptomatic and self-limited, the enlargement can be recurrent and associated with pain or erythema. Focal infiltrates of lymphocytes are also found in the minor salivary glands of the lower lip. Biopsy provides histologic confirmation and quantification of the degree of infiltration.

Extracted from: DHHS Publication No. AHCPR 91-0009.

Xerostomia Associated with Sjögren's Syndrome

Xerostomia may be the result of Sjögren's syndrome, other diseases, medications, or radiation therapy to the head and neck. To determine that the xerostomia has resulted from Sjögren's syndrome, clinicians also confirm the presence of keratoconjunctivitis sicca (dry eye) and a positive lip biopsy with or without the presence of a connective tissue disease. It is estimated that more than one million people, mostly women, suffer from Sjögren's syndrome in the United States.

Xerostomia is usually defined as a symptom that exists when saliva production is less than 0.1 ml/min (or 0.1 g/min). However, the symptom of xerostomia has been reported to appear when normal salivary output declines by approximately 50 percent, regardless of the starting value. Normal saliva production has been estimated to be 600 ml/24h. Patients with chronic xerostomia complain of a continual feeling of oral dryness and find it difficult to eat dry foods. In addition to the subjective complaints, the patient with salivary gland dysfunction is susceptible to increased dental caries, oral pain, frequent infections, and difficulties in speaking, chewing, and swallowing. The biopsy of the salivary glands, usually obtained from the lower lip, is used to differentiate true Sjögren's syndrome from other forms of salivary gland dysfunction.

Confirming Sjögren's Syndrome

The symptoms of dry eyes and dry mouth in the absence of any drug treatment or other disorder likely to be causal suggest a diagnosis of Sjögren's syndrome. According to Talal in the *Cecil Textbook of Medicine* (1985), the diagnosis of Sjögren's syndrome is based upon the confirmed presence of two of the following three criteria:

- a focus score of more than one (1) in the labial salivary gland (lip) biopsy,
- dry eye (keratoconjunctivitis sicca), and
- an associated connective tissue or lymphoproliferative disorder.

The triad of dry eyes, dry mouth, and a connective tissue or collagen disease, usually rheumatoid arthritis, is termed secondary Sjögren's syndrome. Dry eyes and dry mouth in the absence of a collagen disease is referred to as primary Sjögren's syndrome. The use of diuretics, antihypertensive drugs, antihistamines, antipsychotics, and antidepressants may diminish lacrimal and salivary gland function. Because the use of anticholinergic drugs as well as a number of other medications may be the single most frequent cause of xerostomia, it is essential to establish the presence of focal lymphoid infiltrates and autoimmunity in a patient suspected of having Sjögren's syndrome. Supportive serologic data would include the presence of antinuclear antibodies, an elevated erythrocyte sedimentation rate, and the presence of anti-SS-A and anti-SS-B antibodies.

The lip biopsy is a sensitive and specific diagnostic procedure for Sjögren's syndrome. It is well tolerated and causes no disfigurement. The changes in the minor glands of the lower lip show a close correlation with those in the major salivary glands. In addition to confirming the diagnosis, biopsy allows quantification of the degree of lymphocytic infiltration and tissue damage. Aggregates of lymphocytes within the acinar tissue are scored. An aggregate of 50 or more cells represents a focus. The number of foci within 4 mm^2 of glandular tissue is determined and constitutes the focus score. A focus score of more than one (1) is characteristic of Sjögren's syndrome.

Treatment Using Electrostimulation

Electrostimulation has been introduced as a technique for increasing salivary output in the treatment of patients with xerostomia (dry mouth) secondary to Sjögren's syndrome. The procedure uses an electrostimulation device (salivation electrostimulator) to increase salivary production from existing glandular tissue. The device delivers a small electrical stimulus to the mouth via a probe. The electrostimulation device consists of an electric control module, a connecting cord, and a hand-held stimulus probe with two metal electrodes. The device may be battery-powered. Patients with residual salivary tissue in the oral and pharyngeal regions who demonstrate a decrease in the flow rate of saliva are potential candidates for this procedure.

By application of the concept of electrically stimulating nerves to elicit a response, electrostimulation was developed for use in the oral cavity to stimulate the salivary reflex. Investigators have reported that electrostimulation increases salivary output and should be used to treat patients with xerostomia secondary to Sjögren's syndrome. The cost of a battery-operated, hand-held stimulus probe that can provide electrical stimulation to the tongue and hard palate is approximately $1,500.

Proponents of electrostimulation as a method to increase salivary production suggest that this procedure enhances the patient's ability to generate saliva by augmenting normal physiologic salivary reflexes. Salivary secretion is normally controlled by reflex stimulation with effector nerve impulses traveling along sympathetic as well as parasympathetic nerves to the glands. Sympathetic nerve stimulation produces a sparse viscous secretion, whereas the parasympathetic nerve stimulation produces a voluminous watery secretion. The dual secretion (saliva) is a fluid mixture produced from paired major salivary glands (parotid, submandibular, and sublingual) and many smaller aggregations of minor salivary glands imbedded in the submucosa of the cheeks, lips, hard and soft palates, and tongue.

Proponents believe that xerostomia secondary to Sjögren's syndrome can be caused by interruption of the stimulus that elicits salivation at the effector site; such interruption results from loss of glandular tissue with replacement by round cell infiltration, scar, or fatty tissue. They postulate that an electronic device that touches the tongue and roof of the mouth simultaneously will stimulate tactile receptors, taste receptors, and intrinsic muscle mechanoreceptors within the mucosa of the dorsum of the tongue and the roof of the mouth. This produces electrical stimulation to the oral and pharyngeal afferent nervous system resulting in a reflex volley of efferent impulses to all residual salivary tissue, major and minor, in the oral and pharyngeal regions causing salivation.

Conclusion

Electrostimulation has been introduced as a technique for increasing salivary output in the treatment of patients with xerostomia (dry mouth) secondary to Sjögren's syndrome. The procedure uses an electrostimulation device (salivation electrostimulator) to increase salivary production from existing glandular tissue. The device delivers a low-voltage electrical stimulus to the mouth via a probe. Patients with residual salivary tissue in the oral and pharyngeal regions who demonstrate a decrease in the flow rate of saliva are potential candidates for this procedure.

It is estimated that more than one million people in the United States, predominantly middle-aged and elderly women, suffer from Sjögren's syndrome. Patients with chronic xerostomia complain of a continual feeling of oral dryness and have difficulty eating dry foods. These patients are susceptible to increased caries, oral pain, infection, and have difficulty speaking, chewing, and swallowing.

The approach to the treatment of xerostomia in Sjögren's patients is usually determined by the level of severity of the symptoms. Appropriate management of patients with xerostomia requires that those patients whose salivary flow can be increased by means of sialagogues be distinguished from those patients whose salivary flow is either unaffected or insufficiently stimulated. To alleviate some of the complications due to salivary dysfunction in those patients who respond to stimuli, pharmacologic sialagogues as well as sialagogues that include sugarless gums, mints and candies are prescribed in order to increase salivary flow.

Recently, electrostimulation via a hand-held stimulus probe has been introduced as a method of treatment in xerostomia secondary to Sjögren's syndrome. From the single published study as well as data provided to the FDA, it appears that an electrical stimulus applied to the tongue and hard palate (by a battery-operated device) may be useful in the management of salivary hypofunction in certain patients. It appears, however, that there are insufficient data at the present time to determine the clinical utility of electrostimulation, to evaluate the long-term clinical effectiveness of this modality of salivary production, or to identify those xerostomic patients who would benefit from this procedure. Also, electrostimulation is not widely accepted as an effective method of treatment for xerostomia secondary to Sjögren's syndrome. The number of published studies is limited and other less expensive treatments are available. Further research of electrical stimulation of salivary flow is required to determine its role in the treatment of Sjögren's patients with xerostomia.

—by Martin Erlichman

Chapter 29

Oral Health in Scleroderma

From early childhood we have been told how important it is to maintain good habits of cleansing and caring for the teeth.

Not so easy, if one is a scleroderma patient. While these habits become even more important and very necessary to oral health, the disease can make the effort very difficult and discouraging.

Scleroderma literally means "Hard Skin" and may affect hands, fingers, face, and other body parts including the internal organs. It is a chronic disease of unknown cause and with no known cure. It can vary in patients from a mild skin disorder, to a serious, sometimes life-threatening illness.

Persons with scleroderma may have to deal with many varied symptoms. Because the skin tightens, the mouth can develop strictures resulting in a condition called small mouth (MICROSTOMIA). Opening and closing the mouth may be painful or difficult. If the salivary glands become affected, and decrease or discontinue the production of saliva, the mouth may become very dry (XEROSTOMIA). Difficulty in swallowing is increased. The gums may become sore and tender and gum disease (PYORRHEA) is not uncommon. To encourage the production of saliva, fluids and sugar-free candy or gum may be used. Lemon-glycerol swabs applied to gums, tongue and all around in the mouth can combat dryness. With advanced disease there may be a loss of taste or inability to determine the position of food in the mouth.

Hand involvement can add to the problems of maintaining proper oral hygiene. As the skin tightens, fingers can become flexed and ulcerations may appear making it hard to grasp a toothbrush or other oral health aids.

Many scleroderma patients have difficulty chewing. It is important to eat slowly and chew the food well. Intake of fluids can be increased at mealtime to aid swallowing. Particles of food may be left around the teeth, and this increases the need for cleansing the teeth and mouth after every meal. A suggested alternative if unable to floss or brush, is to take a mouth full of water and quietly "swish and swallow."

Almost all scleroderma patients are plagued by dental problems, and sometimes the thought of the discomfort and pain seems a good cause for neglect. Many patients avoid seeing the dentist in the belief that he/she will not understand. Every effort must be made to retain your own teeth. Not only is there great discomfort in having teeth pulled, but false teeth can be very unsatisfactory for scleroderma patients. Tell your dentist about scleroderma and the USF and give him/her the following references:

- Naylor, W. Patrick, D.D.S., M.P.H.: "Oral Management of the Scleroderma Patient." *Journal of American Dental Association.* Vol. 105 (5), pages 814-817, Nov., 1982.

- Melvin, Jeanne L. MSEd, *OTR: Rheumatic Disease-Occupational Therapy and Rehabilitation*, 2nd Edition, F.A. Davis Co., Philadelphia, PA, pages 52-54, 1982.

- Naylor, W. Patrick, D.D.S., M.P.H., R.C. Manor, M.A. "Fabrication of Flexible Prosthesis for the Endentulous Scleroderma Patient with Microstomia." *Journal of Prosthetic Dentistry*, Vol. 50 (4), pages 536-538. October, 1983.

Frequent dental checkups are necessary to insure proper cleansing and to control dental problems before loss of teeth occurs. Patients with gum disease or oral hygiene problems should seek a periodontist (a specialist in the diagnosis and treatment of such problems who is familiar with a wide variety of oral health aids).

Patients should use a soft toothbrush and a gentle motion on teeth and gums. Homecare can start with a visit to an occupational therapist (ask your physician for a referral). The therapist can build up the handle of your toothbrush making it easier to hold. It is wise to have several brushes done at the same time so you will have one whenever it is needed. Electric toothbrush handles can also be made more comfortable.

Cleansing the teeth by flossing is equally as important as brushing, but may be extremely difficult for some scleroderma patients. There are flossing aids available. Ask your dentist to show you the proper way to brush and floss. Fluoride mouth rinses are also beneficial.

It has been recognized that exercise of the mouth and jaws is helpful in combating the small mouth problem. W. Patrick Naylor, D.D.S., M.P.H., who was Project Director of a "small mouth" study undertaken at the Harvard School of Dental Medicine states: "Exercise is a valuable tool when properly applied, used regularly, and above all, monitored carefully by a health professional to assess its effectiveness." To learn facial exercises, ask your physician for a referral to a physical therapist knowledgeable in scleroderma or ask your dentist to offer some exercises or to supervise you in doing the exercises described in Dr. Naylor's articles.

Checklist for Oral Health

- Sugary, sticky, and highly refined carbohydrate foods should be avoided.

- Cleanse mouth and teeth after meals.

- Lubricant for dry lips may be helpful.

- Everyday regular brushing is a must.

- Regular toothpaste may bother your mouth, if so ask dentist to recommend another cleanser.

- Over-the-counter fluoride mouthwash such as "Florigard" or "Act" should he used.

- Dry mouth a problem, inform your physician and dentist.

- Exercises for the face should be learned and performed daily.

- Regular toothbrushes can be made to fit your hand.

- Mouth flossing aids are available if you have a problem flossing conventionally.

- All food must be chewed thoroughly.

Chapter 30

What You Need to Know about Oral Cancer

This chapter summarizes current knowledge of the incidence and mortality, causes and risk factors, prevention, detection and diagnosis, and treatment of cancers of the oral cavity (mouth) and the oropharynx, the part of the pharynx (upper throat) directly behind the oral cavity. Together, cancers of the oral cavity and oropharynx may be referred to as "oral cancers."

Description and Function of the Oral Cavity and Oropharynx

The oral cavity includes the lips, the buccal mucosa (the mucous membrane lining the inside of the cheeks and lips), the gums (gingivae), the retromolar trigone (the area between the teeth and the jaw), the hard palate, the floor of the mouth, and the oral tongue (the mobile, anterior two-thirds of the tongue). The oropharynx consists of the base of the tongue (posterior tongue), the soft palate, the tonsils, and the posterior wall of the throat (oropharyngeal wall).

The lips are covered on the outside by skin and on the inside by the buccal mucosa. Their color comes from blood vessels that show through the thin layer of cells covering the vermilion, located between the surface of the lips and the buccal mucosa. The orbicularis oris muscle allows the lips to close and protrude. The inside of each lip attaches to the gum. The gums end in the retromolar trigone.

NIH Publication No. 92-2876.

Structures of the Oral Cavity

The cheeks form the sides of the oral cavity. At the front of the roof of the mouth is the hard palate, composed of the **maxilla** (upper jaw) and palatine bones. The hard palate separates the mouth from the nasal cavity. The U-shaped floor of the mouth is formed by the **mandible**, the lower, movable part of the jaw.

Extending across the floor of the mouth is the muscular tongue, which is attached by muscles to the mandible. Taste buds, located on the upper surface and sides of the tongue, transmit stimuli to the brain that are interpreted as bitter, sour, salty, or sweet. The tongue aids in swallowing by shaping food into a mass and then pushing it back into the throat. In addition, the tongue forms many of the consonant sounds of speech by pressing against the palate.

Located at the back of the oral cavity, the **oropharynx** is a passageway for both air and food. The base of the tongue, which is not easily seen, extends back to the **epiglottis**, a flap of tissue that covers the air passage to the lungs and that channels food to the esophagus. The soft palate, an arch-shaped muscular structure in the rear roof of the mouth, and its fleshy, V-shaped extension, the **uvula**, separate the oropharynx and oral cavity from the **nasopharynx** (the part

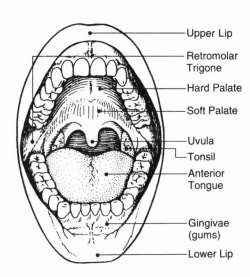

Figure 30.1. *Structures of the Oral Cavity.*

of the pharynx lying behind the nasal cavity). In swallowing, the rear edge of the soft palate swings up against the oropharyngeal wall and blocks the passage to the nose, thus preventing food from entering the nasal cavity. The uvula hangs above the base of the tongue and modifies certain speech sounds. On each side of the entrance to the oropharynx are the almond-shaped tonsils. Their function is believed to be the production of antibodies that help fight infection in the respiratory and digestive systems.

The major **salivary glands** are located within the cheeks and in the floor of the mouth adjacent to the mandible. Throughout the oral cavity and oropharynx, except in the gums and the front portion of the hard palate, are many nests of minor salivary glands. These glands secrete saliva, which moistens the mouth, lubricates food for easier swallowing, and contains an **enzyme** (an **amylase** called ptyalin) necessary for digestion to begin. Saliva also helps to prevent tooth decay by cleaning the teeth and gums of foreign material.

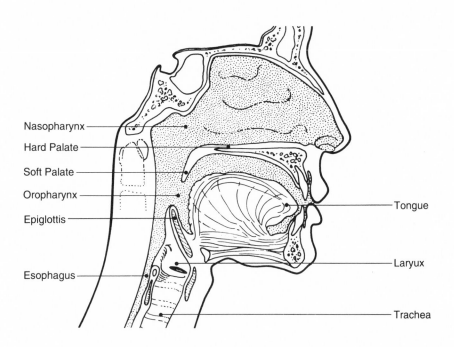

Figure 30.2. *Cross section of upper respiratory and digestive tracts.*

Types of Oral Cancer

All of the oral structures, like other organs of the body, are composed of individual cells. Normally, these cells divide and reproduce in an orderly way to repair worn-out or injured tissues and to allow for cell growth.

Sometimes, though, cell division becomes uncontrolled, leading to an overgrowth of tissue known as a tumor. Tumors can be either benign (noncancerous) or malignant (cancerous). Benign tumors do not invade neighboring tissue, do not spread to other parts of the body, and are seldom a threat to life; however, they may compress adjacent structures and may interfere with body functions. Benign tumors can usually be removed with surgery and are not likely to return.

In contrast, malignant tumors not only compress but also invade and destroy nearby tissues and structures. Moreover, cancer cells can break away from the primary (original) tumor in the oral cavity or oropharynx and metastasize (spread) through the blood and lymphatic

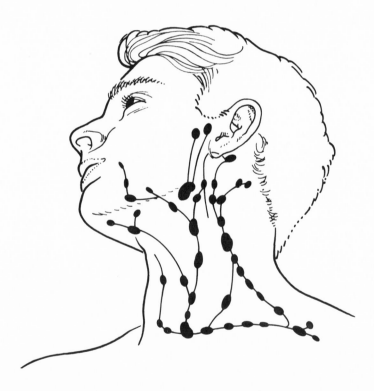

Figure 30.3. Lymph nodes of head and neck.

system to other parts of the body, where they can form metastatic (secondary) tumors.

When oral cancer metastasizes, it most commonly travels through the lymphatic system to the lymph nodes in the neck, also known as the **cervical lymph nodes**. Between 150 and 350 lymph nodes can be found in the head and neck above the collarbone, which is nearly one-third of the total number of lymph nodes in the body. Usually, cervical lymph node metastasis begins high in the neck and progresses to the lower neck just above the collarbone. In general, the risk of spread to the cervical lymph nodes is higher for oropharyngeal tumors than for oral cavity tumors.

Most oral cancers remain confined to the original site or to the cervical lymph nodes for a long time. Approximately 7 percent of oral cavity cancers and 15 percent of oropharyngeal cancers spread to distant parts of the body, most often to the lungs, liver, and bones. Although other organs are affected in both cervical lymph node and distant metastases, the secondary tumors retain many of the characteristics of the original oral cancer. These secondary tumors are known as metastatic oral cancer (rather than lung, liver, or bone cancer) to indicate that they are all part of a single disease and are not new cancers originating in these other organs.

Almost all oral cancers are squamous cell carcinomas, cancers that arise from the tiny, flat cells found in the outermost layer of the skin (the epidermis) and in the lining of the oral cavity and oropharynx. (Carcinoma is cancer that starts in tissue that forms the lining or covering of an organ.) Basal cell carcinomas (cancers that develop in the deepest part of the epidermis) can begin on the skin of the lip and can invade the vermilion. Although rare, melanoma (cancer that affects cells that produce skin pigment) can develop on the gums, the hard palate, the buccal mucosa, and the lip.

Cancer can develop in any part of the oral cavity or oropharynx. The most common sites are the lips, the oral tongue, and the floor of the mouth. Cancers of the hard palate are uncommon in the United States.

Cancers of the oropharyngeal wall are not covered in this chapter. These tumors are similar to those of the **hypopharynx**, the part of the pharynx adjacent to the **larynx** and continuous with the **esophagus**.

Incidence and Mortality

Oral cancer represents about 3 percent of all cancers in this country; in 1991, an estimated 30,800 new cases of and 8,150 deaths from oral cancer occurred in the United States. Oral cancer accounts for about 4 percent of cancers in men and about 2 percent of cancers in women. The disease occurs more frequently in black than in white people, which may be due, in part, to a higher rate of smoking and alcohol use among black people.

Like most cancers, oral cancer is primarily a disease that occurs later in life. However, factors to which we are exposed during adolescence and as young adults largely predict who will develop oral cancer. The incidence increases steadily until about age 65, when the annual rate levels off at about 50 cases per 100,000 population. However, increasing numbers of oral cancers are being diagnosed in younger persons. (See "Causes and Risk Factors.")

The incidence of oral cancer varies widely throughout the world. In Western countries, oral cancers account for 2 to 6 percent of all cancers. For example, in England and Wales, only about 2 percent of all cancers develop in the oral cavity and oropharynx. In contrast, the figure is nearly 50 percent in some parts of India, where many people chew a mixture of tobacco and other substances such as areca nut, catechu, betel nut or leaf, lime, and flavoring agents. Immigrants to the United States have oral cancer rates similar to those in their native countries. However, succeeding generations develop oral cancers at the same rate as other Americans.

Causes and Risk Factors

The primary causes of oral cancer are tobacco and alcohol. Nutritional deficiencies, certain oral conditions, dental factors, and (in lip cancer) exposure to sunlight also are associated with this type of cancer.

Tobacco

Tobacco use—smoking, chewing, and dipping—is the most common cause of oral cancer. The likelihood that oral cancer will develop depends on the type and amount of tobacco used (this may be referred to as the degree or level of risk).

Laboratory studies and epidemiologic research examining disease incidence in various populations show that tobacco use, particularly smoking, is a cause of oral cancer. To date, 43 **carcinogens** (cancer-causing substances) have been identified in tobacco smoke. The level of cancer risk among tobacco users increases with the amount and duration of the behavior. Epidemiologic studies around the world consistently show that male cigarette smokers are at least three times more likely than nonsmokers to develop cancer. Were it not for tobacco use, oral cancer would be almost nonexistent as a cause of death. Cigarette use alone accounts for over 80 percent of all oral cancer deaths in the United States annually. A number of studies indicate that pipe and cigar smokers have the same or a higher risk of developing oral cancer as do cigarette smokers.

Despite the health risks, more than 50 million adults still smoke cigarettes, and each year more than one million teenagers take up the habit. Recent surveys indicate that girls are as likely as boys to become smokers. Smoking begins primarily during childhood and adolescence.

Like cigarette smoking, use of smokeless tobacco (chewing tobacco and snuff) is now recognized as a public health problem. An estimated six million Americans (mostly males) use smokeless tobacco regularly. This habit, which used to be uncommon except in the South, recently has become more popular among teenage and young adult males (under age 30) in all areas of the country. A recent survey of males 16 to 19 years of age revealed a 300 percent increase in the use of snuff and a 250 percent increase in the use of chewing tobacco between 1970 and 1985; a similar pattern of increased use was seen for young adult males.

Smokeless tobacco contains a number of known carcinogens, including tobacco-specific nitrosamines, polycyclic aromatic hydrocarbons, and polonium-210, a radiation carcinogen. N-nitrosonornicotine, a nitrosamine shown to be a powerful carcinogen in laboratory animals, is found in far greater amounts in smokeless tobacco than in other forms of tobacco.

Epidemiologic evidence clearly links smokeless tobacco, especially snuff, with oral cancer. These cancers often develop where the tobacco is placed. Tobacco chewing involves placing a portion between the cheek and gum for extended periods of time. In snuff dipping, the user keeps a small amount (pinch) of powdered or finely ground tobacco tucked between the lip and gum, between the cheek and gum, or beneath the tongue. Some people use smokeless tobacco because they believe it to be a "safe" alternative to cigarettes. However, studies conducted in the southeastern United States indicate that snuff users are four times more likely than nonusers to develop oral cancer; for long-term users, the risk of cancer of the cheek and gum is 50 times greater. Furthermore, studies in the United States and Scandinavia indicate that between 8 percent and 59 percent of smokeless tobacco users develop **leukoplakia**, a lesion that can progress to cancer.

Alcohol

Chronic or excessive alcohol consumption also contributes to the development of oral cancer. It has been difficult to assess the risk of alcohol consumption alone, in part because most heavy drinkers are also heavy smokers. Recent epidemiologic research indicates, however, that the risk of oral cancer is elevated among drinkers even if they do not smoke. The amount of increased risk is proportional to the level of alcohol consumed. In combination, smoking and drinking tend to multiply each other's harmful effects. The largest study of combined alcohol and tobacco use indicated that heavy drinkers and smokers are at least 35 times more likely to develop oral cancer than are people who use neither product.

Another complication in defining the role of alcohol in oral cancer is that the mechanism by which alcohol causes the disease is not fully understood. Because animal studies indicate that pure grain alcohol (ethanol) is not carcinogenic, it may be that nonalcoholic ingredients in alcoholic beverages are responsible for the increased risk. It also is possible that alcohol promotes the carcinogenic potential of other substances, such as tobacco, or it may impair the liver's ability to detoxify potential carcinogens. Nutritional deficiencies also may account for some of the increased risk in heavy drinkers, who commonly get one-third to one-half of their daily calories from alcohol.

Even in the absence of alcohol abuse, certain nutritional deficiencies may increase the risk of developing oral cancer. Several studies have suggested a protective effect of increased fresh vegetable and fruit consumption; however, the constituents of these foods responsible for the apparent decreased risk of oral cancer could not be identified.

Other Causes and Risk Factors

Oral cancer can arise from previously healthy tissues, or the disease can develop in patients with certain oral conditions. Leukoplakia, a condition in which a whitish patch replaces the normal pink mucous membrane of the mouth (due to overproduction of the protein keratin), is a common condition in men over the age of 40. The majority of cases are benign, but some leukoplakias progress into precancerous conditions or oral cancers, particularly when associated with erythroplakia (discussed below).

The appearance of leukoplakia varies; the growth may be flat or elevated, and its edges may be poorly defined or sharply outlined. Tiny cracks may interlace the surface of larger growths. Leukoplakia may be found in several parts of the mouth, or it may be limited to one small area. Any mucous membrane may be affected. The buccal mucosa is the most common site, followed by the tongue, the hard palate, the lips, the gums, and the floor of the mouth.

The causes of leukoplakia are not well understood, but this condition is commonly associated with irritation of the mucous membrane from chronic injury (for example, cheek chewing, sharp teeth, or ill-fitting dentures) and from excessive use of tobacco and alcohol. The condition often occurs in irritated areas, such as the hard palate of pipe or cigarette smokers.

Because cancer may develop in some of these whitish patches, early diagnosis of leukoplakia is important. Scientists do not know exactly what percentage of cases actually progress to cancer. It has been estimated that fewer than 5 percent of leukoplakias become cancerous over a 20-year period. **Biopsy** (removal of all or part of a growth for microscopic examination) is the only way to establish the exact nature of a suspicious-looking patch.

In some cases, identifying and removing the source of irritation will result in complete regression of leukoplakia. Sometimes the growths are surgically removed. **Chemoprevention**, an investigational approach for preventing these growths, is discussed under "Prevention," below.

Lichen planus, generally considered a benign condition, appears as growths that look very similar to leukoplakia. Although these whitish patches can occur anywhere in the mouth, the buccal mucosa is the most common location. Unlike leukoplakia, lichen planus is more common in women than in men and is not associated with tobacco use. Although the cause of the condition is unknown, many researchers believe stress may contribute to its development. There is also some evidence that lichen planus may be caused by problems in the immune system. A biopsy confirms the diagnosis of lichen planus. Although there is no cure for the condition, **steroids**, **retinoids** (forms of vitamin A), and, more recently, **cyclosporine** have been used to treat it.

The most serious oral condition is **erythroplakia**, also called erythroplasia. The red, velvety patch associated with this condition occurs equally in men and women and develops most often in persons 60 to 70 years of age. The most common site in women is the gums; in men, the floor of the mouth is most often involved. Erythroplakia is considered a premalignant (precancerous) condition.

The cause of erythroplakia is unknown; however, as in leukoplakia, the lesion is associated with heavy smoking and drinking. Although less common than leukoplakia, erythroplakia has a much greater potential for becoming cancerous. Erythroplakia is the most common and the earliest sign of oral cancer. Indeed, studies indicate that 80 percent of oral cancers appear as red patches rather than as white ones. (Not all red growths are erythroplakia, however.)

Some dentists and physicians observe erythroplakia for a short period, usually no more than two weeks, to determine whether elimination of irritants improves the condition. If a biopsy proves that cancer is present, surgery is the usual treatment.

Dental factors, such as poor oral hygiene, are sometimes associated with oral cancer. Ill-fitting dentures and bridges, as well as sharp or broken teeth, may produce chronic irritation or infection and increase the risk of oral cancer.

Excessive exposure to the sun can cause cancer of the lip; nearly all cases occur on the lower lip. Often called "farmer's lip" or "sailor's lip," this type of cancer is found most often in white men over 40 years of age. People with light-colored skin and those with prolonged exposure to sunlight (such as outdoor workers) are most prone to developing lip cancer. Some protection from the sun may be offered by lipstick, which may partially account for a low incidence of lip cancer among women.

A person who has had one oral cancer is at increased risk of developing a second oral cancer, especially if that individual continues using tobacco and alcohol. Individuals who have oral cancer also appear to be prone to other primary cancers in the nasopharynx, hypopharynx, larynx, esophagus, and lung.

Prevention

People can reduce their risk of developing oral cancer by minimizing or eliminating their exposure to agents suspected of causing the disease. By far, eliminating all tobacco use is the single most important way to reduce the incidence of oral cancer. Alcohol should be consumed only in moderation, if at all. For people who are outdoors a lot, using a sunblock lotion or a lip balm containing a sunscreen and wearing a wide-brimmed hat can reduce the risk of lip cancer.

Quitting smoking can significantly decrease the chance of developing oral cancer. Recent studies indicate that five years after quitting, former smokers are only half as likely to develop oral cancer as those who continue to smoke.

A number of legislative and public health measures have been taken to inform people (particularly young people) about the dangers of smoking. For example, Federal law requires health warnings on all packages and advertisements of both cigarettes and smokeless tobacco products. Television and radio advertising of these products are prohibited. Moreover, in most states, laws restrict minors' access to tobacco products, although strict enforcement of these laws continues to be a problem.

As part of its prevention efforts, NCI has established a Smoking and Tobacco Control Program, whose goal is to reduce the cancer incidence and mortality caused by or related to the use of tobacco products. The NCI and the American Cancer Society are sponsoring a nationwide program to prevent and reduce tobacco use: this program began in 1991 and will extend through 1998. The NCI also is supporting research in chemoprevention as a way to inhibit the development of oral cancer in people at high risk for the disease, including those already treated for it. Chemoprevention is the use of natural and synthetic substances to prevent cancer.

For example, leukoplakia often recurs after treatment, and surgery frequently is impractical if there are many lesions. Chemoprevention may suppress leukoplakia and, therefore, its potential to progress to oral cancer. Scientists currently are evaluating the effectiveness of 13-cis-retinoic acid (a synthetic form of vitamin A) and beta-carotene (a precursor of vitamin A) in preventing or reversing leukoplakia. Thus far, 13-cis-retinoic acid has shown more promise than beta-carotene in suppressing the formation of new lesions.

Research also is under way in the chemoprevention of second primary cancers in patients already treated for oral cancer. (See "Causes and Risk Factors," above.) Studies to evaluate high doses of 13-cis-retinoic acid have been encouraging; researchers are experimenting with lower, less toxic doses of this drug. In addition, researchers are studying vitamin A and N-acetylcysteine (a drug used to treat some respiratory diseases) in conjunction with intensified screening techniques for detecting second primary cancers in the lung.

Scientists at NCI do not recommend that people take dietary supplements as a way to prevent cancer. Because some substances used in chemoprevention are toxic in high doses, they should be taken only under the supervision of a physician.

Symptoms

General

Early oral cancers usually are asymptomatic (without obvious symptoms of disease, such as pain). These growths may appear in otherwise normal-looking mucous membranes of the mouth or as an area of leukoplakia or erythroplakia. Progression of the cancer may be accompanied by pain and bleeding. Other symptoms include hoarseness, soreness or a sensation of something in the throat, and difficulty in chewing or swallowing. Sometimes, a lump in the neck is the first symptom, which may indicate that the cancer has spread to a cervical lymph node. Finding these or other changes does not necessarily mean that cancer is present, but any problem lasting more than two weeks should be checked by a physician or dentist.

By Site

Cancer of the **lip** occurs most often on the lower lip. The most common symptom is an enlarging growth that is not painful until it ulcerates (becomes an open sore) and becomes infected. Lip cancer may develop slowly, after a long history of leukoplakia.

Early cancer of the **buccal mucosa** is sometimes discovered by a dentist or a physician during a routine examination. The most common symptom is a lump in the cheek that can be felt with the tongue. The lump may not cause pain, even when it grows quite large. However, if a nerve is involved, pain may be felt in the tongue or ear. The growth may bleed if it is irritated by chewing or ulcerated by pressing against the teeth. Muscle spasms of the jaw may make it difficult to open the mouth. A history of leukoplakia, often quite extensive, is common in patients with cancer of the buccal mucosa.

Toothache, loose teeth, or a sore that does not heal may be warning signs of cancer of the **gums**. Ill-fitting dentures caused by progressive changes in the gums also may indicate cancer. Bleeding and pain may occur if the area is injured. If the tumor invades the **mandible**, it may involve a nerve, causing partial or complete numbness of the lower lip. Leukoplakia frequently is present.

Cancer of the **retromolar trigone** may affect nerves, causing earache. Muscle spasms may make opening the mouth difficult.

The most common symptom of cancer of the **hard palate** is a persistent, painless sore. The growth may become ulcerated, causing discomfort. If the tumor involves a nerve, the roof of the mouth may be painful or numb.

Early cancer of the **floor of the mouth** is not painful. It appears as a red, slightly raised area with ill-defined borders. As the cancer grows, a lump can be felt with the tip of the tongue. Eating or drinking may cause discomfort. An advanced tumor produces increased pain, bleeding, bad breath, loose teeth, and a change in speech if the tumor grows at the base of the tongue. Leukoplakia also may be present.

Mild irritation is the most common symptom of cancer of the **oral tongue**. Pain may occur only during eating or drinking. As ulceration develops, the pain becomes progressively worse and may be felt in the ear. Extensive involvement of the muscles of the tongue affects speech and swallowing. An advanced tumor may produce a foul odor.

Early cancer of the **base of the tongue** is often asymptomatic. These tumors are rarely diagnosed early because the base of the tongue is not easily seen. The first symptom often is a sore throat. Some patients experience a sensation of a lump in the back of the tongue. Difficulty swallowing, nasal speech, and earache occur as the tumor grows. An advanced cancer produces bad breath.

The earliest symptom of **soft palate** cancer usually is a mild sore throat that is made worse by eating or drinking. Discomfort may be relieved temporarily if antibiotics are given. As the tumor grows, it interferes with swallowing and may cause a voice change. Food and liquid may be misdirected into the nasopharynx and nose if the soft palate is perforated or destroyed. Earache and headache sometimes occur.

Early cancer of the **tonsil** often produces no symptoms; however, the tumor can be easily seen and is often diagnosed by a dentist or physician during a routine examination. When symptoms do occur, they generally include a sore throat, aggravated by eating or drinking, and earache.

If the tumor involves the hard palate or the upper gum, dentures sometimes fit improperly or cause irritation. An advanced tumor may result in muscle spasms that may make opening the mouth difficult.

Detection and Diagnosis

Detection

Many oral cancer deaths could be prevented by early detection and diagnosis. Tissue changes in the mouth that might signal the beginnings of cancer often can be seen and felt easily.

Monthly oral self-examination, performed in front of a mirror, is effective in detecting oral cancer at an early, more curable stage. In this procedure, the lips, cheeks, gums, and tongue should be checked for color changes. All areas of the mouth should be checked for scabs, cracks, ulcers, swelling, bleeding, or thickenings. The head can be tilted so the front and back of the roof of the mouth can be seen in the mirror. If any abnormalities are found that last longer than two weeks, the patient should see a physician or a dentist.

In addition to evaluating suspicious-looking areas detected by patients, a physician or a dentist should perform oral examinations at regular intervals. A dental mirror is used to inspect areas that cannot be seen directly. Special attention should be given to people who use tobacco and alcohol. All soft and hard tissues of the mouth should be checked.

Irregularities in the shape of the neck can be seen readily by comparing both sides of the neck in a good light. The physician or dentist also will carefully feel (palpate) the inside of the mouth, paying special attention to any area that appears abnormal on visual inspection. Lymph nodes in the front and back of the neck are checked for swelling or changes in consistency.

Toluidine blue, a dye, is sometimes used to help detect oral cancer in people at high risk of developing the disease. Used as a mouth rinse, the dye stains only abnormal tissue and may help identify cancers that are not easily seen.

Diagnosis

A biopsy is necessary to make a definite diagnosis. In an **incisional biopsy**, a sample of tissue from the suspicious-looking area is surgically removed; often, an area of nearby healthy tissue also is taken for comparison. In an **excisional biopsy**, the entire suspicious-looking area is removed, along with a margin of healthy tissue. A pathologist (a physician who diagnoses disease by studying cells and tissue removed from the body) can determine whether the growth is benign or malignant. If the biopsy report is negative but the physician or dentist is still concerned that cancer may be present, the tissue should be examined again by the pathologist. If cancer is found, the pathologist can identify the type and grade (degree of differentiation) of the cancer cells.

Grading is an attempt to predict the aggressiveness of a tumor based on the microscopic appearance of the cancer cells. Well-differentiated (low-grade) cancer cells are abnormal but resemble their normal counterparts; poorly differentiated (high-grade) cancer cells are disorganized and look extremely abnormal. In general, oropharyngeal tumors are more poorly differentiated than oral cavity tumors. Knowing the grade of the tumor may help the physician make treatment recommendations. High-grade tumors are more likely to spread to the cervical lymph nodes than are low-grade ones. Some patients with high-grade tumors have occult (hidden) cancer cells in their cervical lymph nodes; these patients may be treated for cancer in the nodes even when staging procedures have produced no evidence of cancer in them. (See "Treatment," below.)

Even if the cervical lymph nodes show evidence of metastatic disease (such as swelling), the biopsy specimen should always be taken from the primary tumor. However, an enlarged cervical lymph node is sometimes the only symptom of oral cancer. A **needle biopsy** (insertion of a needle into the tumor to withdraw cells for microscopic examination) may be performed on an enlarged node if the primary tumor site cannot be identified. However, its value in diagnosing a neck mass is limited. A needle biopsy produces only a small specimen, which complicates evaluation of the tumor (if, for example, both benign and cancerous elements are present). In a small percentage of cases, cancerous cells in the tumor are not withdrawn, which results in a false-negative biopsy report. Therefore, any negative findings should be confirmed by a surgical biopsy, usually an excisional biopsy, to ensure an accurate diagnosis.

Endoscopy of other parts of the head and neck also may be helpful in identifying the site of the primary tumor if a needle biopsy of a neck mass reveals metastatic disease. An endoscope is an instrument that contains bundles of flexible glass fibers carrying light for visual examination; it has a tweezer-like tool for removing a sample of tissue.

Computed tomography (CT or CAT) scans, specialized x-ray studies, also may be useful in locating the primary tumor. A CT scan involves a series of x-rays taken as an instrument called a scanner revolves around the patient. A computer receives the x-ray images and creates a cross-sectional picture of the body's organs and structures.

Staging

Staging Techniques

If cancer is diagnosed, additional tests are needed to determine the **stage**, or extent, of the disease. This pretreatment evaluation helps the physician plan the best treatment. Staging procedures include a thorough physical examination and laboratory tests. Dental x-rays may identify tumor invasion into the bones of the maxilla or mandible. In addition, chest x-rays may be done to determine whether cancer has spread to the lung.

CT scans can provide important information about the size, density, and extent of the tumor. These scans also are useful in detecting cervical lymph node metastases that may not be found during physical examination; up to 30 percent of lymph node metastases cannot be felt at the time the primary tumor is diagnosed.

A newer technique known as **magnetic resonance imaging (MRI)**, like CT scanning, produces cross-sectional images of internal organs and structures. An advantage of MRI is that it employs a large, very powerful magnet to produce images and, therefore, does not require use of x-rays or contrast agents. Moreover, MRI is often more useful than CT scanning in determining the extent of both the primary tumor and any cervical lymph node metastases.

Liver and bone scans may be performed, especially if the patient has symptoms of metastasis to these sites. These scans involve the intravenous injection of radioactive material that helps highlight areas of tumor growth.

Endoscopy is used to examine other parts of the head, neck, and upper chest, such as the esophagus, the larynx, and the bronchi of the lungs. Simultaneous second primary tumors (other primary cancers occurring at the same time as the tumor under evaluation) can be found in 10 to 15 percent of head and neck cancer patients.

Staging System

The TNM staging system, proposed by the American Joint Committee on Cancer, is the same for all oral cancers. The stage is based on the size of the primary tumor and the extent of invasion into adjacent tissues (T), the presence or absence of cancer cells in the cervical lymph nodes (N), and whether the cancer has metastasized (M) to distant parts of the body.

Oral tumors are classified TX, when the tumor cannot be assessed; TO, when there is no evidence of a primary tumor; Tis (carcinoma *in situ*), when the tumor is very small and confined to its original location; or T followed by a number from 1 to 4, reflecting the size and extent of the tumor. Lymph nodes are classified NX, if they cannot be assessed; NO, if the nodes do not contain cancer; or N followed by a number from 1 to 3, indicating the number and location of the nodes containing cancer. Distant metastases are classified as MX, when the metastases cannot be assessed; MO, when there are no known metastases; or M1, when distant metastases are found.

Using the TNM system, oral cancer can be classified into five different stages:

Stage 0: The tumor involves only the surface cells of the affected area and has not spread to the lymph nodes or to other parts of the body.

Stage I: The tumor is 2 centimeters (cm) (about 3/4 of an inch) or less in diameter and has not spread to lymph nodes or to other parts of the body.

Stage II: The tumor is greater than 2 cm but not more than 4 cm (about 1 1/2 inches) in diameter and has not spread to the lymph nodes or to other parts of the body.

Stage III: The tumor is greater than 4 cm in diameter and has not spread to the lymph nodes, or the tumor is of any size (except massive, as described under stage IV) and involves a single enlarged lymph node that is less than 3 cm (about 1 1/4 inches) in diameter and that is located on the same side of the neck as the primary tumor. In either case, the tumor has not spread to distant parts of the body.

Stage IV: The tumor measures more than 4 cm in diameter, has deeply invaded surrounding tissue, and involves not more than one lymph node (if there is an enlarged node, it is 3 cm or less in diameter) on the same side of the neck as the primary tumor; or the tumor is any size and involves one lymph node more than 3 cm in diameter, multiple lymph nodes of any size on the same side of the neck as the primary tumor, lymph nodes of any size on both sides of the neck, or one or more lymph nodes of any size on the opposite side of the neck from the primary tumor; or the tumor has spread to distant parts of the body.

Treatment

Significant advances have been made in recent years in the treatment of oral cancers because of improvements in surgical techniques, **radiation therapy**, and combination treatment programs. Survival rates are improving, and this trend is expected to continue.

Oral cancers can be treated with surgery alone, radiation therapy alone, or a combination of these therapies. Small tumors (stages I and II) often can be treated successfully with either surgery or radiation therapy alone. Advanced tumors (stages III and IV) usually require the combination of both treatment methods. Treatment for any cervical lymph node metastasis is based on such factors as the number, size, and location of the abnormal nodes.

Chemotherapy, although not curative, has proved useful in relieving symptoms (**palliative treatment**) for patients with recurrent or metastatic disease. In addition, research is under way to evaluate chemotherapy combined with surgery, radiation therapy, or both in patients with advanced cancers (usually stage III tumors and stage IV tumors that have not spread to other parts of the body).

New treatments that have shown promise in laboratory and animal studies are evaluated in **clinical trials** (research conducted with cancer patients). Clinical trials are designed to answer specific questions and to determine whether a new treatment is safe for patients and effective against the disease. Many of the current standard treatments for cancer were developed in such studies. Information about how patients and their physicians can learn about current clinical trials is found under "Clinical Trials and PDQ."

The choice of treatment for a patient with oral cancer depends on many factors, including the site of the primary tumor and the stage of the disease. The age and general health of the patient also are important considerations in planning therapy. Patients with early stage disease usually can be treated successfully with either surgery or radiation therapy. For this reason, treatment decisions may be influenced by the way treatment might affect the patient's appearance and ability to retain oral function, as well as by the patient's occupation, lifestyle, and preferences.

Treatment Planning

The choice of the most appropriate treatment often requires the participation of a team of health professionals. The medical team might include a dentist, oral surgeon, otolaryngologist (a physician who specializes in disorders of the head and neck), medical oncologist (a physician who specializes in treating cancer), radiation oncologist, maxillofacial prosthodontist (a dentist with special training in making **prostheses**, artificial replacements, for facial and oral structures), plastic surgeon, dietitian, speech therapist, and a medical social worker. The composition of the team depends on the patient's needs and on the staff of the hospital or treatment center.

Treatment for oral cancers may injure healthy areas of the mouth, including the teeth, the gums, the soft tissues, and the jaw. All patients, but especially those who will receive radiation therapy, should have a dental evaluation before undergoing treatment. Patients should be informed about techniques for maintaining good oral hygiene both during and after treatment. Further information on dental care can be found under "Side Effects of Treatment," below.

Oral cancers often invade the bones of the maxilla or mandible. In many cases, patients must consult with a maxillofacial prosthodontist before starting therapy so that any necessary prostheses can be made. If extensive surgery must be performed, casts of the mandible and maxilla are necessary for successful rehabilitation.

Often, patients develop malnutrition because they have had trouble eating. Patients who eat well may be better able to withstand the side effects of their treatment. Physicians and dietitians may suggest a variety of ways to get enough calories and protein.

A medical social worker can help the patient understand the treatment and any functional and cosmetic disabilities that are likely to result. The social worker also may provide emotional support to the patient and the patient's family at the time of diagnosis as well as during treatment and rehabilitation.

Methods of Treatment

Surgery

Surgery, also called **surgical excision**, is the usual treatment for many oral cancers. It also may be used to remove leukoplakia and erythroplakia.

All cancer cells must be removed to prevent a recurrence. Surgery involves removal of the primary tumor as well as a margin of normal tissue. The tissue must be examined under a microscope to ensure that the cancer is adequately excised.

Surgery is the preferred treatment for oral cancers located near bone, such as the mandible. The extent of the surgery depends on the size and location of the tumor. Some oral cancers (such as a small tumor on the oral tongue) can be removed completely during biopsy, and no further treatment is necessary. Other tumors require more extensive surgery that may involve removal of portions of the mandible, the maxilla, or the tongue.

Mohs' technique, also called Mohs' micrographic surgery, may be used in the treatment of early oral cancers. Mohs' technique is a precise method of surgically removing a tumor one thin layer at a time, until only healthy tissue remains. This method increases the possibility of removing the entire tumor, while taking as little healthy tissue as possible. Mohs' technique should be performed only by physicians who are specially trained in this procedure.

Other new surgical techniques show promise in the treatment of certain oral cancers. The carbon dioxide (CO_2) laser may be used to remove carcinoma *in situ* (stage 0) as well as some stage I and stage II oral cancers. This technique also may be used to excise leukoplakia and erythroplakia. (A laser is a device that produces a powerful, narrow beam of light at one wavelength. The light beam can be used to cut or vaporize the abnormal growth.) Another technique, cryosurgery, may be used to treat small, superficial oral tumors. (In cryosurgery, liquid nitrogen is applied to the tumor to freeze and kill the abnormal cells. The dead tissue then thaws and flakes away.)

If there is evidence that the cancer has metastasized, the surgeon may remove lymph nodes along with the primary tumor. Removal of the cervical lymph nodes is called neck dissection. The surgeon will attempt to take out only cancerous lymph nodes and a small amount of tissue close to them. If the disease involves muscles and other tissues in the neck, however, the operation may be more extensive.

In radical neck dissection, the surgeon removes a block of tissue from the collarbone to the mandible and from the front to the back of the neck. The large muscle on the side of the neck used in rotating, flexing, and extending the neck also is removed, along with the jugular vein. In another technique, functional neck dissection, the surgeon preserves the muscles of the neck, removing only the lymph nodes and the fibrous tissue surrounding them.

Sometimes, a neck dissection is performed even when staging procedures show no evidence of cancer in the cervical lymph nodes; this is done because some patients are at increased risk of occult metastases in the nodes. This procedure is called prophylactic, or elective, neck dissection. Removing untreated occult cancer in the neck may prevent the recurrence or further spread of the cancer.

The decision to provide prophylactic neck treatment with either neck dissection or radiation therapy is based on a variety of factors. Among these are the site, the size, and the degree of differentiation of cells in the primary tumor (discussed under "Detection and Diagnosis," above).

Surgery also may be used to treat recurrent oral cancers initially managed with either radiation therapy or surgery. (Clinical trials of anticancer drugs and other new treatment approaches are often considered in this case.)

Radiation Therapy

Radiation therapy is the use of high-energy rays to kill cancer cells. The goal is to destroy all tumor cells with minimal damage to normal, healthy tissue. Like surgery, radiation therapy is called local treatment because it affects only the cells in the area being treated.

One type of radiation therapy, external beam, is given using a machine located outside the body; the machine delivers x-rays, gamma rays, or electrons to the cancer site. For very small tumors, an intraoral cone may be used to deliver external beam therapy directly to the tumor. The cone is positioned by a stent (mold) placed in the mouth. The radiation dose is based on the size and location of the tumor. Usually, external beam therapy is administered once a day, five days a week, for several weeks. This schedule helps protect healthy tissues by spreading out the total dose of radiation.

Brachytherapy, a form of internal radiation therapy (also known as **interstitial radiation** or **endocurie therapy**), involves implantation of radioactive material directly into the tumor or close to it. The radioactive implant delivers cancer-killing rays as close as possible to the tumor while sparing most of the surrounding healthy tissue. In brachytherapy, a higher total dose of radiation can be delivered to the tumor than is possible with external beam therapy. Iodine 125, gold 198, radium 226, cesium 137, and iridium 192 are radioactive materials that may be used.

The type of implant and the method of placing it depend on the size and location of the tumor. Often, the radiation is administered through implanted needles, wires, or seeds. Sometimes, special instruments or molds are used to hold the implant in place. An implant usually is left in place for several days; however, a permanent implant is used in some cases. The patient usually stays in the hospital for a few days until the radiation has decreased to a safe level.

Brachytherapy is especially useful in treating small, superficial cancers of the oral tongue and the floor of the mouth. It is less practical for larger tumors and usually does not allow irradiation of cervical lymph nodes, as is often possible with external beam therapy. Treatment of many oral cancers (such as those at the base of the tongue) often requires the use of both external beam therapy and brachytherapy.

Many patients first receive external beam therapy to a wide area that includes the primary tumor, surrounding areas, and the upper cervical lymph nodes. After the initial therapy, a smaller area is treated to minimize the side effects caused by irradiating a large region. The final treatment area is often quite small; radiation here is referred to as a "boost" or "booster treatment." The boost of radiation can be given with either external beam therapy or brachytherapy.

As discussed above, if the primary tumor is treated with radiation, cervical lymph nodes showing evidence of metastases may also be treated with radiation alone in some cases. In addition, prophylactic radiation therapy may be used to eliminate possible occult disease in the nodes. (See "Surgery," above.)

Radiation therapy also may be used to treat recurrent oral cancers initially treated with surgery (Clinical trials evaluating anticancer drugs and other new treatment approaches are often considered for this purpose.) In advanced disease, radiation therapy may be used to relieve symptoms caused by the primary tumor or metastatic tumors.

A number of new approaches to increase the effectiveness of radiation therapy are being evaluated in clinical trials. For example, scientists are comparing conventional external beam therapy with **particle beam therapy**, the use of fast-moving subatomic particles (such as neutrons), for treating patients with locally advanced tumors.

Investigators also are studying **radiosensitizers**, substances that make cancer cells more susceptible to radiation therapy. SR-2508, Fluosol-DA, and the anticancer drugs cisplatin and 5-fluorouracil are some agents being evaluated. Beta-carotene is being studied, both as a radiosensitizer and as a radioprotector (a substance that protects normal cells from radiation damage).

Another investigational therapy is the use of hyperthermia (heat as a cancer treatment) combined with radiation therapy. **Photodynamic therapy** (PDT), also called photoradiotherapy, is a new treatment that uses an interaction between laser light and a substance that makes cells more sensitive to light (photosensitizing agent) to destroy tumor tissue. Researchers are trying to determine whether PDT may be of value in addition to the initial therapy or in the treatment of oral cancers that have recurred after previous treatment.

Researchers also are exploring new **fractionation** schedules of radiation therapy, alone or in combination with chemotherapy. (A fraction is a single dose of radiation, usually given once a day.) Accelerated fractionation involves shortening the overall length of time the radiation therapy is given (for example, administering the same total dose in five weeks instead of seven). In hyperfractionation, the total dose of radiation remains approximately the same as in standard therapy, but it is given in smaller doses two or three times per day.

Chemotherapy

Chemotherapy, treatment with anticancer drugs, has traditionally been used to relieve symptoms in patients with recurrent or metastatic oral cancers. It is a systemic treatment—that is, the drugs enter the bloodstream and travel through the body, affecting cancer cells outside the oral area.

Of the many anticancer drugs available, only a few have proven effective against oral cancers. Three drugs have shown consistent antitumor activity: methotrexate, bleomycin, and cisplatin. Methotrexate has been studied the most and is the agent against which many other drugs are judged. Scientists believe that cisplatin is as effective as methotrexate, but they are looking for related compounds that produce fewer side effects. One promising alternative to cisplatin is carboplatin, a drug similar to but in many ways potentially less toxic than its parent compound. Vincristine, vinblastine, hydroxyurea, cyclophosphamide, doxorubicin, and 5-fluorouracil (also called 5-FU), alone or in various combinations, also are used to treat metastatic or recurrent oral cancers.

Researchers are continuing their search for more effective and less toxic drugs. Agents currently under study include amonafide, ifosfamide (given with mesna, a drug that reduces the side effects of ifosfamide), piroxantrone, and 10-EDAM (a drug similar to methotrexate). Researchers also are testing higher doses of some drugs in an effort to increase their effectiveness. Other work involves the study of new drug combinations.

Intra-arterial chemotherapy, also called regional chemotherapy, is another investigational approach for advanced oral cancers. This is a technique in which a pump delivers chemotherapy directly into an artery that supplies blood to the tumor. This procedure minimizes exposure of healthy tissues to the drugs and increases the concentration of drugs to the cancer.

Combination Therapy

Combination therapy, also called **combined modality therapy**, is used to treat oral cancers that cannot be controlled with either surgery or radiation therapy alone. Radiation therapy can be administered either before or after surgery.

In some cases, preoperative radiation therapy makes surgery possible by shrinking a large tumor. It also has been shown to reduce the risk of recurrence. However, preoperative radiation has disadvantages, such as wound infection and an increased risk of tissue **necrosis** (see "Side Effects of Treatment," below) that have resulted in its declining use.

Postoperative radiation therapy is used to treat tumors that cannot be completely removed surgically. Postoperative radiation also is given to treat rapidly growing tumors and those that have invaded cartilage or bone. Postoperative radiation may decrease the risk of recurrence by stopping the growth of any cancer cells that remain in the body.

In recent years, chemotherapy has been added to the combination therapy approach in an attempt to improve the outlook for patients with advanced oral cancers. These efforts include the following: induction, or neoadjuvant, chemotherapy (chemotherapy given before surgery or radiation therapy); adjuvant, or maintenance, chemotherapy (chemotherapy given after surgery or radiation therapy); and concurrent, or simultaneous, chemotherapy and radiation therapy.

Induction chemotherapy is being studied as a way to shrink tumors, making treatment with radiation or surgery more feasible, and to kill any remaining cancer cells, thereby decreasing the risk of recurrence. Many drug combinations are used in this approach. Some investigators propose the use of chemotherapy to reduce the tumor to a size that could be treated with radiation alone, thus eliminating surgery for some patients.

Adjuvant chemotherapy may prove useful in eradicating any cancer cells remaining after treatment with surgery or radiation. The aim is to reduce the risk of recurrence after therapy. Adjuvant chemotherapy has usually been used following induction chemotherapy and standard therapy.

Treatment with concurrent chemotherapy and radiation therapy is also under investigation. Chemotherapy and radiation therapy each may increase the cancer-killing effects of the other. This role for chemotherapy is based, in part, on the radiosensitizing properties of some anticancer drugs. Chemotherapy also is used to eliminate any remaining cancer cells. Furthermore, researchers are exploring concurrent chemotherapy and radiation therapy as a substitute for surgery in some patients.

Biological Therapy

Biological therapy, also called immunotherapy, is being studied to determine whether it is effective in the treatment of advanced or recurrent oral cancers. This approach involves the use of biological agents to fight cancer. Modern laboratory technology allows researchers to identify and manufacture large amounts of some of the natural substances that the body produces to help boost, direct, or restore its normal defenses (immune system). These substances are called biological response modifiers (BRMs).

In clinical trials, researchers are studying the BRM interleukin-2 (IL-2), a protein that regulates cell growth. In this investigational approach, patients are treated with IL-2 alone or IL-2 combined with lymphokine-activated killer (LAK) cells, white blood cells that have been stimulated by IL-2 to increase their ability to kill cancer cells. Scientists also are exploring IL-2 in combination with cyclophosphamide and with other BRMs (such as interferon, a protein that can kill cancer cells or stop their uncontrolled growth, and bacillus Calmette-Guerin, or BCG, a nonspecific immune system stimulant).

Side Effects of Treatment

Treatment for oral cancer often causes side effects. Some are temporary, but others are permanent and can produce significant cosmetic changes and functional disabilities. Some side effects may be prevented. Others may be corrected with reconstructive surgery or prosthetic reconstruction.

Surgery

Often, surgery to remove small oral cancers leaves only a small scar and minimal, if any, functional disability. Removal of larger, more extensive tumors, however, may involve removal of parts of the oral soft tissue, the maxilla, the mandible, or the tongue. Extensive surgery can result in changes in appearance and can cause problems with chewing, swallowing, and speaking. The patient also may have difficulty moving the shoulder and arm on the affected side. After surgery, the face may be swollen. This swelling usually disappears within a few weeks. However, if the lymph system has been damaged, lymph may collect in the tissues: swelling may last a long time.

Radiation Therapy

Because radiation affects normal as well as cancerous cells, radiation therapy can cause a number of side effects. A dental evaluation before treatment begins is especially important for patients who will receive radiation therapy. (See "Treatment Planning," above.) A number of measures can be taken to prevent complications. Healthy teeth should be preserved. If required, extractions and other dental work usually are performed before treatment begins. Patients should wait at least two weeks, if possible, to allow the mouth to heal before undergoing radiation therapy.

The salivary glands are especially sensitive to radiation therapy. One result is a reduction in the amount of saliva produced. The mouth may become very dry. Use of tobacco and alcohol increases the drying effect. Iced beverages, special chewing gum, and frequent rinsing can help keep the mouth moist. Artificial saliva or salivary gland stimulants may be necessary to relieve dryness. The chance that salivation will return depends on the area treated and the amount of radiation that reached the glands.

Radiation therapy also causes the saliva to become acidic and quite thick. This change, together with the dryness described above, destroys the saliva's protective effect on the teeth. (Dental problems do not result from irradiation of the teeth themselves but from these changes in saliva.) Also, patients sometimes stop routine dental care because the tissues are tender, making it uncomfortable to brush and floss the teeth. The result is that an increased amount of organic material sticks to the teeth. Plaque forms; which rapidly leads to cavities. Dentists encourage patients to clean their teeth and gums thoroughly (using a child's soft toothbrush or a special toothbrush with a soft, spongy tip, if necessary) and to floss between the teeth daily. Patients also should avoid sugar and other foods that contribute to tooth decay. Dentists may recommend a fluoride mouth rinse or gel. In addition, patients may use a salt and baking soda mouthwash to refresh the mouth. It is important for patients to see a dentist regularly for cleaning, fluoride applications, and other procedures that will preserve their teeth.

Some patients are able to wear their dentures during radiation therapy. However, because the gums tend to shrink during treatment and for several months afterward, dentures may not fit properly. Following therapy, dentures may need to be relined or replaced. In any case, patients should not wear their dentures without first consulting their physician or dentist.

Radiation therapy also can cause mouth sores that heal slowly. Often, good oral hygiene can prevent sores.

Many patients have trouble opening the mouth as a result of radiation of the muscles used in chewing and of the temporomandibular joint (where the mandible joins the skull). There is no simple treatment for this condition, but stretching exercises may help prevent it.

Some patients complain that their tongue is sensitive following radiation therapy. This side effect usually disappears with time. Taste also may be altered during treatment (caused by radiation of the taste buds). Some patients report a bitter taste during the early part of radiation therapy. Loss of taste occurs in many patients, but, for most, the sense of taste returns within a week to several months after treatment. For some, however, taste is not as keen as before, although it is usually adequate. A dry mouth, caused by radiation of the salivary glands, may contribute to the loss of taste.

Loss of, or change in, taste often leads to the common and very serious problem of loss of appetite. This side effect, in turn, can cause weight loss. Nutritional guidance is very important in enabling patients to withstand the side effects of their treatment. (See "Treatment Planning," above.)

Radiation therapy can destroy tissue, a side effect called radiation necrosis. Necrosis usually begins with the breakdown of mucous membranes, leaving a small, open sore. Ulceration in soft tissues that have no underlying bone is called soft tissue necrosis. The risk is increased in patients who use tobacco and alcohol. Some patients require antibiotics and a local anesthetic for pain.

Sometimes, areas of the gums shrink, exposing underlying bone. This rare condition, known as bone exposure, may require months or even years to heal. If the gum does not regrow over the exposed area and if a large area is involved, a tissue graft may be necessary to cover the exposed bone.

Large doses of radiation can increase the risk of osteoradionecrosis, destruction of bone tissue resulting from injury to or infection in the jaw. Because osteoradionecrosis is rare, doctors try to ensure that the necessary amount of radiation is given rather than attempting to lessen the risk by reducing the dose of radiation.

Other common problems include hair loss and skin reactions, such as redness or dryness. Patients should not expose treated areas to the sun and should not use skin lotions or creams without consulting their physician. Fatigue is another usual side effect. Resting as much as possible is important.

Chemotherapy

Anticancer drugs circulating in the bloodstream can reach and damage normal as well as cancerous cells. For example, these drugs commonly affect blood-forming cells, cells that line the digestive tract, and other rapidly growing cells. Therefore, chemotherapy can produce a variety of side effects. There may be an increased risk of infection due to reduced numbers of white blood cells, nausea and vomiting, hair loss, and other problems associated with specific drugs. Most of these side effects are temporary and, following completion of treatment, will stop.

271

Rehabilitation

Rehabilitation is a very important part of the overall treatment plan for patients with oral cancer. Various members of the medical team help the patient resume a normal life as soon as possible.

Many surgical techniques are available to restore appearance and oral function. A plastic surgeon may need to repair the defects caused by extensive surgery. Surgery to reconstruct the body's natural contours uses the patient's own tissues, including grafts of skin, cartilage, or bone. **Flaps**, which (unlike grafts) carry their own blood supply, are necessary in some cases.

Frequently, however, a maxillofacial prosthodontist must make a prosthesis to restore appearance and function in patients with oral and facial defects. Intraoral prostheses can be used to restore the teeth, palate, mandible, and other oral structures.

Speech therapy generally begins as soon as possible for a patient who has trouble talking. Often, a speech therapist visits the patient in the hospital to plan therapy and to teach speech exercises. Speech therapy usually continues after the patient returns home.

Periodic consultation with a dentist is necessary to ensure maintenance of good oral hygiene. Prevention of dental disease is necessary for successful rehabilitation.

A medical social worker may provide continued emotional support to help the patient resume normal activities. The social worker also may be able to suggest groups that offer help with rehabilitation, financial aid, transportation, and home care.

Follow-up Care

Because patients who have been treated for oral cancer are at risk for recurrent disease and for new primary cancers, they should be examined regularly by a physician or a dentist. Patients also should follow their doctor's instructions on how to reduce the chance of developing the disease again. (See "Risk Factors" and "Prevention," above.) Furthermore, they may need to consult with a dietitian if eating difficulty or weight loss continues.

Patients should continue to perform monthly oral self-examination. Any suspicious-looking areas should be brought to the attention of a physician or dentist. Early detection and diagnosis are key to successful treatment of oral cancer.

Clinical Trials and PDQ

To improve the outcome of treatment for patients with oral cancer, NCI supports clinical trials at many hospitals throughout the United States. Patients who take part in this research make an important contribution to medical science and may have the first chance to benefit from improved treatment methods. Physicians are encouraged to inform their patients about the option of participating in such trials. To help physicians learn about current trials, NCI has developed PDQ, a computerized resource designed to give physicians quick and easy access to the following:

* descriptions of current clinical trials, including information about the objectives of the studies, medical eligibility requirements, details of the treatment programs, and the names and addresses of physicians and facilities conducting the studies;

* up-to-date information about the standard treatment for most types of cancer; and names of organizations and physicians involved in cancer care.

To access PDQ, physicians may use an office computer with a telephone hookup and a PDQ access code, or they may use the services of a medical library with online searching capability. Cancer Information Service (CIS) offices (1-800-4-CANCER) provide PDQ searches and can tell physicians how to obtain regular access to the database. Patients may ask their physician to use PDQ or may call the CIS at 1-800-4-CANCER themselves. Information specialists at this toll-free number use a variety of sources, including PDQ, to answer questions about cancer prevention, diagnosis, treatment, and research.

Selected References

Available from Libraries

The references listed below can be found in medical libraries, many college and university libraries and some public libraries.

Blot, W.J., et al. "Smoking and Drinking in Relation to Oral and Pharyngeal Cancer," *Cancer Research*, Vol. 48(11), 1988, pp. 3282-3287.

Connolly, G.N., et al. "The Reemergence of Smokeless Tobacco," *New England Journal of Medicine*, Vol. 314(16), 1986, pp. 1020-1027.

Cummings, C.W., et al., eds. *Otolaryngology Head and Neck Surgery*. Saint Louis: C.V. Mosby Co., 1986.

DeVita, V.T., Jr., et al., eds. *Cancer: Principles and Practice of Oncology*. 3d ed. Philadelphia: J.B. Lippincott Co., 1989.

Garewal, H.S., et al. "Response of Oral Leukoplakia to Beta-Carotene," *Journal of Clinical Oncology*, Vol. 8(10), 1990, pp. 1715-1720.

Haskell, C.M., ed. *Cancer Treatment*. 3d ed. Philadelphia: W.B. Saunders Co. 1990.

The Health Benefits of Smoking Cessation: A Report of the Surgeon General. Office on Smoking and Health, U.S. Department of Health and Human Services. DHHS Publication No. 90-8416.

The Health Consequences of Using Smokeless Tobacco: A Report of the Advisory Committee to the Surgeon General. Office on Smoking and Health, U.S. Department of Health and Human Services. NIH Publication No. 86-2874.

Health Implications of Smokeless Tobacco Use. National Institutes of Health Consensus Development Conference Statement, Vol. 6(1), January 1986.

Hong, W.K., et al. "Prevention of Second Primary Tumors with Isotretinoin in Squamous-Cell Carcinoma of the Head and Neck," *New England Journal of Medicine*, Vol. 323(12), 1990, pp. 795-801.

Jacobs, C., et al. "Head and Neck Squamous Cancers," *Current Problems in Cancer*, Vol. 14(1), 1990, pp.1-72.

Laramore, G.E., ed. *Radiation Therapy of Head and Neck Cancer*. Berlin: Springer-Verlag, 1989.

Lee, K.J., ed. *Textbook of Otolaryngology and Head and Neck Surgery*. New York: Elsevier Science Publishing Co., 1989.

McLaughlin, J.K., et al. "Dietary Factors in Oral and Pharyngeal Cancer," *Journal of the National Cancer Institute*, Vol. 80(15), 1988, pp. 1237-1243.

Mashberg, A., and Samit, A.M. "Early Detection, Diagnosis, and Management of Oral and Oropharyngeal Cancer," *Ca-A Cancer Journal for Clinicians*, Vol. 39(2), 1989, pp. 67-88.

Million, R., and Cassisi, N.J., eds. *Management of Head and Neck Cancer: A Multidisciplinary Approach*. Philadelphia: J.B. Lippincott Co., 1984.

Myers, E.N., and Suen, J.Y., eds. *Cancer of the Head and Neck*. 2d ed. New York: Churchill Livingstone, Inc., 1989.

Panje, W.R., et al. "Transoral Carbon Dioxide Laser Ablation for Cancer, Tumors, and Other Diseases," *Archives of Otolaryngology-Head and Neck Surgery*, Vol. 115(6), 1989, pp. 681-688.

Schottenfeld, D., and Fraumeni, J.F., Jr., eds. *Cancer Epidemiology and Prevention*. Philadelphia: W.B. Saunders Co., 1982.

Shopland, D.R., et al. "Smoking-Attributable Cancer Mortality in 1991: Is Lung Cancer Now the Leading Cause of Death Among Smokers in the United States?" *Journal of the National Cancer Institute*, Vol. 83(16), 1991, pp. 1142-1148.

Wang, C.C., ed. *Radiation Therapy for Head and Neck Neoplasms*. Chicago: Year Book Medical Publishers, 1990.

Winn, D.M., et al. "Snuff Dipping and Oral Cancer Among Women in the Southern United States," *New England Journal of Medicine*, Vol. 304(13), 1981, pp. 745-749.

Wright, B.A., et al., eds. *Oral Cancer: Clinical and Pathological Considerations*, Boca Raton, Florida: CRC Press, Inc., 1988.

Available from NCI

The materials listed below are distributed free of charge by NCI. Ordering information is provided at the end of this chapter.

Chemotherapy and You: A Guide to Self-Help During Treatment. Office of Cancer Communications, National Cancer Institute. NIH Publication No. 91-1136.

Oral Complications of Cancer Therapies: Diagnosis, Prevention, and Treatment. National Institutes of Health Consensus Development Conference Statement, Vol. 7(7), April 1989.

"Photodynamic Therapy." Office of Cancer Communications, National Cancer Institute. May 1990.

Radiation Therapy and You: A Guide to Self Help During Treatment. Office of Cancer Communications, National Cancer Institute. NIH Publication No. 91-2227.

Smokeless Tobacco Use in the United States. National Cancer Institute Monograph No. 8. NIH Publication No. 89-3055.

Smoking, Tobacco, and Cancer Program. Division of Cancer Prevention and Control, National Cancer Institute. NIH Publication No. 90-3107.

What Are Clinical Trials All About? Office of Cancer Communications, National Cancer Institute. NIH Publication No. 88-2706.

Additional Information

To obtain additional information on this subject and to order other NCI publications, write to the

Office of Cancer Communications
National Cancer Institute
Bethesda, MD 20892

or call the toll-free Cancer Information Service (CIS) at 1-800-4-CAN-CER.

The CIS is a nationwide telephone service that answers questions from patients and their families, the public, and health professionals. Spanish-speaking staff members are available.

Chapter 31

Oral Cancer on Rise: The Risks of Smokeless Tobacco

The seventh most common cancer—oral cancer—may be on the rise because of the increased use of snuff and chewing tobacco, or "smokeless tobacco," among teenage boys.

Oral cancer occurs on the lip, tongue, or floor of the mouth. Smoking and drinking also increase the risk of oral cancer, but smokeless tobacco is of special concern because of its appeal to teenage boys.

Smokeless tobacco comes in two basic forms: finely ground tobacco or snuff, and loose leaf tobacco sold in pouches or plugs. An estimated 16 million Americans use smokeless tobacco, 3 million of whom are under 21. Sixteen percent of all males between the ages of 12 and 17 used smokeless tobacco in 1985, according to the American Academy of Otolaryngology—Head and Neck Surgery. The habit has filtered down to even younger ages in some localities: A University of North Carolina study showed that one-third of the first-grade boys in rural North Carolina had tried smokeless tobacco. And according to another study, 21 percent of 112 Arkansas kindergartners had indulged.

Chewing tobacco, a habit commonly associated with elderly gentlemen and southern farmers, caught on among teenagers in the mid-1970s when U.S. Tobacco Company (the major manufacturer of smokeless tobacco) began an aggressive ad campaign especially targeted toward young men. Endorsements by such sports heroes as Catfish Hunter (a former New York Yankee pitcher), Earl Campbell (former running back for the Houston Oilers), and Walt Garrison (former running back, Dallas Cowboys) promoted smokeless tobacco

FDA Consumer, Dec 89-Jan 90, December 22, 1989.

and changed its image. In a growing number of youthful circles, smokeless tobacco became a socially acceptable symbol of virility, machismo and coolness.

In a further bid to attract teenagers, U.S. Tobacco Co. offered free samples of smokeless tobacco and concocted low-nicotine and fruit-flavored brands. (One "adult" brand, for instance, has seven times the amount of nicotine as the "junior brands," and most young boys who might first experiment with the adult brand would end up nauseous.)

By 1985, tobacco's opponents began striking back. In that year, Massachusetts became the first state to require warning labels on smokeless tobacco. Other states considered similar action. Federal legislation requiring uniform labeling was passed in 1986. Dentist Greg Connolly, D.M.D., a leading opponent of smokeless tobacco and director of the Office for Nonsmoking and Health in Massachusetts, pressured U.S. Tobacco to stop using current sports heroes to endorse smokeless tobacco products.

Though proponents claim that smokeless tobacco is a safe alternative to smoking, the 1986 Report of the Advisory Committee to the Surgeon General doesn't see it that way. Smokeless tobacco is causally related to oral cancer, says the report. In fact, the report says that the increased risk of cancer of the cheek and gums may reach nearly fifty fold among long-term snuff users.

Nitrosamines, the chief cancer-causing compounds in smokeless tobacco, are contained in the tobacco. Snuff, for instance, delivers 10 times more nitrosamines than a cigarette.

Despite this risk, the habit is attractive for many users. Jared Taylor of Menlo Park, Calif., a fourth-generation chewer who quit after 15 years because of his concern over the link between chewing tobacco and cancer, nevertheless admits he misses his habit. "We were always a very religious family and thought smoking was a sin—it had to be a sin to burn up anything that tasted that good," says Taylor wryly.

Precancerous signs, such as leukoplakia (a white plaque on the gums, cheek or roof of the mouth) may appear after only one year of use. Once oral cancer strikes, it can spread rapidly—and "the first stop is the neck," says Jerome Goldstein, M.D., executive vice president of the American Academy of Otolaryngology.

"Head and neck surgery can mutilate and affect function," says Connolly. "If the cancer is not caught early enough, a person can lose his teeth, salivary glands, portions of his jaw, or sections of the neck or cheek." The tongue may also have to be cut out—and the person is rendered speechless or speaks in a garbled manner, according to Connolly.

Although sports heroes no longer endorse smokeless tobacco products, baseball players remain major users. A recent survey of 282 major league baseball players published in the *New England Journal of Medicine* showed that over half were past or current users of smokeless tobacco. In a baseball tradition going back to Babe Ruth, who was a heavy snuff dipper, the bulge in the back pocket—a tin of snuff or chewing tobacco—is a familiar sight on the baseball field. (Ruth, who also smoked, died of throat cancer.)

The American Academy of Otolaryngology has launched a campaign to warn the public—and especially teenage boys—about the dangers of smokeless tobacco. The academy has also formed an organization called "Athletes Through With Chew," whose spokesmen are all-star pitcher Nolan Ryan of the Texas Rangers and Bobby Brown, M.D., president of the American Baseball League.

The teenage set is at risk. William Frederick McGuirt, M.D., a head and neck surgeon at the Bowman Gray School of Medicine in Winston-Salem, N.C., says he is seeing more and younger smokeless tobacco users with either pre-malignant signs of cancer or dental problems such as receding gums.

Most scientists predict that though it will take 20 or 30 years for the rate of oral cancer to increase due to current smokeless tobacco use, such an increase is inevitable.

As Connolly says, "oral cancer is a time bomb ticking away in the mouths of adolescents."

—by Judy Folkenberg

Judy Folkenberg is a member of FDA's public affairs staff.

Chapter 32

Oral Complications of Cancer Therapies

Introduction

More than one million Americans will develop 228,000 gastrointestinal cancers, 155,000 lung cancers, 143,000 invasive breast carcinomas, 40,000 lymphomas, and 27,000 cases of leukemia. Also included are the estimated 30,000 cases of oral and oropharyngeal cancer.

Management of many malignancies requires local or radical surgical excision. Other forms of cancer treatment may be employed, e.g., radiation therapy, chemotherapy, and bone marrow transplantation. Unfortunately, most cancer treatments affect normal as well as neoplastic cells and tissues. As treatments have become more intensive and therapeutically successful, the effects on normal tissues have increased. The oral cavity is a very frequent site of such side effects. As a result of treatment, as many as 400,000 patients may develop oral complications that may be acute or chronic in nature. The more powerful the treatment modalities, the greater the risk of morbidity.

At a minimum, oral complications are painful, diminish the quality of life, and may lead to significant compliance problems, often discouraging the patient from continuing treatment. Cancer treatments may produce a breach in mucosal integrity, allowing pathogenic organisms to spread systemically, further compromising the patient. At times, levels of oral morbidity may interfere with oncologic therapy, necessitating suspension of therapy until such complications resolve.

NIH Consensus Development Conference Statement, Volume 7, Number 7, April 1989.

Side effects of radiation therapy to the head and neck may be noted as early as the first week. The potentially devastating occurrence of osteoradionecrosis in the irradiated patient has yet to be widely addressed in terms of multicenter, collaborative studies. The prevention and management of this and other oral complications remain as incompletely resolved clinical issues.

Bone marrow transplantation (BMT) is an evolving cancer management with frequent oral complications. Although BMT was once considered desperate and reserved for treatment of end-stage leukemia, it is now used routinely as an effective tool for treatment of several other cancers. Before and after actual transplantation, the possibility of secondary dysfunctions of the oral cavity exists. The stomatotoxicity of chemotherapy and total body irradiation, the associated risk of early septicemia from oral organisms, and the possibility of acute and chronic graft-versus-host disease all may affect the ultimate treatment outcome. Literature on the subject is sparse, and there are few well-documented studies demonstrating the efficacy of treatment of oral complications of BMT.

Pretreatment therapy for oral complications can positively affect the outcomes of cancer treatment. All members of the cancer treatment team should be fully informed of the oncologic treatment plan. Oral care should be initiated at the outset of cancer treatment with the goal of reducing morbidity and in many instances improving compliance.

Oral Complications of Cancer Therapies

Surgical removal of anatomical structures in the head and neck region compromises oral function to varying degrees. In chemotherapy, most complications are the result of myelosuppression, immunosuppression, and direct cytotoxic effects on oral tissues. Major clinical problems in the oral cavity that are associated with chemotherapy include mucositis, local or systemic infection, and hemorrhage. Total body irradiation and radiation for head and neck cancer have both direct and indirect effects on oral and related structures. The oral complications of radiotherapy to the salivary glands, oral mucosa, oral musculature, and/or alveolar bone include growth and developmental abnormalities, xerostomia, rampant dental caries, mucositis, taste loss, osteoradionecrosis, infection, dermatitis, and trismus. It is the recognition of the risk of these complications and their relation to outcome that prompts the discussion and necessitates agreement on the best means of management.

These complications result from the aggressive treatment of cancer; many would not occur if cancers could be detected and treated at an early phase. The emphasis of this conference on the prevention and treatment of complications should not detract from the basic goal of prevention and early detection of cancer.

Role for Pretherapy Interventions Affecting the Oral Cavity in Reducing the Incidence of Oral Complications

Oral complications resulting from anticancer therapies can significantly affect morbidity, the patient's tolerance of treatment, and the quality of life. Death can sometimes result from severe oral complications. There is a role for pretherapy intervention in reducing the incidence and severity of oral complications. Data presented at the conference convincingly demonstrated that appropriate interventions can significantly lessen morbidity and possibly decrease mortality.

There is evidence that preexisting oral disease unrelated to cancer or therapy may increase the risk of oral complications. Before the initiation of cancer therapy, a comprehensive pretreatment dental evaluation is mandated. The following objectives should be fulfilled:

- Establish baseline data with which all subsequent examinations can be compared.

- Identify risk factors for the development of oral complications.

- Develop strategies to avoid treatment complications during and following cancer therapy.

- Perform necessary dental treatment to reduce the likelihood of oral complications induced by cancer treatment.

Which Pretreatment Strategies Are Optimal to Prevent or Minimize Oral Complications?

There are many pretreatment strategies available to minimize or prevent oral complications. These afford the clinician a unique opportunity to ameliorate the side effects induced by cancer therapy. Pretreatment strategies include evaluation, treatment of preexisting dental disease, patient and family education and counseling, prevention of oral mucosal infections, interventions to modify salivary gland dysfunction, reduction of iatrogenic and disease-related neutropenia, and prevention of mucositis.

A comprehensive patient examination is paramount to identify preexisting oral problems that have the potential to affect the course of cancer therapy. To satisfy the objectives of the examination, the following data must be obtained in patients at risk for oral complications: cancer diagnosis, medical history, dental history, dental charting, periodontal charting, appropriate radiographs, and nutritional status. Some clinicians may wish to include volummetric assessment of resting and stimulated whole saliva. Additionally, study models could be obtained where deemed appropriate.

Potentially complicating oral disease should be identified and corrected as early as possible before commencement of anticancer therapy. Significant problems include poor oral hygiene, third molar pathology, periapical pathology, periodontal disease, dental caries, defective restorations, ill-fitting prostheses, orthodontic appliances, and any other potential sources of irritation.

Sources of infection and irritation are important targets for early intervention. At the initial dental evaluation, all cancer patients should undergo thorough oral hygiene procedures, including root planing, scaling, and curettage. These procedures are beneficial in reducing the incidence of oral complications by removing bacteria that can result in local and systemic infection. The neutrophil and platelet count must be considered before any patient undergoes an invasive procedure. This intervention should be supplemented by daily plaque removal including tooth-brushing with a fluoride toothpaste and flossing, if this can be tolerated by the patient. Additionally, the use of topically applied fluorides and chlorhexidine mouth rinse has shown clinical benefit in the prevention and control of dental caries and plaque.

Dental foci may be potential sources for systemic infection and should be eliminated or ameliorated. Treatment may include dental extractions or endodontic therapy. Ideally, dental procedures, but especially dental extractions, should be completed at least 14 days before cancer therapy, if the patient's condition permits.

Most of the pretreatment as well as treatment protocols aimed at preventing or ameliorating oral complications of anticancer therapy require patient adherence to prescribed oral hygiene procedures. Patient and family education, counseling, and motivation are critical to the success of any preventive pretreatment strategy. The patient must be cognizant of the potential side effects of the anticancer regimen. The rationale for pretreatment strategies must be explained to encourage patient adherence to the therapy.

Bacterial and fungal surveillance cultures are not necessary for routine patient management. Suspicious lesions should be cultured. The use of prophylactic acyclovir should be considered in seropositive patients at high risk for reactivating herpes simplex virus infection, i.e., the bone marrow transplant patient and possibly other patients with prolonged, profound myelosuppression. The prophylactic use of acyclovir in patients who are at lower risk probably is not indicated and carries a low risk of development of acyclovir-resistant strains. Although acyclovir is a relatively safe drug, it may have side effects, including renal dysfunction and, rarely, central nervous system toxicity.

Salivary gland dysfunction is one of the most common sequelae of head and neck cancer treatment. At present, there are no agreed-upon pretreatment strategies to prevent or minimize xerostomia. However, studies are being conducted to evaluate various techniques, including radioprotective agents and drugs such as pilocarpine that can maintain or enhance salivary gland function during radiation. The latter approach appears to be the most promising for future clinical applications.

Pretreatment strategies to reduce iatrogenic and disease-related neutropenia in cancer patients are under investigation. A pilot trial of recombinant granulocyte colony stimulating factor (rhG-CSF) administered to patients during chemotherapy resulted in restoration of the neutrophil count and function and a decrease in severity of mucositis. Mucositis is a universal and often painful consequence of chemotherapy and radiotherapy to the head and neck. At the present time, there is no other agent that is effective in preventing therapy-related mucositis. Randomized clinical trials addressing this problem are in progress.

What Are the Most Effective Strategies for Management of Acute Oral Complications Occurring During Cancer Therapy?

Acute oral complications occurring during treatment are related to the type of cancer and forms of therapy. These problems have several different clinical presentations including: mucosal inflammation and ulceration of varying etiologies, oral candidiasis, viral and bacterial infections, dental or periodontal infections, and mucosal bleeding. Treatment of oral infections is important to reduce the debilitating symptoms associated with these lesions and to minimize the risk for developing systemic bacterial or fungal infections.

Mucosal Inflammation and Ulceration

Radiation therapy for head and neck cancer causes mucositis, which can progress from erythema to ulceration. Chemotherapy given in conjunction with radiation may accelerate the onset and increase the severity of radiation mucositis. No currently available drugs can prevent mucositis. Distinguishing radiation-induced mucosal changes from other similar appearing lesions is suggested by their occurrence within the radiation fields. Appropriate cultures and smears may be necessary to diagnose fungal infection in the presence of radiation mucositis. There are several alternative drugs for antifungal therapy; however, prolonged dental contact with nystatin solution, nystatin pastilles, or clotrimazole oral troches may lead to dental caries because they contain large quantities of sugar.

Chemotherapy that does not result in profound myelosuppression can nevertheless cause mucosal ulceration by directly damaging the epithelium. The most commonly associated agents are antimetabolites such as methotrexate, 5-fluorouracil, and purine antagonists. Antitumor antibiotics, hydroxyurea, VP-16, and procarbazine can also cause nonspecific mucosal ulceration.

Oral ulceration may be associated with the underlying cancer, particularly acute leukemias, and with severe neutropenia from any cause. In these cases, the diagnosis is dependent on recognizing the association and ruling out infection. In a high percentage of patients undergoing BMT, oral mucosal lesions may occur as part of acute or chronic graft-versus-host disease. These lesions may take several forms, including erythema, lichenoid change, ulceration, or hyperkeratosis. Therapy depends on management of the underlying disease.

There are also many untested topical oral preparations that claim to reduce the symptoms of oral mucositis. The efficacy and safety of these agents have not been established. Ingredients in these combinations have included: diphenhydramine hydrochloride, kaolin and pectin, magnesium sulfate, antacids, sucralfate, corticosteroids, dyclonine, and lidocaine hydrochloride. In patients having trouble eating because of severe oral mucositis, use of local and/or systemic pain control may be necessary.

Viral Infection

Herpes simplex virus (HSV) is the most common viral pathogen associated with oral lesions in patients receiving myelosuppressive chemotherapy or BMT. A large number of patients have had prior infection with HSV as evidenced by the presence of HSV antibodies in the serum of 30 to 100 percent of adults in the general population. Under conditions of immunosuppression, the latent virus often reactivated, leading to severe oral, and occasionally, disseminated infections. Approximately 50 to 90 percent of BMT patients who are seropositive for HSV will develop HSV infections, usually within the first five weeks after transplantation. Similarly, a large proportion of patients with acute leukemia or others receiving intensive chemotherapy will reactivate HSV during periods of immunosuppression.

In contrast to HSV infection in immune competent individuals, HSV infections in the immuno-compromised host are associated with severe ulcerations that may occur on any oral mucosal surface. In immuno-compromised patients, the mucositis associated with HSV is more painful, severe, and prolonged than mucositis uncomplicated by viral infection. HSV ulcerations may be the portal of entry for bacterial and fungal pathogens. In addition, the virus may cause esophagitis and, rarely, disseminated infection.

Herpes simplex infections are often difficult to diagnose on clinical grounds alone because it may be difficult to differentiate them from mucosal lesions of other etiologies. Due to the morbidity associated with HSV infections and because of the availability of effective antiviral therapy, it is advisable to obtain viral cultures in immuno-suppressed patients. Cytologic and newer diagnostic tests for the presence of viral antigens may be useful for rapid diagnosis of HSV infections. In patients in whom the presumptive diagnosis is oral HSV infection, it is reasonable to initiate therapy with either oral or intravenous acyclovir while awaiting the results of viral diagnostic tests. The intravenous route may be preferred in severe infections and in patients unable to take oral medications.

Oral Candidiasis

Several types of oral mucosal lesions are caused by overgrowth and infection by Candida species, including: *pseudomembranous candidiasis* (removable white plaques), *chronic hyperplastic candidiasis* (leukoplakia-like white plaques that do not rub off), *chronic erythematous candidiasis* (patchy or diffuse mucosal erythema), and *angular cheilitis*. Fungal cultures, potassium hydroxide, and gram-stained smears are helpful diagnostic tools. The white, raised, removable plaques of the pseudomembranous form of candidiasis are most obvious to the examiner. Diagnosis can be confirmed by a potassium hydroxide smear. These organisms may infect other sites in the gastrointestinal tract and cause esophagitis or diarrhea. In neutropenic patients, mucosal infection with Candida may lead to systemic infection.

Topical forms of therapy for oral candidiasis include nystatin and clotrimazole. Pseudomembranous candidiasis can usually be treated with topical nystatin. Lesions of chronic oral candidiasis usually require much longer treatment, especially in patients with severe chronic xerostomia resulting from head and neck radiation therapy. In more extensive infections, such as esophagitis, oral ketoconazole may be effective. For infections not responding to the above measures, a course of low-dose intravenous amphotericin B may be indicated. Disseminated candidiasis should be managed with intravenous amphotericin B.

Bacterial Infections

Bacterial organisms in the mouth can cause localized infections, including acute sialoadenitis of major salivary glands, periodontal abscess, pericoronitis, or other mucosal or dental infection. These problems usually require empirical treatment with selected antibiotics, but gingival and periodontal lesions usually require additional treatment by local debridement of bacterial plaques.

Systemic infection is a major cause of morbidity and mortality in neutropenic patients. In some cases, the oral cavity may be the portal of entry for bacterial pathogens. Whether a source of infection can be identified or not, empiric, broad spectrum antibiotic therapy must be initiated promptly in the febrile neutropenic patient. There are several different antibiotics or antibiotic combinations that may be appropriate in this setting. Because pseudomonas infections are associated with a high mortality rate in neutropenia, the empiric regimen should include antibiotics that adequately treat this organism.

Mucosal Bleeding

Mucositis due to any cause may be accompanied by oral bleeding, especially in severe thrombocytopenia caused by leukemia, lymphoma, or myelosuppression. Disseminated intravascular coagulation is another important potential cause of thrombocytopenia or hemorrhage in immuno-compromised patients. Severe thrombocytopenia may predispose patients to bleeding from routine mechanical oral hygiene procedures. In addition, these procedures may increase the risk of septicemia in patients with severe neutropenia. In these patients, dental plaque can be effectively managed by daily mouth rinsing with a chlorhexidine solution.

Strategies for Management of Chronic Oral Complications Following Cancer Therapy

Therapeutic modalities used in the treatment of malignancy can result in changes in healthy tissues arising long after treatment has been completed. These sequelae must be addressed for the remainder of the life of the patient.

Xerostomia is an example of such a problem in patients receiving therapy for head and neck or other forms of cancer. Total body radiation, and especially local radiation to oral structures, may irreversibly affect the production of saliva by both the major and minor salivary glands. The magnitude of this problem is dependent upon the radiation dose and volume of tissue exposed. Significant xerostomia is not as frequently encountered in patients treated with chemotherapy. Concomitantly administered medications such as psychotropic and antiemetic medications should be evaluated for their xerogenic potential.

Chronic graft-versus-host disease is associated with xerostomia. Painful lichenoid lesions can also develop in these patients and thus compromise therapy unless controlled by immunosuppressive therapy. Long-term cyclosporine can lead to gingival hypertrophy.

There are no widely employed diagnostic criteria to estimate the degree or extent of xerostomia. We are still primarily dependent upon subjective impressions by both patient and clinician. A dry mouth may affect speech, taste, nutrition, and the patient's ability to tolerate dentures or other oral prostheses. Saliva also contains antimicrobial compounds and is important in the mechanical removal of pathogens from the mouth. As a consequence of decreased saliva production, there may be an overgrowth of caries-producing organisms. This may have devastating effects on the dentition, even in individuals without prior history of dental caries. In addition, an increase in the frequency of candidiasis and in the severity of gingival/periodontal infections has been observed in some patients.

Management of chronic xerostomia involves a combination of strategies:

- Continuous maintenance of effective oral hygiene to reduce colonization and proliferation of oral pathogens.

- Use of water or saliva substitutes to keep the mouth moist.

- Stimulation of residual salivary parenchyma to produce more saliva.

Intensive oral hygiene methods and the use of an adequately protective topical fluoride are the most important methods of preventing the dental complications of xerostomia.

In terms of saliva substitutes, several preparations are being tested. Ideally, these should reduce patient discomfort, be long-lasting, and should substitute for salivary components that are necessary for the maintenance of mucosal and hard tissue integrity. There is a need for more effective preparations and more data on the long-term benefits of this form of therapy.

Sialogogues, such as pilocarpine and anetholetrithione, alone or in combination, are being tested to stimulate the formation of saliva. The data suggest that this approach benefits patients who have some residual functional salivary tissue, resulting in a steady increase in salivary flow and symptomatic improvement. These drugs appear to be well tolerated; side effects are minimal and readily controlled. The effectiveness of sialogogues in reducing the long-term ravages of xerostomia (e.g., radiation caries) has not been documented.

The long-term effects of radiation therapy to the head and neck region include obliterative endarteritis with resultant tissue ischemia and soft tissue fibrosis. These changes may progress with time and never resolve. Surgical wounds in the irradiated area heal poorly and chronic radiation ulcers may develop. Fibrosis of the muscles of mastication and the temporomandibular joint, while uncommon, may result in trismus. However, recurrent tumor must be ruled out.

Osteoradionecrosis (ORN), a relatively uncommon clinical event is a consequence of hypovascularity, the cytotoxic effects of radiation on bone-forming cells and tissue, and is associated with hypoxia of the affected bone. As a consequence, when bone is injured, it is unable to heal and becomes susceptible to secondary infection. This process can progress to pathologic fracture, infection of the surrounding soft tissues, and oral-cutaneous fistula formation. It is characterized by severe, constant pain. The risk of developing ORN is lifelong. Chemotherapy does not increase the risk of ORN.

The initiating injury resulting in ORN is frequently the extraction of a tooth from an irradiated mandible. For this reason, all teeth that might have to be removed should be extracted before starting radiation therapy. If clinical conditions permit, at least two weeks, and ideally three weeks, should be allowed for adequate healing between the extraction and the commencement of radiation therapy. Healthy teeth should be preserved. Dentures causing ulceration of the atrophic mucosa over the mandible can initiate ORN. Spontaneous ORN can also occur without any obvious injury to the irradiated mandible.

Traditional treatment of ORN with antibiotics and surgical debridement frequently fails with progressive involvement of the remaining mandible. The keystone of the treatment of ORN is the provision of adequate tissue oxygenation in the damaged bone. This is best done by using hyperbaric oxygen therapy (HBO). Multiple treatments are required. Early stages of ORN without fracture or fistulae may be cured by HBO alone. More advanced cases, in addition to HBO, require sequestrectomy or partial mandibulectomy with eventual bone grafting.

In the event that dental extraction is required following radiation, meticulous surgical technique and antibiotic prophylaxis are necessary. In those patients felt to be at particularly high risk of developing ORN, pre-extraction HBO should be considered. An alternative to postirradiation extraction is endodontic therapy.

Complications in the Pediatric Population

Oral complications arising from the treatment of cancer in children have characteristics in common with those observed in adults. However, because children are actively growing and developing, cancer treatment creates additional long-term problems unique to the pediatric patient. As modern therapy results in increasingly improved survival in a variety of pediatric cancers, long-term sequelae of treatment are beginning to emerge. Some reports indicate that the frequency of oral complications in pediatric patients may be higher than in adults. The nature and severity of these treatment sequelae depend on a number of factors: the type and location of the tumor, the age of the patient, the dose of radiotherapy, the aggressiveness of chemotherapy, the status of oral and dental health, and the level of dental care before, during, and after therapy.

Chronic problems involving target tissues are impaired growth and development of hard and soft tissues, which may result in orofacial asymmetry, xerostomia, dental caries, trismus, and a wide variety of dental abnormalities. The latter include delayed tooth eruption, altered dental root development with shortening and thinning of the roots, enamel opacities, enamel grooves and pits, small teeth, small crowns, and failure of tooth development and eruption. In teeth with underdeveloped roots secondary to cancer therapy, even minimal periodontal disease will result in early loss of teeth. In general, the principles in the preventive and active treatment of xerostomia, dental caries, and trismus in adults appear to be applicable to children. However, evaluation of the efficacy and long-term consequences of these various strategies has not yet been carried out on a large scale.

These children may have lifelong dental problems requiring periodontic, orthodontic, prosthodontic, or orthognathic procedures. Supervised, consistent oral care, meticulous hygiene, and a regular dental recall schedule (to uncover problems early and determine the need for dental intervention) are key to maintenance of dental health care in children cured of their cancer.

In addition, the emotional and psychological consequences of orofacial deformities and oral dysfunction in these children deserve more attention as increasing numbers survive.

The potential for development of secondary malignancies in these survivors is a serious delayed sequela of successful cancer therapy. Although a majority of secondary malignancies reported in children consist of leukemia or lymphomas, soft tissue and bone sarcomas can occur in irradiated sites. The possibility of secondary malignancies arising in these children should heighten the clinician's awareness of this problem.

Providing education and information to the patient and family is essential for maximum treatment compliance. Direct involvement of the family is thought to result in improved adherence to treatment protocols, thereby enhancing the quality of the patient's life.

The therapeutic team should be multidisciplinary and sensitive to the patient's emotional and physical needs related to the illness. Patients traumatized by the loss of normal oral function, the presence of pain, nausea, and impairment of eating, and a life-threatening illness can become depressed. The following preventive measures should be undertaken by the therapeutic team: provide information to increase the patient and family's understanding of the medical/oral condition, the treatment plan, and the consequences of treatment. Methods of educating the patient/family should be individualized based on the diagnosis and needs. Patience and positive reinforcement are important.

Conclusions and Recommendations

- All cancer patients should have an oral examination before initiation of cancer therapy.

- Treatment of preexisting or concomitant oral disease is essential in minimizing oral complications in all cancer patients.

- Prophylactic acyclovir is beneficial in selected patients to prevent herpes simplex virus reactivation.

- Precise diagnosis of mucosal lesions and specific treatment of fungal, viral, and bacterial infections are essential.

- Mucosal ulcerations should alert the cancer team to the risk of systemic infection.

- Currently, the best treatments for chronic xerostomia include regular use of topical fluorides, attention to oral hygiene, and sialagogues.

- Osteoradionecrosis can be prevented. When ORN is present, it is best managed with hyperbaric oxygen alone or with surgery.

- In the pediatric population, it is important to recognize the long-term consequences of radiation therapy that include the dental and developmental abnormalities and secondary malignancies.

- Studies of oral complications should be incorporated into ongoing and future cooperative clinical oncology group protocols.

- Disseminate information concerning oral complications of cancer therapies and develop strategies to assure adherence by health care providers with appropriate preventive measures.

- Develop and implement curricula relevant to oral complications of cancer therapy in schools of medicine, dentistry, dental hygiene, and nursing.

- Direct family involvement in patient care is encouraged for maximum treatment compliance.

Chapter 33

Salivary Gland Dysfunction as a Symptom of Cystic Fibrosis

Cystic fibrosis (CF), the most common fatal genetic disease of Caucasians in America today, affects some 30,000 U.S. children and young adults. Approximately one new case occurs in every 2,000 births, with 1,000 new cases of CF diagnosed every year. Every day, three people with CF die. There is no cure.

This lethal disease causes a buildup of thick, sticky mucus that results in chronic lung and digestive disorders that haunt victims all their lives. Males born with CF are often sterile. Although life expectancy has improved steadily, most victims of CF die of respiratory failure before the age of 30.

Chronic Lung and Digestive Diseases Mark CF

In a healthy person, the exocrine glands (glands with ducts) channel secretions such as sweat, saliva, digestive juices and mucus to different parts of the body. In a person with CF, the transport of sodium and chloride across cell membranes in the exocrine tissues is profoundly altered. Because water moves with salt across the cell membrane, disordered salt transport means lung secretions will contain less water. In addition, scientists have shown that the composition of mucus proteins is altered in CF. A possible new explanation is that transport is defective not only across the cell membrane but also across membranes of organelles, structures within the cells where the secreted proteins are processed. These malfunctions create the thick,

Extracted from: NIH Publication No. 92-3420.

jelly-like mucus that accumulates and clogs the ducts in the lungs, making breathing difficult, and leading to chronic cough and infection. Accumulated mucus in the pancreas interferes with digestive enzymes, often causing malnutrition. Sweat is excessively salty.

Former National Institute of Diabetes and Digestive and Kidney Diseases (NIDDK) researcher Dr. Paul di Sant' Agnese used that characteristic to devise the sweat test, the diagnostic standard for CF for almost 40 years. Genetic tests, recently developed on the strength of increasingly sophisticated techniques in molecular biology, now supplement the sweat test for diagnosis in both newborns and older children.

Looking at Salivary Function Relative to CF

The National Institute of Dental Research (NIDR) supports research relevant to cystic fibrosis through studies of factors involved in tissue inflammation and through research on saliva and salivary glands. The abnormal glandular secretions characteristic of CF include thick, sticky saliva that blocks salivary ducts, making them susceptible to infection. By studying normal salivary processes, NIDR investigators hope to determine the defective secretory mechanisms in persons with CF.

Investigators are focussing on the role of macrophages in the development of fibrous tissue and inflammation in the lungs, processes that are associated with cystic fibrosis. Macrophages are white blood cells that participate in certain immune functions and defend against infectious agents. The scientists showed that the alveoli (small sacs) in the lungs of CF patients contain large numbers of highly activated macrophages. These cells secrete increased amounts of inflammatory products such as interleukin 1 and transforming growth factor beta, which promote inflammation by recruiting other white blood cells to the lungs. The macrophages also enhance the development of fibrous tissue by stimulating connective tissue cells to grow and produce increased amounts of collagen, the protein of fiber. Understanding how inflammation occurs in the lung will enable scientists to develop improved agents for preventing or treating the inflammatory and fibrotic changes that damage the lungs of individuals with CF.

Like many body fluids, salivary secretion results from the equalizing forces of osmosis. Specialized sac-like acinar cells in the salivary glands pump salt from the blood into the gland and water follows osmotically. This fluid then flows down the salivary ducts to the mouth. In recent years, NIDR scientists have investigated the mechanism by which salt is secreted by the acinar cells. They have shown that a specific ion transport system located in the acinar cell membrane is mainly responsible for this process. The transporter pumps salt into the acinar cell, and this accumulation ultimately results in salt and fluid secretion.

In current studies, NIDR scientists have shown that activity of this transporter can be stimulated by chemical agents secreted by certain nerves. They suggest that drugs could be designed to mimic or enhance the effects of these naturally occurring agents and thus increase salivary excretion. Such drugs would be useful in patients suffering from decreased salivary flow caused by disease or by the many medications that affect saliva production. Significantly, these studies identifying the ion transport events that underlie the secretion of salt and, therefore, water in the salivary glands may also be helpful in defining the mechanisms by which mucus accumulates in the lungs of CF patients.

Cystic fibrosis is a disease of epithelial cells—cells that line both the internal and external surfaces of the body including the salivary glands. NIDR scientists are also focussing on how the movement of fluid through the salivary glands is regulated. During the past year, they carried out an extensive study of the characteristics of one type of cell receptor, the muscarinic receptor, that stimulates movement of fluid through the many types of epithelial cells. This study was conducted using acinar cells from rat parotid salivary glands, an excellent model of human parotid glands, one of the three pairs of salivary glands.

The study showed that a single muscarinic receptor in the cell of the parotid gland can link up with two distinct proteins, G proteins, involved in generating the message to move fluid (saliva) through the cells. One signal from the receptor controls two cell processes (driven by the two proteins): these allow for an increase in saliva flow and a simultaneous limitation in specific exocrine proteins released into the saliva. These exocrine proteins, which are present to protect oral tissues from harm, are found at high levels under resting conditions but are not as necessary during food consumption when large volumes of saliva are secreted to help form a food bolus and move it into the esophagus. By limiting the release of exocrine proteins, these signalling events enable the cell to concentrate its energy on producing the additional saliva needed when the food is ingested. Because the basic process of fluid movement is similar for all exocrine glands, these findings in the salivaries not only expand knowledge of normal secretory function, but also offer insight into what goes wrong in these glands of CF patients.

Chapter 34

Fever Blisters and Canker Sores

Fever blisters and canker sores are two of the most common disorders of the mouth, causing discomfort and annoyance to millions of Americans. Both cause small sores to develop in or around the mouth, and often are confused with each other. Canker sores, however, occur only inside the mouth—on the tongue and the inside linings of the cheeks, lips and throat. Fever blisters, also called cold sores, usually occur outside the mouth—on the lips, chin, cheeks or in the nostrils. When fever blisters do occur inside the mouth, it is usually on the gums or the roof of the mouth. Inside the mouth, fever blisters are smaller than canker sores, heal more quickly, and often begin as a blister.

Both canker sores and fever blisters have plagued mankind for thousands of years. Scientists at the National Institute of Dental Research, one of the federal government's National Institutes of Health, are seeking ways to better control and ultimately prevent these and other oral disorders.

Fever Blisters

In ancient Rome, an epidemic of fever blisters prompted Emperor Tiberius to ban kissing in public ceremonies. Today fever blisters still occur in epidemic proportions. About 100 million episodes of recurrent fever blisters occur yearly in the United States alone. An estimated 45 to 80 percent of adults and children in this country have had at least one bout with the blisters.

NIH Publication No. 92-247.

What causes fever blisters?

Fever blisters are caused by a contagious virus called herpes simplex. There are two types of herpes simplex virus. Type 1 usually causes oral herpes, or fever blisters. Type 2 usually causes genital herpes. Although both type 1 and type 2 viruses can infect oral tissues, more than 95 percent of recurrent fever blister outbreaks are caused by the type 1 virus.

Herpes simplex virus is highly contagious when fever blisters are present, and the virus frequently is spread by kissing. Children often become infected by contact with parents, siblings or other close relatives who have fever blisters.

A child can spread the virus by rubbing his or her cold sore and then touching other children. About 10 percent of oral herpes infections in adults result from oral-genital sex with a person who has active genital herpes (type 2). These infections, however, usually do not result in repeat bouts of fever blisters.

Most people infected with the type 1 herpes simplex virus became infected before they were 10 years old. The virus usually invades the moist membrane cells of the lips, throat or mouth. In most people, the initial infection causes no symptoms. About 15 percent of patients, however, develop many fluid-filled blisters inside and outside the mouth three to five days after they are infected with the virus. These may be accompanied by fever, swollen neck glands and general aches. The blisters tend to merge and then collapse. Often a yellowish crust forms over the sores, which usually heal without scarring within two weeks.

The herpes virus, however, stays in the body. Once a person is infected with oral herpes, the virus remains in a nerve located near the cheek bone. It may stay permanently inactive in this site, or it may occasionally travel down the nerve to the skin surface, causing a recurrence of fever blisters. Recurring blisters usually erupt at the outside edge of the lip or the edge of the nostril, but can also occur on the chin, cheeks, or inside the mouth.

The symptoms of recurrent fever blister attacks usually are less severe than those experienced by some people after an initial infection. Recurrences appear to be less frequent after age 35. Many people who have recurring fever blisters feel itching, tingling or burning in the lip one to three days before the blister appears.

What causes a recurrence of fever blisters?

Several factors weaken the body's defenses and trigger an outbreak of herpes. These include emotional stress, fever, illness, injury and exposure to sunlight. Many women have recurrences only during menstruation. One study indicates that susceptibility to herpes recurrences is inherited. Research is under way to discover exactly how the triggering factors interact with the immune system and the virus to prompt a recurrence of fever blisters.

What are the treatments for fever blisters?

Currently there is no cure for fever blisters. Some medications can relieve some of the pain and discomfort associated with the sores, however. These include ointments that numb the blisters, antibiotics that control secondary bacterial infections, and ointments that soften the crusts of the sores.

Is there a vaccine for fever blisters?

Currently there is no vaccine for herpes simplex virus available to the public. Many research laboratories, however, are working on this approach to preventing fever blisters. For example, scientists at the National Institute of Dental Research and the National Institute of Allergy and Infectious Diseases have developed a promising experimental herpes vaccine. In tests on laboratory mice, the vaccine has prevented the herpes simplex virus from infecting the animals and establishing itself in the nerves.

Although these findings are encouraging, the scientists must complete more animal studies on the safety and effectiveness of the vaccine before a decision can be made whether to test it in humans. The vaccine would be useful only for those not already infected with herpes simplex virus.

What can the patient do?

If fever blisters erupt, keep them clean and dry to prevent bacterial infections. Eat a soft, bland diet to avoid irritating the sores and surrounding sensitive areas. Be careful not to touch the sores and spread the virus to new sites, such as the eyes or genitals. To make sure you do not infect others, avoid kissing them or touching the sores and then touching another person.

There is good news for people whose fever blister outbreaks are triggered by sunlight. Scientists at the National Institute of Dental Research have confirmed that sunscreen on the lips can prevent sun-induced recurrences of herpes. They recommend applying the sunscreen before going outside and reapplying it frequently during sun

301

exposure. The researchers used a sunblock with a protection factor of 15 in their studies. Little is known about how to prevent recurrences of fever blisters triggered by factors other than sunlight. People whose cold sores appear in response to stress should try to avoid stressful situations. Some investigators have suggested adding lysine to the diet or eliminating foods such as nuts, chocolate, seeds or gelatin. These measures have not, however, been proven effective in controlled studies.

What research is being done?

Researchers are working on several approaches to preventing or treating fever blisters. As mentioned earlier, they are trying to develop a vaccine against herpes simplex virus. Several laboratories are developing and testing antiviral drugs designed to hamper or prevent fever blister outbreaks. Researchers also are trying to develop ointments that make it easier for antiviral drugs to penetrate the skin.

Acyclovir is an antiviral drug that prevents the herpes simplex virus from multiplying. The U.S. Food and Drug Administration has approved the drug for use in treating genital herpes, and is considering its approval for use in treating oral herpes. Researchers have found that acyclovir taken in pill-form reduces the symptoms and frequency of fever blister recurrences in some patients. In one study, 50 percent of patients who took four acyclovir pills daily for four months had no fever blister outbreaks. Before taking the drug, they had an average of one recurrence every two months. In separate studies, pills taken at the onset of symptoms or acyclovir cream applied to the blisters or to areas of the lip that tingled or itched were found to be only minimally effective. The long-term effects of daily oral doses of acyclovir are not known, nor are the effects the drug might have on an unborn child.

Basic research on how the immune system interacts with herpes simplex viruses may lead to new therapies for fever blisters. The immune system uses a wide array of cells and chemicals to defend the body against infections. Scientists are trying to identify the immune components that prevent recurrent attacks of oral herpes.

Scientists are also trying to determine the precise form and location of the inactive herpes virus in nerve cells. This information might allow them to design antiviral drugs that can attack the herpes virus while it lies dormant in nerves.

In addition, researchers are trying to understand how sunlight, skin injury and stress can trigger recurrences of fever blisters. They hope to develop methods for blocking reactivation of the virus.

Canker Sores

Recurrent canker sores afflict about 20 percent of the general population. The medical term for the sores is *aphthous stomatitis*.

Canker sores are usually found on the movable parts of the mouth such as the tongue or the inside linings of the lips and cheeks. They begin as small oval or round reddish swellings, which usually burst within a day. The ruptured sores are covered by a thin white or yellow membrane and edged by a red halo. Generally, they heal within two weeks. Canker sores range in size from an eighth of an inch wide in mild cases to more than an inch wide in severe cases. Severe canker sores may leave scars. Fever is rare, and the sores are rarely associated with other diseases. Usually a person will have only one or a few canker sores at a time.

Most people have their first bout with canker sores between the ages of 10 and 20. Children as young as 2, however, may develop the condition. The frequency of canker sore recurrences varies considerably. Some people have only one or two episodes a year, while others may have a continuous series of canker sores.

What causes canker sores?

The cause of canker sores is not well understood. More than one cause is likely, even for individual patients. Canker sores do not appear to be caused by viruses or bacteria, although an allergy to a type of bacterium commonly found in the mouth may trigger them in some people. The sores may be an allergic reaction to certain foods. In addition, there is research suggesting that canker sores may be caused by a faulty immune system that uses the body's defenses against disease to attack and destroy the normal cells of the mouth or tongue.

British studies show that, in about 20 percent of patients, canker sores are due partly to nutritional deficiencies, especially lack of vitamin B_{12}, folic acid and iron. Similar studies performed in the United States, however, have not confirmed this finding. In a small percentage of patients, canker sores occur with gastrointestinal problems, such as an inability to digest certain cereals. In these patients, canker sores appear to be part of a generalized disorder of the digestive tract.

Female sex hormones apparently play a role in causing canker sores. Many women have bouts of the sores only during certain phases of their menstrual cycles. Most women experience improvement or remission of their canker sores during pregnancy. Researchers have used hormone therapy successfully in clinical studies to treat some women. Both emotional stress and injury to the mouth can trigger outbreaks of canker sores, but these factors probably do not cause the disorder.

Who is susceptible?

Women are more likely than men to have recurrent canker sores. Genetic studies show that susceptibility to recurrent outbreaks of the sores is inherited in some patients. This partially explains why the disorder is often shared by family members.

What are the treatments for canker sores?

Most doctors recommend that patients who have frequent bouts of canker sores undergo blood and allergy tests to determine if their sores are caused by a nutritional deficiency, an allergy or some other preventable cause. Vitamins and other nutritional supplements often prevent recurrences or reduce the severity of canker sores in patients with a nutritional deficiency. Patients with food allergies can reduce the frequency of canker sores by avoiding those foods.

There are several treatments for reducing the pain and duration of canker sores for patients whose outbreaks cannot be prevented. These include numbing ointments such as benzocaine, which are available in drug stores without a prescription. Anti-inflammatory steroid mouth rinses or gels can be prescribed for patients with severe sores.

Mouth rinses containing the antibiotic tetracycline may reduce the unpleasant symptoms of canker sores and speed healing by preventing bacterial infections in the sores. Clinical studies at the National Institute of Dental Research have shown that rinsing the mouth with tetracycline several times a day usually relieves pain in 24 hours and allows complete healing in five to seven days. The U.S. Food and Drug Administration warns, however, that tetracycline given to pregnant women and young children can permanently stain youngsters' teeth. Both steroid and tetracycline treatments require a prescription and care of a dentist or physician.

Patients with severe recurrent canker sores may need to take steroid or other immuno-suppressant drugs orally. These potent drugs can cause many undesirable side effects, and should be used only under the close supervision of a dentist or physician.

What can the patient do?

If you have canker sores, avoid abrasive foods such as potato chips that can stick in the cheek or gum and aggravate the sores. Take care when brushing your teeth not to stab the gums or cheek with a toothbrush bristle. Avoid acidic and spicy foods. Canker sores are not contagious, so patients do not have a worry about spreading them to other people.

What research is being done?

Researchers are trying to identify the malfunctions in patients' immune systems that make them susceptible to recurrent bouts of canker sores. By analyzing the blood of people with and without canker sores, scientists have found several differences in immune function between the two groups. Whether these differences cause canker sores is not yet known.

Researchers also are developing and testing new drugs designed to treat canker sores. Most of these drugs alter the patients' immune function. Although some of the drugs appear to be effective in treating canker sores in some patients, the data are still inconclusive. Until these drugs are proven to be absolutely safe and effective, they will not be available for general use.

Chapter 35

Oral Thrush: A Type of Candidiasis

What is candidiasis?

Candidiasis is a name for several types of infection caused by germs (yeast) called *Candida*. When infection occurs in the mouth and causes creamy white, curd-like patches on the tongue or other oral surfaces, it is called **thrush**. If infection spreads deeper into the throat and affects the feeding tube (esophagus), it is termed **esophagitis**. *Candida* infection in the vagina is often called a **yeast infection** or **vaginitis**. Candidiasis of the skin affecting the armpits or groin has also been described.

Candida organisms are often present in small numbers in the mouth, gut, vagina, and skin of normal, healthy persons but may not cause symptoms of infection. A damaged immune system makes it easier for *Candida* to grow, as do many antibiotic medicines (for example, ampicillin) that kill bacteria which normally compete with *Candida* for growth. Diabetes mellitus and steroid therapy are other risk factors for candidiasis.

National Aids Treatment Information Project. Kaiser Family Foundation. http://www.kff.org/natip/candi.html/. The Henry J. Kaiser Family Foundation, based in Menlo Park, CA, is an independent health care philanthropy and is not associated with Kaiser Permanente or Kaiser Industries. The Foundation's work is focused on four main areas: health policy, reproductive health, HIV policy, and health and development in South Africa. The foundation also maintains a special interest in health policy and innovation in its home state of California. Contact: The Henry J. Kaiser Foundation, 2400 Sand Hill Road, Menlo Park, CA 94025. Telephone 415-854-9400. Fax 415-854-4800.

What is its significance in HIV disease?

Candidiasis affecting the mouth, vagina, foreskin of the penis, or moist creases in skin folds is a very common early sign of weakening of the immune system from HIV disease and is most often first seen when the T-cell count is between 200-500. *Candida* infection of the esophagus may occur in more advanced HIV disease.

What are the symptoms and signs of candidiasis?

Candidiasis in the mouth may look like creamy white patches similar to cottage cheese, red spots, or large areas of redness on the tongue and other surfaces. It may cause soreness or a bad taste or be without any symptoms altogether. Cracks and redness of the skin at the corners of the mouth may also occur. *Candida* esophagitis often produces discomfort or pain in the chest, especially when swallowing, and difficulty swallowing. *Candida* vaginitis typically causes irritation and swelling of the vaginal lips (labia), a thick white discharge, and discomfort at the front of the vaginal opening during urination. Candidiasis in skin folds may result in itching, redness or darkening, and discharge.

How is it diagnosed?

Most surface forms of candidiasis such as thrush are diagnosed by their typical appearance and response to treatment with antifungal medications. Clinicians can determine if vaginitis is caused by *Candida* by looking at vaginal discharge under the microscope. Discharge in the mouth or skin folds can also be examined in this manner. Occasionally cultures (growing *Candida* in the laboratory from samples of discharge or tissue) are performed, especially if treatment does not seem to be working. If candidal esophagitis does not respond to treatment, then diagnosis may require examination with an endoscope, a flexible instrument that is placed into the esophagus to visualize it and grasp small pieces of tissue for microscopic examination and culture.

How is candidiasis treated?

Since *Candida* is present throughout the environment, it is difficult to eliminate the organism completely from the body. The goal of treatment is to suppress *Candida* growth so that it does not cause symptoms or tissue damage.

Candidiasis treatment can be **topical** or **systemic**. Topical treatment means applying medication directly to the infected area using a **cream, suppository** (type of medicine that is inserted into the rectum or vagina), **liquid suspension**, or **troche/lozenge** (medicine that comes in a tablet that is dissolved in the mouth). For most forms of candidiasis, topical treatment will usually work well and should be tried before resorting to systemic treatment. **Nystatin, clotrimazole**, and **miconazole** are commonly prescribed topical drugs. Systemic treatment means taking pills or getting medicine through the vein (intravenous) in order to distribute it through the blood to all body tissue and organs. It is necessary for *Candida* esophagitis and other severe internal infections. **Ketoconazole** and **fluconazole** are commonly prescribed systemic drugs taken by mouth, and intravenous **amphotericin** is used to treat serious and resistant cases.

Often, especially in earlier stages of HIV infection, candidiasis will not recur after treatment is stopped. However, as HIV disease progresses and the immune system weakens, recurrences of candidiasis become more likely. It may be possible to control these by having topical medication at home and using it at the first sign of recurrence, or it may be necessary to use the topical medication daily to prevent recurrence. Systemic treatment of candidiasis may need to be started if topical medication does not effectively treat episodes and control recurrences. Resistance (infection that does not improve with treatment) may occur with the long term use of any of the topical or systemic medications.

Some patients have found that certain other treatments may help control candidiasis. These include gargling daily with an antiseptic mouthwash, using large amounts of garlic, drinking acidophilus bacteria culture or eating yogurt that contains live acidophilus, and applying yogurt directly into the vagina.

Chapter 36

HIV and Oral Health

Why Is Dental Care Important?

If you are infected with HIV, good oral health and regular dental care become more important. Many of the first signs of HIV appear in your mouth. Simple dental problems may become more serious when you have a weak immune system. These problems may be treated more easily when found early.

You should:

* Examine your face, neck, and mouth weekly
* Inform your dentist or physician of any changes in your face, neck, or mouth
* Inform your dentist of your medical history and HIV status
* Have frequent dental exams, cleanings, and prompt care
* Brush and floss daily or as recommended by your dentist.

Signs of HIV Infection in the Mouth

The more common oral problems found in persons with HIV or AIDS are described as follows. If these or any other oral problems occur, see your dentist.

Candidiasis (Thrush) is a fungal infection that most often occurs on the roof of the mouth and/or tongue. It may go down the throat. Features include:

- white, yellow, red, or red and white patches (may be wiped off)
- may occur as a split in corners of the mouth
- may have an odor
- may have pain on swallowing.

Treatment is with topical or systemic antifungal drugs. Candidiasis patches may return after treatment.

Hairy Leukoplakia is a painless and harmless rough, whitish area that is usually on the sides of the tongue and is seen mostly in persons with HIV. Unlike candidiasis, this area does not wipe away. This condition generally does not need to be treated and may go away by itself and reappear.

Kaposi's Sarcoma (KS) is a type of cancer that occurs most often in the roof of the mouth, gums, or skin of some persons with HIV. Features include brown, red, blue or purple, flat, raised or swollen areas which may vary in size from small to large (usually growing). KS is usually painless, unless infected. This condition may not need treatment. If treatment is required, antibiotics may be used if infected, or the condition may need chemotherapy, radiation, or surgery.

HIV Gingival (Gum) and Periodontal Problems

Gingivitis is inflamed, infected, or swollen gums that may not heal with routine dental cleanings. Features include a fiery red band of color along the gum line in an otherwise healthy mouth, and gums that may be sore and bleed easily.

Necrotizing Gingivitis is a painful infection which may destroy gums. This infection is characterized by gums that bleed easily, often between the teeth, very bad odor and bad taste in the mouth and the formation of ulcers or sores.

Necrotizing Periodontitis is a more severe form of necrotizing gingivitis in which the bone beneath the gum is exposed or destroyed. This usually affects one area of the mouth, but may occur in the whole mouth. The gums recede, exposing parts of normally covered teeth or bone.

Treatment for gingival (gum) and periodontal problems includes thorough, frequent, and deep scaling of the teeth, proper home care and brushing, and antimicrobial rinses by prescription. These problems must be treated or they will become more severe, and may need antibiotics and/or surgery.

Other Oral Problems

The following oral problems often appear in persons without HIV infection, but are more common or severe in persons with HIV.

Oral warts may occur in groups anywhere in the mouth and are caused by a virus. The warts appear as white or pink in the mouth, may vary from a small raised cauliflower-like growth to a larger raised area and may or may not be painful.

Herpes is a common contagious viral infection in persons with HIV that may occur anywhere in the mouth or on the lips (fever blisters), heals slowly and may reappear in the same area. It may occur as a group of small ulcers or sore that together form a large, painful ulcer. Treatment is topical or systemic antiviral medications by prescription.

Recurrent oral ulcers (canker sores) commonly occur on the inside of the cheeks and lips, but may be almost in the mouth or throat. They are round or oval sores with a bright red halo. These ulcers are painful and may take weeks or months to heal if not treated. Treatment includes topical cortisone-like ointment by prescription; or in severe cases, a systemic cortisone-like drug may be prescribed.

Examine Your Face, Neck and Mouth Weekly

As a person with HIV, you need to pay close attention to your face, neck and mouth. Once you learn how they normally look and feel, you will notice any change more easily.

- Feel for bumps on your face, neck or in your mouth.
- Note anything that seems different, unusual or painful.
- Check for puffy or bleeding gums.
- Look for red, white or purple spots in your mouth.
- Be aware of bad or funny tastes or odors, problems in chewing, swallowing or loose teeth.
- See your dentist or physician if you notice any changes or have any concerns.

Examine Your Face and Neck

Do both sides appear the same? With your hands, feel the right and left sides of your neck and under your jaw. Feel for any bumps.

Examine Your Mouth

Floor of Mouth: Touch the tip of your tongue to the back of the roof of your mouth and look at the floor of your mouth and underside of your tongue. Feel this area using your forefinger.

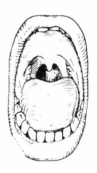

Figure 36.1. Examining the floor of your mouth.

Roof of Mouth: Say "AH" and tilt your head slightly backward to see roof of mouth. Use the forefinger to feel entire area.

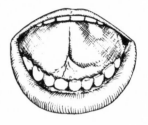

Figure 36.2. Examining the roof of your mouth

Tongue: Stick out the tongue and grasp end with a gauze square. Look and touch the top surface. Pull the tongue to the right and then to the left. Observe and touch each side.

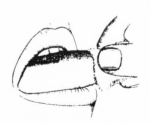

Figure 36.3. Examining your tongue

Cheeks: Pull your cheek away from the teeth. Keeping your mouth slightly closed, look at each cheek and feel them with your fingers.

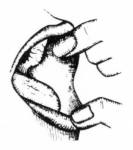

Figure 36.4. Examining your cheeks

Lip and Gums: Inspect your lips and gums by first looking at and feeling the outside. Pull the lower lip down and feel the inside and outside of your lip and gums. Repeat for the upper lip and gums.

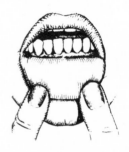

Figure 36.5. Examining your lips and gums

Remember, if you notice any changes, see your dentist.

Confidentiality

You should inform your dentist of your HIV status. This information is important for treatment decisions, the use of prescription drugs, and watching for changes in the mouth. If your dentist needs to discuss your oral problems with your physician, the dentist needs your written informed consent. There are laws to protect your confidentiality. Remind your dentist about keeping your HIV status confidential.

Discrimination

It is against the law to deny dental care to persons with HIV or believed to have HIV. If you have been treated unfairly or denied care because of your HIV status and live in the greater Boston area, call the HIV Dental Ombudsman Program.

The HIV Dental Ombudsman Program is a comprehensive dental access program for persons with HIV/AIDS in Greater Boston. The program is designed to remove or reduce barriers to oral health services for persons with HIV/AIDS by providing education, advocacy, referrals, and payment for treatment. This program is funded by Title I of the Ryan White CARE Act.

If you need a dentist, free telephone consultation or more information call or write:

HIV Dental Ombudsman Program
Division of Public Health
Boston Department of Health and Hospitals
1010 Massachusetts Ave.
Boston, MA 02118
(617) 534-4717

Other Important Resources Outside of the Greater Boston Area:

AIDS Action Committee of Massachusetts
(617)437-6200 or (800)235-2331

U.S. Public Health Service
Centers for Disease Control and Prevention (CDC)
National HIV/AIDS Hotline
(800)342-AIDS

—by Myron Allukian, Jr., DDS, MPH, Helene Bednarsh, RDH, MPH, and Lee Thornhill, Bureau of Oral Health Programs, Boston Department of Health and Hospitals, Joseph L. Konzelman, Jr., DDS, Henry M. Jackson Foundation, Walter Reed Medical Center, and assistance from Drs. David Rosenstein, Murray Bartley, and Gary Chiodo, Oregon Health Sciences University.

Chapter 37

Tongue Troubles: Strange Appearances Can Point to Problems in Your Health or Lifestyle

Stick out your tongue. What do you see? Chances are you see a velvety-pink muscular organ that helps you taste, chew, swallow and talk. But if you ever looked at your tongue and noticed red and white patches or what appeared to be black hair, no doubt you were surprised—maybe even a little frightened. Fortunately, most changes in the color or texture of your tongue aren't serious, and few adults may ever develop irregularities. Tongue disorders typically result from nutritional deficiencies, poor oral hygiene or use of some medications. Once the source of the problem is identified, simple treatment usually clears up the discomfort and unsightly appearance.

Most Common Conditions

Here are four of the most common problems that can affect your tongue, and how they're managed:

- **Geographic.** Normally, the surface of your tongue is dotted with tiny areas of raised pink tissue called papillae (puh-PIL-e). In geographic tongue, smaller papillae become white and less visible while other areas are smooth and red. The resulting appearance resembles a "map" of white and red patches that may change size and configuration daily. Although geographic tongue

©1995 Reprinted from October 1995 *Mayo Clinic Health Letter* with permission of Mayo Foundation for Medical Education and Research, Rochester, Minnesota 55905. For subscription information, call 1-800-333-9038.

is one of the most common tongue irregularities, only 2 percent of adults may ever develop it. Those that do may also have an inflamed and sore tongue. Others may have no symptoms at all except for the change in appearance. The cause is unknown. But it tends to occur in people with family histories of eczema, asthma or hay fever. The red and white patches usually disappear on their own in a few weeks to months. When necessary, a prescription anesthetic ointment and topical corticosteroid can help relieve the discomfort and inflammation.

- **Smooth.** Papillae shrink or disappear, making your tongue look shiny and thin. Your tongue may also be tender and sensitive to spicy foods. **Bald or atrophic** (uh-TROF-ik) are other descriptions of the wasting away appearance. The problem often occurs because of a prolonged nutritional deficiency of folic acid, iron, riboflavin or vitamin B-12. With adequate nutrition, symptoms generally begin to improve within two weeks. Your tongue should regain its normal appearance in a month. In the meantime, a prescription anesthetic ointment can help relieve the discomfort. Avoiding irritants such as spicy foods, alcohol and tobacco can also help.

- **Furred.** Instead of shedding naturally, dead skin cells build up on the papillae. The result is a white coating over most of your tongue that feels like fur. Poor oral hygiene is a common cause. Furring also tends to develop from use of antibiotics or tobacco, high fever of dry mouth associated with fasting. In some people with poorly fitting dentures or an inability to wear them, furring may be related to eating a low-fiber diet. You can eliminate the coating by gently brushing the surface of your tongue daily with toothpaste applied to a soft-bristled toothbrush.

- **Black hairy.** As in furred tongue, dead skin cells accumulate on the papillae. But in black hairy tongue, the matting is colored black by bacterial overgrowth down the middle of your tongue. Poor oral hygiene and dry mouth can cause excessive bacterial growth. But often, the buildup of bacteria is a side effect of medications, especially antibiotics, which may disrupt your mouth's balance of naturally occurring organisms. If so, black hairy tongue should improve once you finish your prescription. If you're on long-term antibiotic therapy, your doctor may be able to substitute another antibiotic that won't cause similar symptoms. Other factors that may discolor your tongue but not cause a hairlike appearance include tobacco and the metallic salt (bismuth) in Pepto-Bismol. Sensitivity to some mouthwashes and breath mints or enzymes in certain fruits, candies and red wine may also turn your tongue brownish-black. Brushing your tongue daily with a soft-bristled toothbrush and toothpaste or a solution of one part hydrogen peroxide to two parts water helps remove the buildup.

Be Reassured . . .

Tongue troubles usually aren't serious. Most of the time, the only treatment needed is tongue brushing. In fact, brushing your tongue daily along with your teeth is generally a good practice. It may just prevent your tongue from giving you trouble in the first place.

Chapter 38

Halitosis:
Battling Bad Breath

'Tis the season for crowded parties. Don't let bad breath spoil the small talk. Occasional bad breath is usually due to bacteria, certain foods or a dry mouth. To battle bad breath:

- **Brush and floss** after you eat. Good dental hygiene is the best way to prevent odor.

- **Brush your tongue.** Dry mouth that develops while you sleep allows dead cells to collect in your mouth and coat your tongue. Brushing your tongue is one more way to tame "morning breath."

- **Chew sugar-free gum.** The action stimulates flow of saliva to prevent dry mouth and to wash away food particles and bacteria.

- **Rinse your mouth with water.** Periodically swish your mouth with water to keep saliva flowing.

- **Avoid odor-causing foods and beverages.** Most likely offenders are garlic, onions, fish, milk, eggs, legumes, cabbage, broccoli, Brussels sprouts, coffee and alcohol.

©1994 Reprinted from December 1994 *Mayo Clinic Health Letter* with permission of Mayo Foundation for Medical Education and Research, Rochester, Minnesota 55905. For subscription information, call 1-800-333-9038.

- **Carry mouthwash or breath mints.** Not all mouthwashes fight bacteria, but they disguise bad breath. The strong oils in peppermint, spearmint or wintergreen also cover up odor.

When bad breath doesn't respond to self-care, ask your dentist to check for gum disease or poor-fitting dental work. See your doctor for a possible medical cause.

Part Five

The Jaw and
Other Structural Problems

Chapter 39

Temporomandibular Disorders: Aches and Pains from Flaws in the Jaws

Though an unseemly nickname, "The Great Impostor" aptly describes the jaw-motion maladies known as temporomandibular (TM) disorders. Indeed, the clicks, earaches, headaches, facial pain, and restricted jaw use that point to these disorders mimic symptoms of such other conditions as pinched nerves, sinusitis, mumps, and ear infections.

A decade ago, the Impostor was scarcely heard of. But today, hardly a week passes without a news story on this emerging facet of dentistry as cases are diagnosed and treated in increasing numbers. Also increasing, however, is concern about over- diagnosis and over-treatment, sometimes with unproven therapies. This is not a small concern: Temporomandibular (named for the bones that form the hinges of the jaw) disorders may afflict as many as 60 million Americans, says the American Dental Association (ADA).

Women between 15 and 44 appear to be most susceptible, though reported cases include both sexes in all age groups. About 5 percent of patients have severe, even disabling, symptoms that require extended care and, infrequently, highly specialized surgery. Fortunately, symptoms are usually mild and often disappear, even without therapy. To treat every noisy, aching TM joint would be "clinical overkill," as one researcher put it.

Disagreement over definitions, diagnosis, causes and treatments—and whom to treat—has prompted several national meetings. ADA,

FDA Consumer, June 1988, and extracts from NIH publication 94-3487, *TMD: Temporomandibular Disorders*.

for example, convened a consensus conference of experts in 1982 to develop preliminary guidelines for the screening, diagnosis and treatment of TM disorders.

TM Structures

A complex network of bones, ligaments, joints and muscles make up the specialized system by which we chew, yawn, and otherwise move the jaw.

"Temporomandibular" refers to the temporal bones and the mandible, or jawbone, which form the hinges that allow the jaw to move. The temporal bones join the jawbone at the sides of the head via fibrous tissue called ligaments, which form a capsule around the joint. Inside the capsule, firmly attached to the jawbone and the capsule, is a thin, cartilage-like, pliable oval disk. This disk separates the bones and forms compartments between itself and the bones: one compartment on its temporal-bone side and another on its jawbone side.

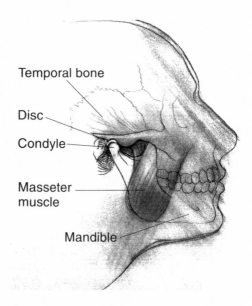

Figure 39.1. *The temporomandibular joint connects the lower jaw, called the mandible, to the temporal bone at the side of the head. If you place your fingers just in front of your ears and open your mouth, you can feel the joint on each side of your head. Because these joints are flexible, the jaw can move smoothly up and down and side to side, enabling us to talk, chew and yawn. Muscles attached to and surrounding the jaw joint control its position and movement.*

Within each compartment is a fluid-filled membrane or sac. The disk and membranes absorb shocks and lubricate the joint.

The TM joints can be felt at the front of the earlobes when the mouth is opened. Some jaw-moving muscles can be felt at the temples and cheeks when the teeth are clenched. Other muscles attached to the jawbone can be felt at the back of the roof of the mouth when the jaw is moved.

Opening and closing the mouth and moving the jaw forward, backward, and side to side require different types of motions in different joint compartments with different sets of muscles. These are essentially hinging and gliding actions.

Anything that interferes with the proper functioning of any part of this complex system of structures could result in a TM disorder.

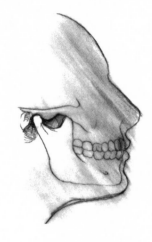

Figure 39.2. *When we open our mouths, the rounded ends of the lower jaw, called condyles, glide along the joint socket of the temporal bone.*

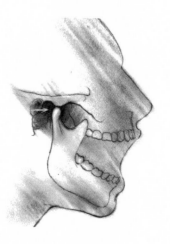

Figure 39.3. *The condyles slide back to their original position when we close our mouths. To keep this motion smooth, a soft disc lies between the condyle and the temporal bone. This disc absorbs shocks to the TMJ from chewing and other movements.*

Symptoms

Pain is the most frequently reported complaint with a TM disorder. "Usually it is a dull ache and often it is worsened or brought on during or after eating or yawning," writes Joseph Marbach, D.D.S., in *Executive Health Report*(September 1986). He notes:

- About 85 percent of patients feel pain on only one side—usually in the temple, cheek, and front of the ear.
- Half have pain in the neck muscles.
- More than a quarter have pain in the shoulder muscles.
- Nearly half feel the pain constantly or at least once a day.

Theories as to what produces the pain include pressure on nerves from misaligned bones in the TM joint, inflammation of the joint capsule, and muscle spasm. The fact that a spasm in one muscle, Marbach writes, can prompt chain-reaction spasms in nearby muscles "helps explain how an initial problem in the TM joint could spread to the neck, shoulders, and back."

Limited jaw movement, the other dead giveaway of a TM disorder, may result from such defects as disk displacement (nearly always forward of the jawbone) or abnormal tissue growth in the joint. Some experts cite the width of the first three fingers as the extent to which a normally functioning jaw should be able to open.

Also commonly reported are various joint noises, which may or may not be signs of a TM disorder. A click when opening the jaw may indicate a displaced disk, but many people have noises without having a TM disorder. A grating or crackling noise more likely signifies arthritis. Moreover, not all TM patients have joint noises. Joint noises without pain or restricted jaw movement would not be enough evidence for a diagnosis of a TM disorder.

It's unclear yet which symptoms are important as far as the need for treatment is concerned. "About a third of the general population have clicking," says Glenn Clark, D.D.S., M.S., co-director of UCLA's Temporomandibular Joint Facial Pain Clinic; "but only a few of these go on to develop locking or disk problems."

Complicating the difficulty in diagnosing a TM disorder is that symptoms may fluctuate: They may worsen, improve, recur or disappear completely. "Opening too wide to bite into a triple-decker sandwich or yawning," explains D. Gregory Singleton, D.D.S., of the Food and Drug Administration, "can overstretch the ligaments and muscles. But within a few weeks, they'll return to normal and the pain will simply go away." Singleton heads the review of dental devices, including those used to treat TM disorders, at the agency's Center for Devices and Radiological Health.

Causes

Clark attributes symptoms of TM disorders to causes that fall into five main areas: arthritis in the joints, clicking that develops into locking or disk disorders, muscle hyperactivity and strain, breakdown of the support provided by the teeth, and injury—as from an accident or even simply grinding the teeth.

Some researchers believe that TM disorders are the result of misaligned teeth. The guidelines from the 1982 consensus conference state: "Although the scientific literature has not shown that occlusal [bite] problems cause TM disorders, clinical data do confirm the two conditions frequently coexist, but the nature of the relationship between them is unclear at this time." In the February 1988 *Journal of the American Dental Association*, Stephen Vincent, D.D.S., M.S., and Gilbert Lilly, D.D.S., report that while "some studies have shown that malocclusion can cause bruxism [grinding the teeth], malocclusion might not correlate with TMJ disorders."

Some believe improperly applied orthodontic treatments, such as braces, can cause TM disorders. But as Vincent and Lilly state "There appears to be no *definitive* [emphasis added] correlation between orthodontic therapy and the signs or symptoms of TM dysfunction."

Types of TM Disorders

Despite unclear definitions—the use of different groups of symptoms, for instance, in different studies—and incomplete understanding about the natural course of most TM disorders, experts at the 1982 conference agreed on this "working" system to differentiate the disorders:

- **Chewing muscle problems.** This category includes the most common disorder, technically named myofascial pain dysfunction (MPD) syndrome. Muscle spasms, often from grinding teeth, create facial pain that may spread to nearby muscles. Among reported cases, women outnumber men by 3 to 1.

- **Disturbances in the joint's functioning.** The most common of these is said to be disk displacement due to stretching or tearing of the fibrous tissue attaching it to the joint capsule.

- **Problems due to injury.** An example is jawbone dislocation from a blow during a car accident. This is our only joint that can be dislocated without force from outside the body (from strained opening of the mouth, for example) notes Donald Rinchuse, D.M.D., M.S., M.D.S., Ph.D., in the June 1987 American Journal of Orthodontics and Dentofacial Orthopedics.

- **Degenerative joint disease.** (Called osteoarthrosis in its noninflammatory stage and osteoarthritis in its later inflammatory stage.) Fibrous and cartilage-like tissues wear away from the TM joint for reasons not fully understood. This can alter movement and create a crackling sound. Results of a study reported in the *British Dental Journal* in 1973 suggest untreated MPD syndrome is somehow related to subsequent osteoarthrosis in some people. Nearly half the participants previously had MPD in their osteoarthrotic joints.

- **Inflammatory joint disorders.** The membranes on the sides of the disk can become inflamed due to rheumatoid arthritis.

- **Chronic restricted jaw movement.** An example is fibrous ankylosis, in which fibrous tissue forms in the joint to reduce jaw movement. Untreated, it can eventually "freeze" the jaw.

- **Growth disorders of the joint.** The jawbone may continue to enlarge after growth should have stopped. This causes the bite and joint movements to become abnormal.

Diagnosis

An accurate, specific diagnosis requires thorough dental and medical histories. In 1982, ADA cited the dentist as the "primary therapist" to manage TM-disorder patients. (It is reasonable to ask about your dentist's experience in treating TM disorders and to get a second opinion before treatment is begun.)

The question "Do you grind your teeth?" will likely come up. Non-chewing gnashing, a common sign of stress, tires the muscles to set the stage for a spasm-pain-spasm cycle that can result in a TM disorder. A patient describes her case: "My new job was so stressful that I was literally grinding chips off my teeth. Then one morning, I woke up with an earache. I didn't connect the pain with my teeth. But when I went to my dentist about the grinding, he asked if I'd had any pain. He had me wear a custom-made mouth-piece day and night for nearly two months. Now I wear it just at night. If the aching comes back, I wear it more often until the pain goes away."

The patient may be asked whether the jaw gets "stuck," whether the bite feels uncomfortable or unusual, whether arthritis has been a problem, whether the pain seems to follow a pattern, and whether there was a blow to the jaw or head (joint inflammation from injury might not show up right away).

Gently feeling (palpating) the TM joints and muscles helps pinpoint areas with incoordinations or tenderness. Listening at the joints with a stethoscope during jaw movement helps differentiate noises. Casts of the teeth show the actual bite.

Radiological tests can provide useful information about the positions of the bones and other parts of the TM joints. (See "Radiological Tests for TM Disorders" below.) The decision to order such tests is a judgment call, thus emphasizing the importance of visiting a professional experienced in treating TM disorders. The 1982 consensus guidelines advise that X-rays are appropriate for initial screening and that, if additional tests are ordered, they should be "to rule out or confirm specific diagnoses."

Depending on the findings, further examination by a physician, orthodontist, oral surgeon, or TM specialist may be advised. A biopsy may be warranted if a tumor is suspected.

Beware of dubious diagnostic tests. One procedure of doubtful worth that is being promoted for diagnosing TM disorders is applied kinesiology, or muscle-strength testing. But the 1982 guidelines state that no scientific evidence supports the idea that applied kinesiology is a "reliable indicator of jaw dysfunction" or is useful to establish "proper jaw position or vertical dimension" or to help determine a patient's health status.

Radiological Tests for TM Disorders

More than one type of radiological examination may be needed to accurately diagnose a temporomandibular (TM) disorder. Ordinary X-rays, for instance, outline bones clearly, but they don't show soft tissue, such as ligaments. Computed tomography (CT) shows bones even better, but it isn't used initially because it's much more expensive and can expose the patient to considerably more ionizing radiation. Other tests(arthrography and magnetic resonance imaging (MRI))have their special benefits and drawbacks, too.

331

Ordinary X-rays

Views are taken to show the TM joint in several positions: with the teeth clenched, with the joint relaxed, and with the mouth fully opened. Estimated cost: $75.

- **Benefits**: Useful for initial screening to help detect obvious abnormalities when there is reason to believe that organic disease may exist.

- **Drawbacks:** Not definitive. Doesn't show soft tissue. Exposes the patient to ionizing radiation.

Arthrography

A dye is injected into the TM joint spaces so that, when a conventional X-ray picture is taken, certain parts of the joint show up in contrast. Estimated cost: $500.

- **Benefits:** Guidelines from a 1982 consensus conference convened by the American Dental Association advise using arthrography in two situations: when surgery is being considered because a disturbance to a joint's functioning has not responded to prolonged conservative treatment and when a displaced disk is the suspected cause of painful limited opening of the mouth.

- **Drawbacks:** Requires a high degree of skill to perform. Uncomfortable for the patient because it may cause momentary pain and tenderness and swelling afterwards. Allergic reaction to the dye is possible. A surgical procedure. Exposes the patient to ionizing radiation.

Computed Tomography (CT)

The picture-taking part of a CT machine moves around the patient to take views of the bones and muscles from many different angles. The information is entered into a computer, which creates an image of a cross-sectional "slice" of the area. Estimated cost: $500.

- **Benefits:** Shows bone detail better than X-rays and MRI. Can be manipulated to show some soft tissue, such as the TM joint disk. Does not involve surgery.

• **Drawbacks:** May be misinterpreted. In several patients, for example, an increased joint space seen with CT and interpreted to be a displaced disk was shown with arthroscopy to be, in fact, abnormal tissue on the temporal bone due to degenerative joint disease. Can expose the patient to more ionizing radiation than conventional X-rays.

Magnetic Resonance Imaging

Using giant magnets and radiowaves, MRI involves taking views of the desired area from different angles that are then entered into a computer to produce a picture "slice" of the area similar to a CT scan. The patient is actually moved via a table inside the machine. Estimated cost: $800.

• **Benefits:** Clearly displays details of the disk and other soft tissue. Involves neither surgery nor ionizing radiation.

• **Drawbacks:** Most costly. It may not be available locally.

Most insurance companies offer plans that cover these diagnostic tests for TM disorders, according to the Health Insurance Association of America, but whether an individual's plan includes such coverage depends on whether that person's employer has contracted for it.

Treatments

More than 26 therapies are in use, by one estimate, and treatment is given not only by dentists, physicians, and oral surgeons but also by persons outside traditional dentistry and medicine, such as psychologists and chiropractors. The consensus guidelines call for "a *scientific* [emphasis added] basis for establishing a treatment . . . and testing its efficacy." And they state that no scientific evidence supports the effectiveness of osteopathic and chiropractic manipulations for TM disorders.

Whenever possible, state the guidelines, TM-disorder therapies should be conservative and reversible. Such measures bring symptomatic relief to 80 percent of the patients. Therapy usually lasts about three months.

Treatment of muscle spasms may include a prescription relaxant drug such as diazepam (trade name: Valium), moist heat, massage, and a soft diet. Over-the-counter aspirin, ibuprofen or acetaminophen may be given for the pain. Aspirin and ibuprofen are also anti-inflammatory drugs and, so, are used for arthritis, too. FDA's Center for Drug Evaluation and Research has approved a number of prescription analgesic and anti-inflammatory drugs for patients requiring stronger treatment. If inflammation persists, corticosteroids may be injected into the joint, provided there is no infection.

When grinding causes the spasms, a bite appliance can be used to help the patient hold the upper and lower teeth apart. The plastic device may be formed from a cast of the person's teeth so it fits precisely to reposition the jaw, allowing the muscles and ligaments to rest. Wires on each side fasten the appliance over the teeth and allow it to be attached and removed easily.

If chewing patterns become altered from damage caused by the grinding, the bite may become skewed. To restore alignment, the dentist may file selective teeth, fill or crown damaged teeth, or replace missing teeth.

Counseling, relaxation training, or biofeedback may help if stress is a problem. In biofeedback, electrodes taped to the skin transmit impulses made by the tensing muscles to a computer screen. The idea is that relaxing the muscles is easier when the patient can see the impulses diminish with the tension.

Surgery

When surgery is advised, it's reasonable to seek a second or even a third opinion. A good place to ask about TM specialists, says Clark of UCLA, is the nearest university with a dental or medical program.

"Surgery is appropriate initial treatment when a tumor must be removed," he says, "or when there is severe jaw immobility, which may mean the joint has fused. But these are uncommon occurrences."

If nonsurgical therapies have failed to give relief and if the cause of the problem can indeed be corrected or reduced by surgery, other operations are appropriate, says Clark. "A disk that has caused the jaw to lock may be repaired or repositioned." If the disk can't possibly be repaired and it's causing severe pain or locking the jaw, it can be removed,' he says, "but this would be a last resort."

An outpatient surgical procedure called arthroscopy is being investigated for use on the TM joint. A specially trained surgeon makes a tiny incision and inserts a very thin, lighted tube called an arthroscope. Through this tube, the surgeon can visually examine the area, flush it out, perform a biopsy, remove scar tissue called adhesions, or manipulate a locked displaced disk back where it belongs.

This was already being done in larger joints, says Clark, "but the knee, for instance, is 8 to 10 times larger than the TM joint, and we just haven't had the smaller instruments until now. We need more trained people to do this "

Reversible and Conservative Treatment

The key words to keep in mind about TMD treatment are "conservative" and "reversible." Conservative treatments are as simple as possible and are used most often because most patients do not have severe, degenerative TMD. Conservative treatments do not invade the tissues of the face, jaw or joint. Reversible treatments do not cause permanent, or irreversible, changes in the structure or position of the jaw or teeth.

Because most TMD problems are temporary and do not get worse, simple treatment is all that is usually needed to relieve discomfort. Self-care practices, for example, eating soft foods, applying heat or ice packs, and avoiding extreme jaw movements (such as wide yawning, loud singing and gum chewing) are useful in easing TMD symptoms. Learning special techniques for relaxing and reducing stress may also help patients deal with pain that often comes with TMD problems.

Other conservative, reversible treatments include physical therapy you can do at home, which focuses on gentle muscle stretching and relaxing exercises, and short-term use of muscle-relaxing and anti-inflammatory drugs.

The health care provider may recommend an oral appliance, also called a splint or bite plate, which is a plastic guard that fits over the upper or lower teeth. The splint can help reduce clenching or grinding, which eases muscle tension. An oral splint should be used only for a short time and should not cause permanent changes in the bite. If a splint causes or increases pain, stop using it and see your practitioner.

The conservative, reversible treatments described are useful for temporary relief of pain and muscle spasm-they are not "cures" for TMD. If symptoms continue over time or come back often, check with your doctor.

There are other types of TMD treatment, such as surgery or injections, that invade the tissues. Some involve injecting pain relieving medications into painful muscle sites, often called "trigger points." Researchers are studying this type of treatment to see if these injections are helpful over time.

Surgical treatments are often irreversible and should be avoided where possible. When such treatment is necessary, be sure to have the doctor explain to you, in words you can understand, the reason for the treatment, the risks involved, and other types of treatment that may be available.

Scientists have learned that certain irreversible treatments, such as surgical replacement of jaw joints with artificial implants, may cause severe pain and permanent jaw damage. Some of these devices may fail to function properly or may break apart in the jaw over time. Before undergoing any surgery on the jaw joint, it is very important to get other independent opinions.

Other irreversible treatments that are of little value-and may make the problem worse-include orthodontics to change the bite; restorative dentistry, which uses crown and bridge work to balance the bite; and occlusal adjustment, grinding down teeth to bring the bite into balance.

Although more studies are needed on the safety and effectiveness of most TMD treatments, scientists strongly recommend using the most conservative, reversible treatments possible before considering invasive treatments. Even when the TMD problem has become chronic, most patients still do not need aggressive types of treatment.

Vitek Recall

The Food and Drug Administration has recalled artificial jaw joint implants made by Vitek, Inc., which may break down and damage surrounding bone. If you have these implants, see your oral surgeon or dentist. If there are problems with your implants, the devices may need to be removed. Persons who have Vitek implants should call MedicAlert at 1-800-554-5297 for more information.

The Bottom Line

Expert after expert calls for long-term, controlled studies toward more conclusive information about TM disorders, including why most reported cases are among women 15 to 44.

Meanwhile, how can a person guard against the Great Impostor?

Good dental care is a start. Problems related to the teeth and how they fit together should be identified and treated early on. An example is when a missing tooth such as a molar isn't replaced, says FDA's Singleton. "The muscles will ultimately overpower the teeth," he says, "causing the molar behind to tip into the space. Then the tooth above gradually changes the way it meets the lower tooth, which can stress the chewing muscles. This can cause a spasm, or cramp, which causes pain, which can lead to further spasms. To regain the original relationship, the tipped-over tooth must be straightened with braces and a bridge made to fill the space."

Being aware that there are different TM disorders and that most cases will improve or go away with little or no treatment helps, too. But if symptoms persist more than three or four weeks, says Singleton, "it's a good idea to seek professional advice from someone experienced in the field. Most important is an accurate diagnosis. Minor temporary ailments, like stretched ligaments, must be differentiated from chronic problems, like arthritis or muscle spasms associated with bruxism. Every possibility must be explored to correctly identify contributing factors and to rule out others, so that any treatment given is both necessary and specific to the diagnosis."

— by Dixie Farley

Dixie Farley is a member of FDA's public affairs staff.

Chapter 40

Jaw Pain: How to Navigate the Treatment Mine Field

Introduction

A tiny hinge between the jaw and the skull has become a battle-ground for practitioners who can't agree on how to treat it when it acts up. And for many patients with an aching or balky jaw, the temporomandibular joint, as it's called, has become a field of agony both physical and financial.

Embedded in an intricate web of nerves and muscles, the jaw joint, like any other, is vulnerable to disease or injury; it must also absorb the enormous forces created by chewing and teeth gritting. Because the mouth is part of the emotionally expressive muscle system of the face, tension tends to funnel itself into that region. Sometimes the alignment of the teeth and jaw interferes with the joint's smooth operation, or the cartilage disk that cushions the joint is displaced or wears out. It's estimated that 10 to 20 million Americans, mostly women, report a wide array of distressing symptoms: pain in the jaw muscles or in front of the ear, clicking or popping sounds in the joint, locking, difficulty chewing or talking, dizziness, headaches, neck pain, even backaches.

Treating orofacial pain has become a big business; consumers spend $32 billion annually seeking relief, and temporomandibular disorder (TMD) accounts for much of this. But TMD, also known as TMJ (temporomandibular joint) syndrome, is also often misdiagnosed and overtreated.

©1993 *American Health*. Reprinted with permission.

As many as 25 different types of practitioners, including general dentists, orthodontists, oral and maxillofacial surgeons, chiropractors, nutritionists, physical therapists, pain specialists and psychologists, treat TMD. Yet many disagree about what causes it and what to do about it. "About 40 percent of Americans have some form of TMD," says Dr. James Fricton, co-director of the TMD and orofacial pain division at the University of Minnesota, "but only 5 percent to 10 percent have a problem that warrants treatment."

The widely divergent views of how to treat this complex disorder are an open invitation to inadequately trained or even disreputable practitioners, who have found TMD to be a veritable gold mine. According to Dr. John Dodes, president of the New York chapter of the National Council Against Health Fraud, "TMD still remains the hottest area of out-and-out quackery in dentistry. Patients with vague pain in remote parts of the body have been erroneously diagnosed with TMD; they've even been told that a bad bite causes menstrual cramps or impotence."

Most practitioners treat TMD in good faith, says Dr. Z. Annette Iglarsh, a physical therapist affiliated with the University of Maryland Dental School in Baltimore. "Yet many patients walk out traumatized by the experience. They end up with enormous bills and are a physical mess."

What Causes TMD

Ever since ancient times, doctors have had theories about the ills that afflict the hardworking jaw. Even today, a person seeking help may still encounter an array of practices dating from the 1930s, when the characteristic clicking and popping sounds in the joint led to the theory that TMD was entirely a mechanical problem, caused by a bad bite. Back then, dentists went to work altering the dental landscape by capping or grinding down the teeth or even breaking and resetting the jaw to "re-balance" the mouth.

Then came the explanation that TMD was just a behavioral problem, generally affecting stressed-out career women who grind and clench their teeth. In the 1980s, magnetic resonance imaging (MRI) offered a clear view of the joint and gave impetus to surgery to repair the disk, whether needed or not. (One often overused form of TMD surgery is arthroscopy, a minimally invasive procedure that enables surgeons to reach and repair the disk via tiny scopes). Postural and hormonal imbalances are among other fashionable explanations for the disorder. Today, all these approaches continue to have proponents and, unhappily, consumers in search of pain relief may bounce about among various experts, each devoted to his own school of thought.

In fact, according to Dr. Harald Löe, director of the National Institute of Dental Research in Bethesda, MD, the term TMD actually encompasses a wide range of neurological, muscular, behavioral and mechanical disorders with no single cause or single treatment. These disorders can be broadly divided into three categories.

- Disorders of the muscles used for opening and closing the jaw and for chewing clenching or grinding the teeth (bruxism) can cause muscle spasm or strain, as can pencil chewing, poor dental work (ill-fitting fillings or crowns), singing or yawning.

- Disorders in and around the joint, including inflammatory conditions, degenerative diseases such as arthritis and dislocated or worn jaw disks. If untreated, the ligaments and tissue surrounding the joint can become inflamed.

- Disorders of the cranial bones and jaw, ranging from fractures to congenital and developmental deformities, such as a severe overbite.

Other symptoms—general stress, a bad bite or posture that strains the neck and facial muscles—are now thought in many cases to be secondary problems caused by TMD. There is one exception; people who grind or clench their teeth often do so because they are tense. If the underlying stress is treated, these bad habits usually disappear along with the muscle problems they cause.

Current research tends to focus on the joint itself. Scientists report that some TMD patients have low levels of the natural lubrication fluid that keeps all the body's joints in working order. They've also found suspiciously high levels of pain transmitters in the jaw joints of TMD patients, as well as enzymes and other substances that cause inflammation and destruction. And because roughly 85 percent of those who seek treatment for jaw pain are women in their childbearing years, some researchers have suggested that hormones such as estrogen may stretch the ligaments that operate the jaw.

Treatment

No matter the cause, once jaw pain starts, patients may find themselves in a diagnostic tangle. When do tense jaw muscles lead to changes in the joint? And how does a chronic joint problem affect jaw muscles? "That's the $64,000 question," says Dr. Steven Syrop, director of the TMD clinic at the Columbia University School of Dental and Oral Surgery, "and it has created continued controversy over how we diagnose and treat these disorders."

Syrop and other experts advise patients to take a team approach, including consulting a dentist, a neurologist, a physical therapist and a psychologist. A TMD workup should include a thorough medical history and physical exam, a psychological/behavioral questionnaire and, when necessary, x-rays, as well as CT or MRI scans, to examine the disk and rule out a tumor.

But many critics are particularly skeptical of costly electronic diagnostic machines that purport to establish the correct position for the jaw as a prelude to orthodontic treatment to adjust the teeth to match it. A patient's jaw position, in fact, may be incorrect, says Dr. Norman Mohl, a professor of oral medicine at the State University of New York at Buffalo, but the machine cannot provide accurate information about what the correct position should be.

Once a diagnosis is made, Syrop recommends "comprehensive, conservative and reversible" therapy, which initially rules out such irreversible procedures as jaw surgery (repairing or replacing the disk or joint with synthetic or cartilage implants, for example) or orthodontics to alter the bite; A sizable number of people with clicking jaws and other symptoms have no need of major treatment; many need no treatment at all. As for children, only a tiny percent require treatment; any work that will alter the bite should wait until the child's facial bones and teeth have fully developed.

Reversible Methods of Treatment

In general, muscular problems can be safely treated with simple jaw exercises, heat packs, muscle-relaxing drugs and anesthetic sprays to stop spasms, a soft diet to ease muscle strain, and stress reduction to ease tooth grinding and clenching. Inflammation responds to corticosteroids and other anti-inflammatory drugs; pain can often be controlled with low doses of anti-depressants.

Many dentists prescribe plastic mouth guards, or stabilization splints, which fit over the upper or lower teeth. These devices, usually worn at night, keep the jaws apart and decrease grinding and clenching. Today a key part of treatment is physical therapy. Patients are taught jaw and tongue exercises to retrain stressed muscles, and they are given relaxation and posture exercises to eliminate strain on the head, neck and facial muscles.

Some physical therapists use transcutaneous electrical nerve stimulation, known as TENS, or various forms of electrogalvanic stimulation to help relax muscles, as well as ultrasound treatment to promote tissue healing. "Unfortunately," says Iglarsh, "these devices are commonly mis-prescribed by dentists, who use them as a single treatment, instead of incorporating them into a comprehensive program of exercise and stress reduction."

Irreversible Treatment Methods

If the jaw pain is caused by a displaced disk, the dentist may try to realign it and retrain stretched muscles and ligaments with a re-positioning splint made of hard plastic. One type of device used for this purpose is known as a MORA (mandibular orthopedic repositioning appliance). MORA's come in many varieties and should be worn for only a few months. But often they're prescribed inappropriately, adjusted improperly or worn too long. Such misuse misaligns the jaws and wears down the teeth so that expensive corrective dental work or braces may be required.

If the disk or the ligaments holding the disk are torn, an oral surgeon may recommend surgical repair. But before going ahead, get a second opinion, advises Dr. Larry Wolford, a clinical professor of oral and maxillofacial surgery at Baylor University in Dallas. Sometimes if you wait three to six months, the joint will adjust itself, developing scar tissue in place of the injured disk. But in other cases, says Wolford, surgery may turn out to be the most appropriate solution.

Consumers in search of treatment may find out that practitioners differ even on how they define conservative or comprehensive care. "It depends on whom you talk to," says Terrie Cowley, co-director of the TMJ Association a patient advocacy group in Milwaukee. "Even the experts don't agree on who's an expert."

One reason for the diagnostic confusion and the many treatments is that the American Dental Association has not established guidelines for diagnosis and therapy. In addition, the overall quality of TMD dental research is poor. Dr. Alexia Antczak-Bouckoms, an assistant clinical professor of dentistry at Harvard's School of Dental Medicine, says that of more than 4,000 international reports she examined for the upcoming NIH report, she found that fewer than 1 percent were based on randomized controlled studies, and that even many of these were flawed in design. In fact, she adds, "there was no consensus on diagnosis or even on what getting better means."

Even the Food and Drug Administration (FDA) admits that monitoring dentistry has been a low priority with the agency until now, though this policy may change. Pressure from advocacy groups such as Ralph Nader's Public Citizen, together with the airing of congressional hearings last summer about unsafe Teflon and silicone jaw joint implants, has led the FDA to warn manufacturers not to market synthetic dental implants until long-term studies have been completed.

Meanwhile, consumers are left to protect themselves from unnecessary, expensive and possibly harmful treatment. "Remember," says Columbia's Syrop, "in matters involving a painful jaw, less may be best." Syrop offers consumers the following advice:

• Avoid any practitioner who believes in only one approach.

• As a rule of thumb, seek help from practitioners affiliated with a university dental or medical school.

• Choose a multidisciplinary team (a dentist, a neurologist, a physical therapist and, if necessary, a psychological counselor). If other specialists are recommended, make sure they share the same TMD philosophy. Different approaches can produce mixed results.

• Get a specific diagnosis.

• Ask your practitioners about the goal of each treatment.

• Don't hesitate to get a second opinion, or even a third, if you're uncertain of your practitioner or the treatment prescribed.

• Try reversible treatments first: physical therapy, heat packs, eating soft food, cutting stress and eliminating bad habits like chewing pencils or grinding teeth. You might also consider wearing a stabilizing mouth guard at night to rest your jaws and muscles (the device should be checked periodically).

• If you use a mouth repositioning appliance, remember that it should be used for only three or four months at a time and then reassessed.

• Keep written records and copies of your file and x-rays.

One Woman's TMD Nightmare

Paula Beaulieu's ordeal began in 1978 with a simple set of braces to close a gap in her front teeth. Over time, she developed painful clicking in her jaw and severe headaches, subsequently diagnosed as temporomandibular joint disorder (TMD). After years of treatment and 20 surgical procedures, including two jaw implants, Beaulieu, now 40, is unable to wrinkle her forehead or raise her eyebrows; one eye closes with difficulty; her smile is lopsided—and sometimes she is in severe pain. "I'm lucky—at least I have a face," Beaulieu says.

Beaulieu is one of an estimated 150,000 people who received synthetic (often Teflon or silicone) implants to replace the jaw disk or the entire joint between 1973 and 1990. In 1989, the Food and Drug Administration (FDA) declared Teflon implants unsafe. In 1991, the products were seized and the patients notified.

When first diagnosed with TMD, Beaulieu went to a dental clinic at the University of Colorado, where a variety of therapies were prescribed. "Splint therapy was a total failure. It only made my pain worse," she says. "Biofeedback was a joke." In 1981, she had surgery to repair dislocated right and left disks. It didn't work.

In 1985, blinding headaches forced her to seek help from a TMD "expert" who sent her to a psychiatric pain specialist. "He made me feel like my father was to blame for my jaw problems," says Beaulieu. Eventually, an oral surgeon determined that the right disk was torn and suggested replacing it with a Teflon-coated device. "My doctor said this implant would revolutionize TMD treatment and that I'd never need surgery again," Beaulieu recalls. When the pain persisted over the next three years, her surgeon told her, "it's healing pain."

But x-rays told a different story. The Teflon portion of the implant had disintegrated into a fine powder and had lodged in the surrounding tissue and bone. By 1988, her surgeon had replaced the broken device on her right side with muscle grafts from her temple and inserted a silicone implant into the left side to "balance" the jaw. Over the next 13 months, Beaulieu required five more operations to replace failed muscle grafts and clean out mysterious growths caused by the Teflon powder. "I began contemplating suicide," she says.

In 1989 Beaulieu started studying to become a dental assistant. "I couldn't beat the doctors, so I decided to join them." Reading the medical literature, she learned what her own oral surgeon had failed to tell her: many patients' Teflon implants were disintegrating, and patients' immune systems were destroying the body's own tissue and bone in response to foreign material. Similar problems, though to a lesser degree, were occurring with silicone jaw implants.

In 1990, unable to open her mouth wider than the width of a fingertip, Beaulieu found a small study reporting success with an all-metal joint and disk implant. After complete replacements of both joints with metal devices and reconstructive surgery, her teeth now touch and she can talk clearly for the first time in years. But she still needs nightly treatment with pain-killers, anti-inflammatory drugs and mouth-stretching devices; her bills have topped $200,000.

In June of 1992, Beaulieu testified at congressional hearings on dental devices. Both Teflon and silicone devices had slipped through an FDA loophole that exempts from testing products similar to those already on the market.

Today few people know that Teflon implants may disintegrate and should be removed before they do; broken silicone implants should also be taken out. Many oral surgeons, fearful of litigation, simply aren't telling their patients, says Jeanine Gisvold, a California attorney who organized a lawsuit against the implant manufacturer.

Beaulieu, who now lives in Oregon, sees no end to her problems. "As long as Teflon is in my body—and experts say it's unlikely it can be completely removed—my problems will continue. Still," she adds, "I'm 100 percent better than I was."

People with Teflon or silicone implants who want more information should call Medic Alert, the FDA's implant registry (800)554-5297, the TMJ Implant Patient Support Network (504)TMJ-7400, or contact TMJ Association, which you can do by writing to:

TMJ Association
6418 W. Washington Blvd.
Milwaukee, WI 53213

(414) 259-3223.

—*by Cathy Sears*

Cathy Sears edits the Dental Care Section at *American Health*.

Chapter 41

Orthognathic Surgery

Orthognathic surgery refers to the surgical repositioning of the maxilla (upper jaw), mandible (lower jaw), and the dentoalveolar segments (teeth) to achieve facial and occlusal balance. One or more segments of the jaw(s) can be simultaneously repositioned to treat various types of malocclusions and jaw deformities. This type of surgery requires a thorough preoperative analysis and detailed treatment plan. The preoperative evaluation includes a photographic analysis and a complete orthognathic work-up including cephalometric and panorex radiographs, dental impressions, and models. This is done by the Pedodontist/Orthodontist in coordination with the Craniofacial Surgeon. All findings are analyzed and pre-surgical model surgery performed to ascertain the feasibility of various treatment options. Additionally, computer analysis may be done pre-surgically by the Craniofacial Surgeon to simulate surgical results, thereby facilitating proper planning of the case and to help educate the patient and family. Computer analysis can provide the craniofacial team with visual information and numerical data that is the compilation of many time-consuming calculations such as those used in various cephalometric analyses.

Usually, pre-surgical orthodontics are necessary to straighten the teeth and align the arches so that a stable occlusion can be obtained postoperatively, while orthodontics following surgery are frequently required to revise minor occlusal discrepancies. Orthognathic surgery is often delayed until after all of the permanent teeth have erupted unless, medical conditions necessitate that the surgery be performed earlier. In adult patients, orthognathic surgery can be combined with soft tissue contouring to improve the aesthetic results.

Maxillary advancement is a type of orthognathic surgery that may be necessary to improve the facial contour and normalize dental occlusion when there is a relative deficiency of the mid-face region. This is done by surgically moving the maxilla (upper jaw) with sophisticated bone mobilization techniques and fixing it securely into place. For most patients, the use of screws and miniplates have replaced wiring of the bone and teeth required to hold the jaw stable. Inlay bone grafts can be utilized for space maintenance and secured with screw and plate fixation, while onlay bone grafting is used to augment the bony skeleton and improve facial soft tissue contour.

Depending on the soft tissue profile of the face, or the severity of an occlusal discrepancy, problems with the lower face may require surgery on the mandible (lower jaw). This can be done in conjunction with or separate from maxillary surgery. The mandible can be advanced, set back, tilted or augmented with bone grafts. A combination of these procedures may be necessary. Preoperative planning is crucial to the success of the procedure and evaluates the surgical and orthognathic options. The surgeon chooses the type of mandibular surgery based on his experience, evaluation of the photographic and cephalometric analysis, and model surgery. Following any significant surgical movement of the mandible, fixation may be accomplished with miniplates and screws or with a combination of interosseous wires and intermaxillary fixations (IMF— wiring teeth together). Rigid fixation (screws and plates) has the advantage of needing limited or no IMF. However, if interosseous wiring is used, IMF is maintained for approximately six weeks. Nutritionally balanced, blenderized diets are important for proper healing in the patient in IMF.

The chin is an important component of the facial profile as well as the attainment of aesthetic balance. The position and projection of the chin should be evaluated in patients considering orthognathic and facial soft tissue contouring procedures. Photographic and cephalometric analysis help determine the amount of change necessary to obtain a well-balanced face. The chin can be augmented with such alloplastic materials as silicone, polyethylene or hydroxyapatite. However, most craniofacial surgeons prefer a sliding horizontal osteotomy genioplasty. This procedure gives a natural contour to the chin when larger changes are needed and avoids the risk of infection with extrusion that goes along with alloplastic implants.

Orthognathic surgery not only improves function but can change the soft tissue contour and balance of the cheek, nose, lips and chin. This type of surgery can make dramatic improvements in facial appearance and self esteem.

—by Larry A. Sargent, M.D.

Larry A. Sargent is Professor of Plastic Surgery, and Director, Tennessee Craniofacial Center at the University of Tennessee, Chattanooga, TN.

Chapter 42

Information about Treacher Collins Syndrome (Mandibulofacial Dysostosis)

What Is Treacher Collins Syndrome?

Treacher Collins syndrome is the name given to a birth defect which may affect the size and shape of the ears, eyelids, cheek bones, and upper and lower jaws. The extent of facial deformity varies from one affected individual to another. A physician named Treacher Collins was one of the first to describe this birth defect. "Syndrome" refers to the group of deformities which characterizes affected individuals. Another commonly used medical name for this syndrome is "mandibulofacial dysostosis."

Questions and Answers about Treacher Collins Syndrome

What causes it?

This syndrome is caused by an abnormality in the genes. If both parents are normal, that is showing no signs of the syndrome themselves, this abnormality is the result of a change in the genetic material at the time of conception. The exact cause of this change is not known. If one parent is affected, the abnormal gene is then known to have been contributed by that parent.

©1991 Cleft Palate Foundation. Reprinted with permission.

Does this mean that this can happen again in my family?

If both parents are normal, the chances of a second child being born with this syndrome are extremely small. However, if one parent is affected, the chance that any pregnancy will result in a child with Treacher Collins is one out of two (50 percent risk). For this reason, it is very important that both parents of an affected child be thoroughly examined before any recurrence risks are quoted to them.

If my child, who has Treacher Collins, marries and has children, will all the children have it too?

No. The risk is 50 percent for each pregnancy.

What are the risks that my other children will transmit this syndrome to their own children?

If your other children are normal (showing no signs of the syndrome), there is no increased risk to their children. If another family member shows any feature of the syndrome, the occurrence risk for each pregnancy is 50 percent.

Will my child be mentally retarded?

There is no evidence that mental retardation is a feature of this syndrome. Hearing loss, however, is present in most affected individuals, to some degree. Early diagnosis and treatment of the hearing loss can prevent associated developmental and educational handicaps.

Will my child be deaf?

The term "deaf" applies only to very severe hearing losses in which the nerves for hearing, in the ear or the brain, do not function properly. The hearing loss in Treacher Collins syndrome is due to abnormalities in the structures of the outer and middle ear which conduct sound to the nerve endings in the inner ear. Thus, the loss in Treacher Collins syndrome is usually termed "conductive" and in the majority of affected children it is not of sufficient severity to be termed "deafness." However any degree of hearing loss may affect the development of speech and language and ability to succeed in school.

Problems Associated with Treacher Collins Syndrome

First, Treacher Collins syndrome, like nearly all birth defects, varies in severity from patient to patient. In fact, some cases are so mild that they are never recognized unless they are seen by specialists experienced in making such a diagnosis. In other children, the physical abnormalities of the face and ears are much more obvious and functional problems may develop.

Second, both the oral cavity (mouth) and the air passage (nose and throat) tend to be small in persons who have this syndrome. This may produce problems for the affected infant with breathing and feeding. You should be on the alert for such problems. If your infant has difficulty breathing or feeding, or has weight loss or poor weight gain, discuss your observations and concerns with your child's primary care provider or craniofacial center. Some children who have severe breathing difficulties require an operation to improve breathing and/or feeding.

Third, cleft palate is a frequently associated conditions this syndrome. Cleft palate itself sometimes can cause feeding problems and increase the risk of middle ear problems. Your child's primary care provider or cleft palate or craniofacial center can assist you with management of feeding problems

The next concern after breathing and feeding is hearing. The hearing loss in Treacher Collins syndrome is usually bilateral (meaning that both ears are affected) and, while it is not severe enough to be termed "deafness," it is severe enough to affect the ability to hear the human voice. Hearing levels can and should be measured. Depending upon the results of the testing, your child may be fitted with a hearing aid to restore his/her access to the world of sound. An early childhood program of speech and language therapy may also be recommended.

The fact that a hearing loss is present does not mean that your child will be dependent upon sign language. The great majority of children with this syndrome do learn to talk. However, there are several features of the syndrome, besides the hearing loss, which can affect speech and language development. Particularly in the severely affected child, the size and position of various structures inside the month (e.g., the relationship of the upper and lower teeth) may affect the ability to learn certain speech sounds will be delayed until the cleft is closed and its function restored.

You can facilitate your child's speech and language development by:

- seeking early evaluation by a specialist in hearing (an audiologist) and a specialist in communication development (a speech/language pathologist), and

- following their advice with regard to the need for a hearing aid and for early therapy programs.

The specialists most prepared to evaluate and manage your child are those who are members of a multidisciplinary craniofacial team.

Other Areas of Development: Social, Educational, Etc.

The facial deformity and need for treatment of Treacher Collins syndrome may create problems in family and social relationships, in school adjustment, and so on. The craniofacial center may have a psychologist or social worker, or the center can refer you to someone for evaluation and counselling if needed. Remember that children with Treacher Collins syndrome, like all other children, are individuals. They vary in social adjustment, academic achievement, and in their ability to cope with adults. The professionals of craniofacial centers try to maximize each child's potential by offering early diagnosis and treatment when indicated.

Treatment

- First, as explained above, your child may need a hearing aid and this can be determined in the first few months of life.

- Second, an early childhood program for speech and language stimulation may be recommended.

- Third, if a cleft palate is present, the craniofacial team will advise you on the optimum timing for surgical closure of the cleft.

- Fourth, reconstructive surgery is available to improve the appearance of the face. The craniofacial center will advise you on what to expect from such surgery and on optimum timing. Since not all children are affected to the same degree, both the necessity and the outcome of reconstructive surgery vary from child to child.

What Should I Be Doing for My Child Now?

Be certain that the diagnosis is correct. Treacher Collins syndrome shares some features with other syndromes, and not all physicians are aware of this. For this reason, you are best advised to locate a craniofacial center where genetic consultation, evaluation, and treatment planning will be provided by an experienced multidisciplinary staff composed of representatives from a variety of medical, dental, and other health care specialties. You may not have such a center in your locality, but the care your child will receive will be more than worth the inconvenience of traveling to another city. Finally, meet other individuals with similar deformities and their families by joining a parent patient support group.

To obtain a list of craniofacial centers and/or parent/patient support groups in your region, please contact the:

Cleft Palate Foundation
1218 Grandview Avenue
Pittsburgh, PA 15211

(412)481-1376
(800)24-CLEFT

Chapter 43

Facial Reconstruction in Treacher Collins Syndrome

Treacher Collins syndrome (also called mandibulofacial dysostosis and Franceschetti Syndrome) is a highly complex disease process. The basic etiology is unknown, but it is generally thought to be inherited as an autosomal dominant trait with variable penetrance. It is characterized by hypoplasia of the facial bones, especially the zygoma and the mandible. Facial clefting causes this hypoplastic appearance, with possible deformities or deficiencies of the ear, orbital, mid-face, and lower jaw regions. The clinical appearance is a result of the zygoma (malar bone) failing to fuse with the maxilla, frontal, and temporal bones. Highly variant degrees of involvement (complete, incomplete, and abortive forms) can be seen, but common facial features may include:

- Hypoplastic cheeks, zygomatic arches, and mandible,
- Microtia with possible hearing loss,
- High arched or cleft palate,
- Macrostomia (abnormally large mouth),
- Anti-mongoloid slant to the eyes,
- Colobomas,
- Increased anterior facial height,
- Malocclusion (anterior open bite),
- Small oral cavity and airway with a normal-sized tongue,
- Pointed nasal prominence.

The craniofacial team's geneticist should evaluate all Treacher Collins patients and their families to determine if the disease has been caused by inheritance of a family trait or as the result of a spontaneous gene mutation. If the disease has been inherited by one child in a family, there is a 50 percent chance that the parents will give birth to another involved child. If neither parents nor other family members are affected and a child is born with the condition, then a mutation has occurred. There is a 50 percent chance that this child will pass the trait on to future generations. Fortunately, genetic advances and careful prenatal screening have made Treacher Collins syndrome extremely rare.

An extensive array of complications can affect treatment. Because of the small jaw and airway, combined with the normal size of the tongue, breathing problems can occur at birth and during sleep for a child with Treacher Collins syndrome when the base of the tongue obstructs the small hypopharynx. This situation can cause serious problems during the induction of general anaesthesia. Consequently, a tracheostomy may be required to adequately control the airway. Learning and speech difficulties can also occur depending on the degree of conductive hearing loss common in the syndrome. Learning disabilities can potentially create a significant social stigma for the child. As with other disfiguring conditions, assessing and treating the psychological needs of the Treacher Collins patient is a vital function of the true craniofacial center.

Treatment of the hard and soft tissues of the face can require a number of surgical interventions, the first being the correction of the eyelid coloboma in the first years of life (depending on the severity). The next stage is orbital reconstruction with calvarial bone grafts and correction of the lateral canthal displacement. Multi-stage ear reconstruction follows at about 5-7 years of age. Correcting the lower face and jaws involves close coordination between the craniofacial surgeon and the pedodontist/orthodontist, with orthodontic intervention beginning with the eruption of the patient's permanent teeth. After the teeth are aligned to their proper axis (or as closely as is possible), treatment of the lower face then involves orthognathic surgery to reposition the mandible and the maxilla, usually done during the patient's teen years. This can be a one- or two-step procedure. The combined procedure involves rotating the mid-facial segment around a transverse axis at the frontonasal angle (for severe maxillary hypoplasia) and lengthening the mandibular ramus. For less severe cases, a LeFort I type osteotomy technique is used to lower the maxillary tuberosities along with a ramus lengthening procedure for the mandible. As the child's face continues to grow, additional procedures may be required to correct any developing deformities. Complimentary procedures such as rib cartilage grafts on the zygoma, closure of the macrostomia, and secondary genioplasties are performed according to individual cases. A well-planned treatment regimen can produce excellent results with the ultimate goal being the complete restoration of form and function, thus enabling the patient to adapt to a "normal" way of life.

—by Larry A. Sargent, M.D.

Larry A. Sargent, M.D. is Professor of Plastic Surgery, Chattanooga Unit, University of Tennessee College of Medicine Medical Director, Tennessee Craniofacial Center Chattanooga, Tennessee.

Chapter 44

Information about Pierre Robin Sequence

What Is Pierre Robin Sequence?

The term Pierre Robin Sequence is given to a birth defect which involves an abnormally small lower jaw (micrognathia) and a tendency for the tongue to "ball up" and fall backward toward the throat (glossoptosis). Robin Sequence patients may or may not have cleft palate, but they do not have a cleft lip. While the current complete name is "Pierre Robin Malformation Sequence," it has also been known as "Cleft Palate, Micrognathia and Glossoptosis," "Robin Anomalad," "Pierre Robin Complex," and as "Pierre Robin Syndrome." The condition was first described in 1822 and is named after the French physician who associated the above problem with breathing problems in affected infants.

What Causes the Condition?

The immediate cause of Robin Sequence seems to be the failure of the lower jaw to develop. During prenatal development the small jaw seems to prevent the tongue from descending into the oral cavity and so the palate may not close completely. This sequencing of events leads to the classification of this condition as a malformation sequence. The exact reason for the failure of development of the lower jaw remains unknown. To date there is no evidence that it is due to abnormalities of genes or chromosomes or to factors such as drugs, x-rays, or maternal diet.

Pierre Robin Sequence is an uncommon condition. It occurs no more frequently than once in every 8,000 live births and may occur as infrequently as once in every 30,000 live births. In contrast, cleft lip and/or palate occurs once in every 700 to 800 live births.

Will Future Children Be Affected?

The parents' risk of having another child with this or other similar condition is commonly considered to be within the 1 percent to 5 percent range for parents who already have one child with this condition. However, there have not been enough large scale family studies for geneticists to provide exact risk predictions. There are a number of conditions, most commonly Stickler Syndrome, that also includes the features of Robin Sequence. The recurrence risks for these syndromes are not the same as for Robin Sequence. Consequently it is extremely important that the diagnosis of Robin Sequence is confirmed by an experienced medical geneticist, preferably one associated with a multidisciplinary craniofacial team.

Problems Associated with Pierre Robin Sequence

It is important to remember that Pierre Robin Sequence, like most birth defects, varies in severity from child to child. Thus some children may have many more problems than other children with the same diagnosis. Problems in breathing and feeding in early infancy are most common. Parents are advised on how to position the infant in order to minimize problems (i.e., not place the infant on his/her back). For severely affected children, positioning alone may not be sufficient and the pediatrician may recommend specially designed devices to protect the airway and facilitate feeding. Some children who have severe breathing problems require a surgical procedure to ease their breathing.

Other problems include possible congenital heart murmur and eye defects. The pediatrician will also carefully monitor the baby for ear disease. Virtually all babies with clefts of the palate are prone to build-ups of fluid behind the eardrum. If untreated this could lead to mild or moderate (but reversible) loss of hearing. Since this could affect speech and language development, the baby needs to have his/her hearing monitored from early infancy by audiologists who specialize in testing infants and small children.

Treatment

Fortunately the small mandible (lower jaw), that is so noticeable when the infant is born, grows rapidly during the first year of life. In some children the jaw may grow so rapidly that by the time the child is approximately six years of age, the profile looks normal. Some minor differences in the shape of the jaw do remain, but are not noticeable except on x-rays of the head. Because of this "catch-up" growth, some children do not require surgery on their jaw. The cleft palate, however, needs to be surgically closed. In some children this surgery is delayed to take advantage of growth which may tend to narrow the opening in the palate. Because children with a cleft of the palate are at higher risk for delayed or defective speech development, their speech development should be monitored by a Speech Pathologist during their early years. If speech is not progressing adequately then the child can be enrolled in speech therapy.

Since children with Pierre Robin Sequence may have problems in a number of areas, parents are well advised to locate a craniofacial center where evaluation and treatment planning will be undertaken by an experienced multidisciplinary staff composed of health care professionals from many different specialties. If such a center is not located in your city or town, it may be well worth the inconvenience to travel to another city for your child's appointments. To obtain a list of Teams treating Craniofacial Anomalies, contact the:

Cleft Palate Foundation
1218 Grandview Avenue
Pittsburgh, PA 15211

(412)481-1376
(800)24-CLEFT

Chapter 45

Information about Crouzon Syndrome (Craniofacial Dysostosis)

What Is Crouzon Syndrome?

Crouzon syndrome, also called craniofacial dysostosis, is one of many birth defects in which there is abnormal fusion (joining between some of the bones of the skull and of the face). This fusion does not allow the bones to grow normally, affecting the shape of the head, appearance of the face and the relationship of the teeth. Crouzon was a doctor who described a patient with a characteristic group of deformities (syndrome) which were then observed in other individuals.

Crouzon syndrome is caused by an abnormality in the genes. If both parents are normal, that is showing no sign of the syndrome themselves, this abnormality is the result of a change in the genetic material at the time of conception. The exact cause of this change is not known. If one parent is affected, the abnormal gene is then know to have been contributed by that parent.

If both parents are normal, the chances of a second child being born with Crouzon syndrome are extremely small. However, if one parent is affected, the chance that any pregnancy will result in a child with this syndrome is one out of two (50 percent risk). For this reason, it is very important that both parents of an affected child be thoroughly examined before any recurrence risks are quoted to them.

Questions and Answers about Crouzon Syndrome

If my child, who has Crouzon Syndrome, marries and has children, will all the children have it too?

If your other children are normal (not showing signs of the syndrome), there is no increased risk to their children. If another family member has the syndrome, the occurrence risk for each pregnancy will be 50 percent.

Will my child be retarded?

There is no data to indicate that mental retardation is a regular feature of this syndrome. Development should be evaluated periodically and if any concerns regarding mental function arise, appropriate referral for testing should be made.

What to Expect

Like most birth defects, Crouzon syndrome varies in severity from patient to patient causing more problems in some than others. For a complete evaluation, optimum treatment planning, and comprehensive services, we advise you to contact a craniofacial center. At such a center, an experienced multidisciplinary staff composed of representatives from different health care specialties will assist you with care as well as in anticipating and meeting problems.

You should watch for any sign of ear disease and hearing loss, since research indicates that individuals with Crouzon syndrome may be quite vulnerable to ear problems. For an infant, the specialists at the craniofacial center can assess hearing in the early months of life. Hearing should be monitored as your child grows. While many children with Crouzon syndrome develop speech and language normally, some do not. The speech pathologist at the craniofacial center assesses speech and language development at regular intervals and will advise you if therapy is indicated.

Some individuals with Crouzon syndrome have problems with dry eyes, excessive tearing, or muscle balance (strabismus). A screening eye examination by an ophthalmologist (eye doctor) should be obtained and any problems treated as they arise.

The major problem for individuals with Crouzon syndrome is underdevelopment of the upper jaw. This produces facial deformity (bulging eyes and sunken middle third of face) and malocclusion (abnormal relationship between the upper and lower jaws). Dental and plastic surgery specialists monitor facial growth and correct deformities.

The facial deformity and need for treatment of Crouzon syndrome may create problems in family and social relationships, school placement, and so on. The craniofacial center may have a psychologist or social worker, or can refer you to one for evaluation and counselling if needed. Remember that children with Crouzon syndrome, like all other children are individuals. They vary in social adjustment, academic achievement, and in their ability to cope with adults. The professionals at craniofacial centers try to maximize each child's potential by offering early diagnosis and treatment, when indicated.

Other specialties represented on the team vary somewhat from center to center. If your child has needs or problems requiring other specialties, you will be referred to them as needed.

Treatment

The need, extent and timing for treatment of the deformities of Crouzon syndrome depend upon how severely the individual is affected and the age. For the infant, surgery may be required to release and reshape the bones of the skull, so that they may grow more normally. Orthodontics, to straighten the teeth, and jaw surgery, to place the teeth in a more normal position, may be done in childhood, the teens or even the adult years. These are complicated operations which are usually performed by specially trained craniofacial surgeons associated with major craniofacial centers.

What Should I Be Doing for My Child Now?

First, be certain that the diagnosis is correct. Crouzon syndrome resembles several other syndromes, and not all physicians are aware of this. A geneticist can provide the necessary evaluation and information. Second, locate a craniofacial center. You may not have a center in your city but the care your child will receive will be more than worth the inconvenience of travelling to another city. Third, meet other individuals with similar deformities and their families by joining a parent/patient support group.

To obtain a list of craniofacial centers and/or parent/patient support groups in your region, please contact the:

Cleft Palate Foundation
1218 Grandview Avenue
Pittsburgh, PA 15211

(412)481-1376
(800)24-CLEFT

Chapter 46

Information about Choosing a Cleft Palate or Craniofacial Team

Throughout the United States there are many qualified health professionals caring for children with cleft lip and palate as well as other craniofacial defects. However, because these children frequently require a number of different types of services which need to be provided in a coordinated manner over a period of years, you may want to search for an interdisciplinary team. Such a team can coordinate and implement all or most of these services through one central facility. When you are selecting a team, here are some points to consider:

1. Number of different specialists actually participate in the team.

    The more extensive the group of specialists who participate on the team, the more likely every aspect of treatment can be considered during the team evaluation. You should ask how many of the following are represented on the team:

    *   Plastic Surgeon
    *   Pediatrician
    *   Otolaryngologist
    *   Geneticist/Dysmorphologist
    *   Audiologist
    *   Speech Pathologist
    *   Orthodontist

Cleft Palate Foundation 1990.

- Pedodontist
- Prosthodontist
- Oral Surgeon
- Psychologist
- Social Worker
- Nurse

If your child has a craniofacial defect, then the team you choose may also include the following:

- Neurosurgeon
- Ophthalmologist

2. Qualifications of the individual members on the team.

You should inquire if all the members of the team are fully trained and appropriately certified in their areas of specialty, as well as licensed. This may become an issue that will also affect insurance coverage.

3. Experience of the team.

In general, the quality of care increases with the amount of experience the team has. You should ask how often the team meets and approximately how many patients are seen at each meeting. You may also want to try to determine how long this group of professionals has been meeting as a team and also how much experience the various individual professionals have had.

4. Location of the team.

The distance of the team from your home may NOT be an important consideration in choosing a team, in general, the team will be seeing your child only periodically throughout his/her growing years. Usually routine treatment such as general dental care orthodontics, speech therapy, and pediatric care will be provided by professionals in your own community who will be in regular contact with professionals on the interdisciplinary team. Thus; your travel to a team will usually be limited to several trips a year or even once a year. If a larger, more experienced team is available a few hours away, this may be preferable to a less experienced local team.

5.   Affiliation of the team and its members.

You may want to ask if the Team is registered with the American Cleft Palate-Craniofacial Association and how many of the individual members of the Team are also members of the American Cleft Palate-Craniofacial Association. Staying current with recent developments in the field is one sign of a conscientious and concerned health care professional. You may also want to determine whether the team has any relationship to an established hospital or to a medical school or university. Facilities for diagnostic studies and treatment frequently are better with such an affiliation.

For a list of cleft palate or craniofacial teams in your state or region, or for further information, you may contact:

Cleft Palate Foundation
1218 Grandview Avenue
Pittsburgh, PA 15211

Chapter 47

Information about Financial Assistance

Financial resources to help pay all or part of the costs of treating a person with a cleft lip and/or palate fall into three general categories: health insurance, federal and state resources, and private and non-profit agencies, foundations, and service organizations. The most important thing to remember is there are many sources of funds available to help you get the care you need.

Health Insurance

Private and Group Health Insurance will usually cover at least a portion of the cost of the treatment of a cleft lip or palate after a deductible is met. Check your health care plan or call the insurance company for specific coverage information. When choosing health insurance policies, check into coverage of not only surgery and medical care but also dental care and services such as hearing testing, speech and language testing and treatment, and psychological testing and/or counselling. If you have reason to think you are not being covered according to your policy, call your State Insurance Board.

Federal and State Resources

Champus is a program of medical benefits provided by the Federal Government for members and their dependents who are in the uniformed services. Persons covered by Champus should contact the

Health Benefits administrator at the nearest military installation for more information.

Medicaid (Title XIX of the Social Security Act of 1966) is a federal assistance program that covers most of the cost of medical care for people with low incomes who require hospital or physician services, or certain laboratory and x-ray procedures.

In some states, services such as treatment for speech or hearing defects may be covered. Application can be made in the county offices of the Social Services, Welfare, or Human Resources Office.

Recently Medicaid was expanded to include a new program entitled Medical Assistance Pregnant Women and Children's Program (MAPWC). This nationwide program was mandated by Federal legislation to provide medical/dental care for pregnant women and for children from birth to six years of age. The financial eligibility requirements for children under six years of age differ from Medicaid requirements and include children from working families who might otherwise be excluded from Medicaid benefits. The application form is much shorter and simpler than the forms for Medicaid and income limits are higher. Application can be made in the county offices of the Social Services, Welfare, or Human Resources Office.

Children's Special Health Services (formerly called the Crippled Children's Program) provides comprehensive medical care to children under the age of 21 who have congenital or acquired physically handicapping conditions. Specific medical and financial criteria have to be met by the applicant before financial assistance is approved. Applications are available through the Director, Children's Special Health Services of each state. You may contact your State Department of Health for further information or you may receive information from an agency or medical facility in your community that provides these services.

Vocational Rehabilitation Services are designed for persons 16 years of age and older with emotional, mental, physical/medical and/ or developmental disabilities that hinder their prospects for employment. Assistance in obtaining local office telephone numbers can be secured by contacting the State Department of Human Resources or the Welfare Office.

The **Hill-Burton Act** provides funds for indigent care at hospitals where federal monies were used for construction. The hospital admissions office has information on the availability of these funds and the guidelines for eligibility.

Private and Non-profit Agencies/foundations and Service Organizations

The **Easter Seal Society**, a non-profit organization, serves physically or developmentally disabled children and adults. Although their primary focus is on patients with cerebral palsy and similar neurological conditions, local chapters provide a variety of other services including speech and hearing services. For a description of services in your area, contact your state office or the national office: The National Easter Seal Society, (312)726-6200.

The **March of Dimes Birth Defects Foundation** supports programs designed to prevent birth defects, and promotes research, professional education and treatment. Each local chapter determines how its local funds are to be allocated. While chapters are not encouraged to use funds for treatment of individuals, the local chapter may assist families when no other funds are available in meeting the costs of treatment. The local chapters are usually listed in the telephone directory.

The **Grottoes of America** provide dentistry to the handicapped. The patient must be under 18 years of age to receive assistance from this organization. In addition they must have one of the following conditions: cerebral palsy, muscular dystrophy, mental retardation or myasthenia gravis. National Headquarters are in Columbus, Ohio; and their telephone number is (614)860-9193.

The **National Association for the Craniofacially Handicapped (FACES)** provides financial assistance for supportive services, i.e., transportation, food, and lodging, to families of individuals who are receiving treatment for craniofacial deformities resulting from birth defects, injuries, or disease. The Foundation office is located in Chattanooga, Tennessee; and their telephone number is (615)266-1632.

Local service organizations such as **Lions**, **Sertoma**, **Kiwanis**, and **Civitan Clubs** sometimes provide emergency one-time financial aid if funds are available. Local churches and church groups, e.g., the **Knights of Columbus**, **Masons**, etc., may also serve as resources. Telephone numbers for these organizations can usually be found in the yellow pages of the telephone directory under Clubs, Fraternal Organizations, and Religious Organizations.

Remember to discuss your financial needs with the team coordinator, social worker or other appropriate member on the local cleft palate team. They may be aware of other funding sources not mentioned above.

The Cleft Palate Foundation can refer you to local cleft palate teams and to parent support groups. They can also refer you to insurance advocates in your region and provide you with brochures and fact sheets about various aspects of clefting. Contact the:

Cleft Palate Foundation
1218 Grandview Avenue
Pittsburgh, PA 15211

(412)481-1376
(800)24-CLEFT

Part Six

Braces, Implants, and Dentures

Chapter 48

Orthodontic Brace: Perfect Smile Replaces Tin Grin

When her four children, ages 9 to 16, all had braces at the same time several years ago, Wanda Brown of Knoxville, TN, always knew what she'd be doing on her days off work.

"I knew it was Tuesday because we were at the orthodontist," she says with a laugh.

Today her children smile at the results of all those appointments: The three oldest have straight, perfect teeth, while the youngest has had some treatment but still awaits full braces.

"I really wanted braces," says daughter Diana, 17. "I'm glad I had them because I feel a whole lot better about myself. I'm always smiling now."

Years ago, few teens had such a positive attitude about braces. Orthodontic appliances triggered taunts like "metal mouth" and "tin grin." But today, braces are almost a status symbol among middle-class American teenagers. About three million teenagers in the United States and Canada have braces, an increase of about 30 percent in the last 10 years, according to the American Association of Orthodontists.

Teeth aren't any more crooked than in the past. It's just that more teenagers want the perfect smiles that braces can give them, and more parents are willing to foot the bills. Today there are more orthodontic devices than ever before, allowing more choices in how braces look and how long the patient must wear them.

"In general, people get braces for aesthetic reasons," says D. Gregory Singleton, D.D.S., a senior dental officer with FDA's Center for Devices and Radiological Health and an orthodontist in private practice.

FDA Consumer, March 1995.

"But that doesn't mean they won't get a functional benefit in the process," he adds. A better bite and fewer jaw problems are often the by-products of what begins as a cosmetic procedure.

The "Crooked" Smile

Anyone who's spent time in an orthodontist's chair has seen pictures and plaster molds of the "ideal" mouth. The top front teeth extend over the lower front teeth slightly, while the molars line up and meet on both sides of the mouth, top and bottom. The teeth are straight and not crowded, spaced together like a string of pearls.

But in most mouths, variations on this theme are more common. Some problems affect chewing or speaking, but most are simply cosmetic issues.

Improper tooth alignment is called malocclusion. Malocclusion is not a disease, but crooked teeth can decay faster than straight ones because people have more trouble keeping them clean. Severe misalignments may require extra flossing and brushing. But malocclusion doesn't always cause jaw problems or pain, and many people have lived long and healthy lives with misaligned teeth.

Nevertheless, malocclusions can be embarrassing. There are three types of malocclusions, and a number of other bite problems. The malocclusion types are:

- **Class I:** Teeth line up correctly top to bottom, but they are spaced too far apart or are crooked, crowded or turned.

- **Class II:** Upper teeth protrude and the lower teeth are too far back. This is also called an "overbite."

- **Class III:** Lower teeth are too far in front and the upper teeth are too far back. This is also called an "underbite." This is the most difficult problem to correct, says Singleton, and may require surgery.

Other orthodontic problems include:

- Open bite: Front teeth stay open even when biting down with back teeth. This can make chewing food difficult or impossible.

- Closed bite: When biting down, upper teeth cover the lower teeth completely. This is also called a "deep bite."

- Crossbite: When biting down, some upper teeth close inside or outside lower teeth.

Types of Malocclusions

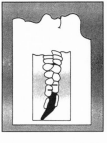

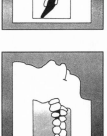

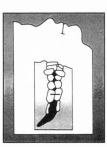

Class III
Lower teeth are too far in front, or upper teeth are too far back. Also called an "underbite."

Class II
Upper teeth protrude and lower teeth are too far back. Also called an "overbite."

Class I
Teeth line up correctly, but they are crooked, crowded, turned, or spaced too far apart.

Other Orthodontic Problems

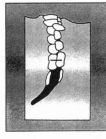

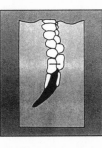

Cross Bite
Upon biting down, some upper teeth close inside lower teeth.

Closed Bite
Upon biting down, upper teeth cover lower teeth.

Open Bite
Upon biting down with back teeth, front teeth stay open.

Figure 48.1.

381

Causes

Bite problems stem from a number of causes. Most are inherited, but others are behavioral.

Habits such as a reverse swallow, tongue thrust, or sucking the thumb, fingers or the lower lip can apply pressure to teeth. Over time, teeth spread. If these habits aren't corrected before treatment, the teeth may spread even after the braces are removed.

Babies who suck their thumbs or pacifiers aren't generally at risk, says Singleton. As long as they break those habits by age five or six, they usually don't cause malocclusion in their permanent teeth.

Baby teeth can greatly affect the look and health of permanent teeth. If a baby tooth falls out too early or decays, the other teeth may move to fill in the space, blocking permanent teeth from coming in when they are ready. Similarly, if a baby tooth does not fall out soon enough, the bigger tooth behind it may come in crooked. And if a permanent tooth is lost to decay or trauma and is not replaced, the other teeth will drift to fill the space, sending them out of alignment.

The size of teeth can affect their alignment as well. Teeth that are too small can drift, and teeth that are too large will crowd. Mouth size can also cause drifting or crowding.

Bands and Brackets

Braces and other orthodontic appliances can solve most bite problems. Braces apply gentle pressure to teeth, moving them slowly over a period of 12 to 36 months. As teeth move, the jaw bones around them grow to fill in spaces left by the tooth roots. The main advancement for braces in the last 15 years has been the elimination of metal bands around front teeth. Today, small brackets are bonded onto the front teeth instead, greatly reducing the "metal mouth" look.

The brackets are tiny devices that attach each tooth to an archwire. The wire acts as a track to guide teeth along. Metal bands are now used only around the back teeth, which are stronger and more difficult to move.

Today's brackets can also be made of more aesthetically pleasing materials. Clear or tooth-colored materials can be used to create almost invisible braces, although they tend to be more expensive and difficult to work with. Some braces can even be hidden on the inside of the teeth, although these are more difficult for the orthodontist to place and adjust. They can also irritate the patient's tongue, which may hit them repeatedly. Most teens and children get stainless steel brackets because they're durable and less expensive than other kinds.

Another development has been "space age" wires. These wires, made of nickel titanium alloys developed through the NASA space program, hold their shape better than stainless steel wires. As a result, they require fewer replacements and trips to the orthodontist, often shortening treatment time.

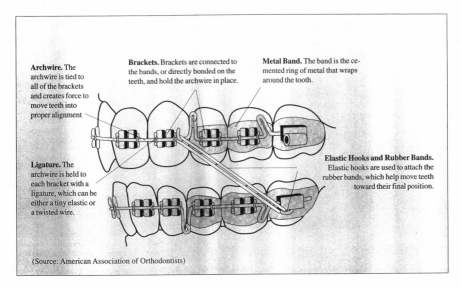

Archwire. The archwire is tied to all of the brackets and creates force to move teeth into proper alignment

Brackets. Brackets are connected to the bands, or directly bonded on the teeth, and hold the archwire in place.

Metal Band. The band is the cemented ring of metal that wraps around the tooth.

Ligature. The archwire is held to each bracket with a ligature, which can be either a tiny elastic or a twisted wire.

Elastic Hooks and Rubber Bands. Elastic hooks are used to attach the rubber bands, which help move teeth toward their final position.

(Source: American Association of Orthodontists)

Figure 48.2. *Components of Braces*

Other appliances include "elastics," small rubber bands that apply extra pressure between the jaws. "Headgear," which fits around the head or neck, helps move jaws into a new position, and "functional appliances," worn sort of like a football player's mouth guard, help align jaws and chewing muscles. "Retainers" help keep teeth straight after treatment. Special-purpose appliances can correct specific problems, such as the roof of the mouth being too small. Most patients wear a combination of two or more appliances over the course of treatment.

Some patients can even make a fashion statement with their braces, getting multicolored ligatures—the small wires or elastics that hold the arch wires to the brackets. Elastics and retainers also come in an array of colors. It's even possible to put a logo or mascot on a retainer.

The latest development, although not widely used, is magnets attached along the archwire to the upper or lower molars. Encased in stainless steel and placed with opposing or attracting forces, the magnets can help create or close spaces between teeth. In some cases, they can replace headgear, one of the most conspicuous orthodontic appliances.

FDA reviews all new materials and orthodontic devices before they go on the market. Manufacturers must file a pre-market notification, showing through laboratory or clinical tests that their device is substantially equivalent to others already in use. Most older orthodontic devices were already on the market in 1976, the year device regulations went into effect. Unless FDA receives evidence to the contrary, those devices are assumed to be safe and effective.

Not Just for Kids

Just because braces weren't fashionable or affordable when you were a kid doesn't mean you have to go through life with a major malocclusion. In 1979, 17 percent of orthodontic patients were adults. By 1992, that number had risen to 23 percent. Of those, 70 percent are women.

Orthodontists have made adult braces more palatable by fashioning them out of plastic and ceramic, which are clear or tooth-colored. Some appliances can fit on the inside of teeth, completely out of sight. Called "lingual braces," these devices may not be appropriate for everyone. They are not as strong as traditional braces so they usually have to be worn longer. They are also more difficult to adjust, and they can be uncomfortable because the patient's tongue hits them.

FDA has found new appliances to be substantially equivalent to older stainless steel brackets. Many of them, however, are more expensive. Nevertheless, braces are increasingly popular among adults. They have even gotten good press from famous patients: Cher, Diana Ross, and Phyllis Diller have all sported "tin grins" and beautiful smiles later.

Keeping Braces Clean

Perhaps the biggest challenge of living with braces is keeping them clean. The nooks and crannies formed by braces create ideal hiding spots for bacteria that lead to cavities and gum problems.

Patients who don't take care of their teeth risk even more dental decay than they would have without the braces. "This is a problem especially for patients around 11 and 12 years old," says Single-ton. Flossing and brushing for them are often not a priority, he explains.

Orthodontic patients should brush thoroughly after every meal and before bed. Flossing is more of a challenge because the wires make maneuvering difficult. A floss threader, available from an orthodontist or pharmacy, helps the floss slip behind the archwire and get to the gums.

Certain foods can damage braces. Sticky food, hard food, crunchy food, and sweets are the four troublemakers for those who wear braces. Sticky foods like gum, taffy and caramels can loosen cement and damage the brackets. Hard food like apples and carrots must be cut into bite-sized pieces so they won't break appliances. Crunchy foods like corn chips, popcorn and nuts should be avoided for the same reason. And sweets, because they feed bacteria when caught between braces, should be avoided as much as possible. Teeth should be brushed soon after eating sweets to prevent decay.

In fact, many orthodontists say that much of the success of braces depends on the willingness of the patient to stay away from harmful foods, keep teeth clean, and wear appliances faithfully.

What Cost Beauty?

The cost of braces varies with the patient, but typically treatment runs from $1,800 to $4,500. Some insurance plans cover a portion of the cost.

"It wasn't as high as I'd expected," Wanda Brown remembers. "I guess I thought we'd have to sell the house to pay for it. The cost was absolutely worth it— without question."

Aside from cost, braces can be physically uncomfortable. A day or two of soreness is not unusual after every visit to the orthodontist because of adjustments to the archwire. Also, some patients must have teeth extracted to make room for others.

Fifteen-year-old Michael Brown, for example, had to have 11 teeth extracted before getting braces. Most of them were baby teeth that hadn't come out on their own. "That was pretty painful," he remembers. "Compared to that, the braces weren't bad."

In addition to pain and expense, orthodontic patients must keep track of extra equipment daily. Elastics, retainers, headgear—school lockers are full of orthodontic devices. More than a few teens make the mistake of wrapping their retainers in paper napkins while they eat and then accidentally tossing them out.

"We've been through a few restaurant trash bins," Brown remembers. Did they find the missing retainer? "Oh yes!" she says. "I'm sure some people thought we were crazy, but we always searched till we found it."

—by Rebecca D. Williams

Rebecca D. Williams is a writer in Oak Ridge, TN.

Chapter 49

Mouth Jewelry:
A Glossary of Orthodontic
Devices

Introduction

You're wearing braces? So do millions of other people. This chapter provides lots of interesting information for people with braces.

Orthodontic Appliances:

You're getting a Bionator? An Activator? Or some kind of retainer? I bet you want to know more about it:

Anterior Bite Plate: has a little shelf just behind the top front teeth that the bottom teeth hit on so the rear teeth will grow out to the same length as the front ones.

Bionator I: pulls the mandible forward and spreads it so it will grow that way and keeps the front teeth from growing vertically so the back ones can catch up.

Bionator II: holds the mandible forward so it will grow and has plastic over the back teeth keeping them from growing so the front teeth can catch up.

Bonded Retainer: for the bottom teeth.

The BoWoW Kids! Jeff and Tommy Bower. Website http://www.world-net/ home/flyingbb/ Special thanks to **The BoWoW Kids** for all the descriptions. Reprinted with permission.

Celb Nightguard: keeps you from bad habits at night.

Class II Activator: pulls the mandible forward and makes it grow, makes the teeth grow flat.

Coil Springs: are wired in to move one jaw toward the other like rubber bands do; most times they are for kids who won't wear their rubber bands.

Fan Expander: has an expander screw in front and a hinge in back; as you crank the screw it spreads only the front teeth wider but keeps the back ones in place.

Fränkel I Appliance: teaches the mandible to stay more forward where it's supposed to be and so the muscles pull on your front top teeth to move them back.

Fränkel II Appliance: uses the mouth muscles to advance the mandible and make it grow. It also has a screw on each side to advance it further.

Fränkel V Appliance: uses the muscles and a headgear to move the mandible forward so it will grow; stops the maxilla from growing and flattens an open bite.

Habit Crib ("Habit Rake"): keeps kids from sucking their thumb—*Ouch!*

Habit Crib & Retainer: a removable habit crib and retainer, for kids who suck their thumb; like the other habit crib but you can remove it.

Hawley Retainer: an upper retainer but can be used for upper or lower. There's a bunch of different ones really for minor teeth movement but is supposed to be worn most times right after you get your brackets off.

Herbst Appliance: a splint with tubes and hinges to hold the mandible forward so it will grow and push the maxilla back so it won't grow. It's for kids that won't wear their headgears or to help headgears work better.

Hyrax Rapid Palatal Expander: splits your palate and moves the back teeth apart to make the arch wider.

Lingual Arch: keeps the mandible from moving while baby teeth fall out and get replaced with adult teeth. It's called removable, but only the ortho can remove it, not the patient.

Nance Appliance: holds the molars from rotating or moving forward while kids are waiting for their bicuspids to grow in.

Quad Helix W Expander: spreads the back teeth apart with a spring.

Ricketts Retainer: a retainer often used for Black people and some Hispanics because the top of their mouth is supposedly taller and it's supposed to work better. *Remark: This description is quoted from an orthodontics book. We do **not** intend to offend anyone!*

Saggital Appliance: makes space to fix overcrowding in places in the mouth by cranking a screw to push individual teeth to different places they need to go.

Space Maintainer (on the right): keeps space between teeth so an adult tooth can grow in when it's ready.

Space Regainer (on the left): has a crank to push teeth apart for an adult tooth to grow there.

Teuscher Activator: pushes the mandible back to keep it from growing and makes the maxilla grow.

Woodside Activator: pulls the mandible forward and makes it grow.

Chapter 50

Dental Implants:
The Latest in False Teeth

Implanting materials and methods now make it possible to implant anchors in the bones of the jaw to hold permanent dentures. Implanting small titanium sockets, or one of the other types of implant fixtures holds promise of more closely approximating the look, feel and function of natural teeth for some people who are facing the loss of their own teeth. There are limitations, however, and many things to consider before asking for dental implants.

After the dentist tells you the state of things in your mouth means the teeth you call your own will not be with you for long, wouldn't it be nice if he or she could just screw in replacements? There'd be no need for dentures—no worrying about those tiny seeds the TV pitchman says are bound to become trapped behind a dental plate. No need to know about the holding power of dental adhesives or the special washes for false teeth that soak away all those stains the ads assure you are inevitable.

And there are millions of Americans who do endure the hassles of dentures. A 1985-1986 survey by the National Institute for Dental Research found that Americans 65 and older had lost an average of 10 teeth, and those 35 to 64 had an average of nine teeth missing. Four out of 10 (42 percent) of Americans 65 and older have lost all their teeth, as have 4 percent of those 35 to 65 years of age.

Ordinary dentures, generally made of plastic, are custom-fitted to match and adhere to the upper or lower jaw or made to clamp on to remaining teeth with metal supports or bridges.

FDA Consumer, December 1988.

But today there are dental implants, which add a method of attaching the denture with metal anchors directly and permanently to the jaw bone with no need to ever be removed by the wearer.

Dental scientists have discovered materials that will bond with bone and withstand the pressure created by biting and chewing. The bonding process is called "endosseous [within the bone] integration." Refined surgical techniques and follow-up have reduced the likelihood of the implant loosening, breaking, or being rejected by the body.

As many as 100,000 Americans will undergo surgery to be fitted with dental implants by 1992, according to a report of a June 1988 National Institutes of Health consensus development conference on dental implants. That compares with an estimated 24,500 implants done before 1985.

At least 10,000 dentists implant dental prostheses today, compared to 1,000 or so five years ago, the conference report stated. Dental implants are now being done at a rate of about 6,000 to 7,500 a year, adds Paul J. Mentag, a dentist and assistant professor of prosthodontics at the University of Detroit.

"We have the ability to functionally and aesthetically rehabilitate the oral invalid to a state of excellent dental health," says Paul H.J. Krogh, a Washington, D.C., oral and maxillofacial (jaw) surgeon and president of the Academy of Osseointegration, which represents 1,150 oral surgeons, other dental professionals, assistants, technicians, physicians and scientists.

"Not every patient is a candidate for implants," cautions the American Dental Association (ADA), headquartered in Chicago, which represents 146,000 dental professionals and students.

ADA points out there is no substitute for natural teeth, that implants will never function as well as the real thing. And the association's position is that implants are not suggested for cosmetic purposes alone.

"The best implant is a natural tooth," echoes Albert Guckes, a prosthodontic consultant at the dental clinic of the National Institute of Dental Research, Bethesda, Md. "With today's technology we can salvage badly damaged teeth, and that's the way to go," he says.

ADA says an individual's decision whether or not to have a dental implant should be made only after a careful examination and consultation with the person's dentist. A second professional opinion can add perspective.

If You Are Thinking of Having Dental Implants, Consider the Following:

- Determine if it is possible to save your own teeth.

- Will you be able to keep the schedule required for implant surgery and follow-up? Some implants require many visits and a second stage of surgery. It may take as long as four to six months or more before the implant is completed.

- Know what to expect in the way of pain, soreness, and possible long-term restrictions to your diet. You also may have to wear temporary devices.

- Will you be able to follow special oral hygiene instructions and maintain a schedule of regular dental checkups that may go on for years?

- Your body might reject the implant after a few months or a few years. Are you prepared to accept that possibility?

- Medical risks are inherent in implant surgery, just as in any surgical procedure. In implant surgery, risks include sinus perforation, local and systemic infection, and paresthesias (abnormal or impaired skin sensation).

The Cost of Implants

Dental implants are expensive. The cost of surgery, prosthesis, and associated professional services for a single implanted tooth is approximately $1,000 in Augusta, Ga., according to Ralph McKinney Jr., chairman of the department of oral pathology of the Medical College of Georgia in Augusta. In Washington, D.C., patients can expect to pay from $4,000 to $6,000 for a permanent lower bridge and up to $10,000 to $12,000 for a full fixed upper denture bridge or $18,000 to $24,000 for both upper and lower implants. Elsewhere, dentists and surgeons doing dental implants report that charges range up to $30,000.

Don't expect financial help from health or dental insurance plans. Since the implant devices are considered experimental by insurance companies, they will probably not be covered until they are proven effective, according to the Health Insurance Association of America.

Who are the people most skilled in doing this relatively new form of dental surgery? According to Phillip Worthington, M.D., professor of oral and maxillofacial surgery at the University of Washington in Seattle, 90 percent of American oral surgeons and approximately 40 percent of periodontists (specialists in gum disease) have done implants. The number of general practitioners and prosthodontists (specialists in bridges and dentures) who have done the procedure could not be determined.

Twenty thousand dentists have trained for implant work in the United States, Worthington's research determined. The scope of their training varies from having viewed instructional videotapes to having invested years in apprenticeship to others experienced in the procedure. The procedure is not regulated, and there are no accepted criteria for skill or experience that must be met to perform the procedure. ADA has not formally recognized implant surgery as a specialty.

D. Gregory Singleton, D.D.S., of FDA's Center for Devices and Radiological Health, in Silver Spring, Md., suggests talking with others who have had implants when making a decision about going to a particular dentist or oral surgeon.

Types of Implant Methods

Four general designs of devices are in use in implant dentistry today. The two most frequently used, according to Barry E. Sands, biomedical engineer at the Center for Devices and Radiological Health, are:

- **One- and two-stage cylindrical implants.** These are inserted directly into holes drilled into the jawbone as sockets for screws to anchor a single false tooth, groups of false teeth, or entire rows of replacements. In two-stage implants, the cylinder is fitted into the bone and the gum is sutured closed over the device until the area heals and the device bonds to the bone around it. Then the surgical site is reopened to allow abutments to be placed in the cylinders, and the prosthesis is attached.

- **Blade types.** Shaped to fit channels cut lengthwise into the jaw bone, blades have openings to accept bone regrowth through their framework. Tiered vanes above the gum line allow attachment of the prosthesis, which is generally done at the same time as the surgery.

394

The other types of devices: pin- and tooth-shaped, are less frequently implanted today and are generally used only for replacing
individual teeth.

Most implant hardware in use today is made from titanium alloys.
Coatings of calcium phosphates, carbon compounds, and titanium are
sometimes added to promote successful bonding of the implant to
bone. However, the coatings have not been shown to improve the bonding of the implant to bone, according to Sands.

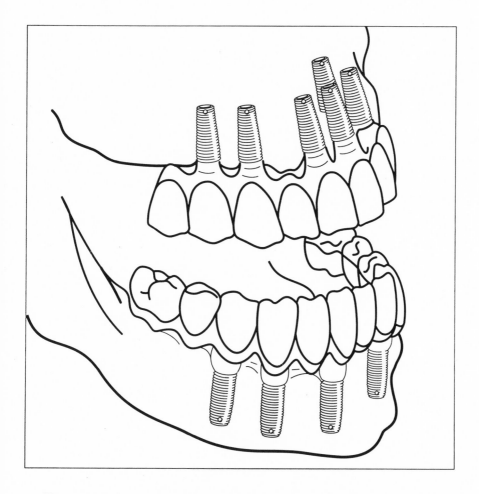

Figure 50.1. Cylindrical Implants (Drawing courtesy Nobelpharma USA, Inc.)

The Risks

Blade-Shaped Implant

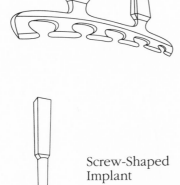

Screw-Shaped Implant

Tripodal Pin Implant

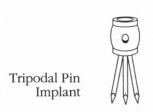

Due to the routine presence of bacteria in the mouth, there is a risk of infection of the tissue or bone surrounding the implant. There also is some risk that the additional stress of the implant on bones in the jaw will speed up bone resorption and lead to implant failure and possibly a toothless future. Persistent pain or discomfort, speech problems, nerve injury, and damage to adjacent teeth are rare but possible complications of implants.

Conditions that can rule out dental implants include hypertension, heavy smoking, alcohol and drug abuse, chronic illnesses such as diabetes, bone deterioration, and bruxism (habitual tooth grinding), according to the University of Detroit's Dr. Mentag.

Endosseous implants are medical devices, regulated by FDA to ensure their safety and effectiveness. They are Class III devices, a category that covers life-supporting, life-sustaining, and implanted items. Under the 1976 Medical Device Amendments, FDA will require manufacturers of dental implants to submit data from controlled clinical studies to demonstrate the safety and effectiveness of their products or stop marketing them as early as 1990, according to FDA's Singleton.

FDA wants to know of problems consumers have with dental implants. "All the consumer needs to do

Figure 50.2. Other Types of Implant Methods

is call the nearest FDA office and explain the nature of the problem. A report will get back to us. But we can't do anything until we hear about it," Sands says. Post-marketing surveillance is a way to detect and correct problems or remove a harmful or ineffective device from use as quickly as possible. (See "Looking for Trouble in Medical Devices," in the September 1987 issue of *FDA Consumer*.)

Dental implants have arrived. They may not be the solution for every case of tooth loss, but for those who are candidates, implants promise an alternative to dentures.

—by Vern Modeland

Vern Modeland is a member of FDA's public affairs staff.

Chapter 51

Dental Implants: More Trouble than They're Worth?

The need to wear removable dentures can distress people as much as losing their teeth does in the first place. Full-jaw dentures—bulky devices that grip the gums—can slip, reduce the ability to chew, and irritate gum tissue. Partial dentures, which clip onto the neighboring teeth, are also bulky, and their clasps can promote decay or loosen the teeth they're attached to.

A fixed bridge can help people who are missing only a few teeth without causing those problems. But to attach the bridge, the dentist must cut down and cap adjacent healthy teeth; and a wide bridge can loosen those teeth.

It's no wonder that dental implants—artificial teeth attached firmly to the jawbone—have intoxicated manufacturers, dentists, and patients alike. The number of dentists doing implants and the number of people getting them have both jumped tenfold in the past decade.

Aggressive marketers and dentists eager to cash in on this innovation have fueled the boom. For example, a recent ad in Reader's Digest, placed by the American Association of Oral and Maxillofacial Surgeons, called implants "the next best thing to natural teeth," and claimed they would allow you to "Smile, Talk, Eat, Live, Laugh, Naturally."

Despite such enthusiastic claims, dental implants have formidable disadvantages. These very expensive devices sometimes simply fail, even when a skilled practitioner does the work; and many dentists installing implants lack the skills and the training to do it well. Many of those dentists have taken only one or two weekend courses offered by a manufacturer. Few dental schools offer anything more than brief courses in implantation, and the American Dental Association has no standards of training or experience for dentists doing the procedure.

Down in the Mouth

If you're considering implants, you need to be exceedingly cautious, well informed, and assertive. First, be aware of these factors:

- **Treatment is long and hard.** Implantation usually requires two operations, each lasting one to three hours, depending on how many implants you're receiving. Most people can get by with local anesthesia, often with an intravenous sedative. If you prefer general anesthesia, be sure someone other than the implanter administers it and that emergency support systems are available.

  The first surgery usually involves drilling into the jawbone and inserting one or more artificial roots—a metal screw, cylinder, or blade—that will anchor the false teeth. (When the patient has lost too much bone or when the implanted root would jut into a sinus cavity or hit a nerve, dentists can try to anchor the teeth with a frame that sits under the gum, directly on the bone.) For the next three to six months, you wear a temporary tooth or denture while the bone bonds to the metal root. The dentist then reopens the gum and attaches a metal post to each anchor. (In some cases, the anchor and post can be installed in a single procedure.) Finally, the dentist attaches anything from a single artificial tooth to a full set of dentures onto the posts.

  The entire procedure generally requires 10 to 15 office visits over a period of six to nine months. In contrast, dentists can usually install partial dentures in two to three visits, and full dentures or fixed bridges in about half a dozen visits.

- **Implant surgery may be risky.** In addition to the usual risks of any surgical procedure—even a relatively minor one like this—implantation can cause infection of the gums or bone and can damage the roots of neighboring teeth, the nerves leading to the lip, or the sinus cavity. Skilled implanters rarely encounter those complications, but you face significant risks in the hands of an inexperienced practitioner. Some people may not be healthy enough to undergo the procedure: heavy drinkers or smokers, people with a weakened immune system, and people with a chronic disease—particularly high blood pressure, heart disease, or diabetes.

- **Implants may fail.** The biggest risk of this procedure is loosening or fracture of the implant. The device may not fit snugly into the socket drilled in the bone, or it may fail to bond with the bone. Infection after surgery can destroy the supporting bone. Or there may have been too little bone in the first place to withstand the stress of chewing.

  Bone tends to be less supportive in the back of the jaw than in the front, and chewing puts far more stress on the rear teeth than on the front teeth. The bone in the upper jaw is also less supportive than that in the lower jaw. So you're most likely to lose your original teeth in the upper rear. Unfortunately, that's where implants are most likely to fail, for the same reasons. Conversely, implants do best in the lower front, where you're least likely to need them.

  While reliable statistics are hard to come by, the five-year survival rate for implants installed by reasonably experienced implanters seems to be better than 90 percent in the front of the lower jaw— between 80 and 90 percent in the lower rear and upper front, and between 70 and 80 percent in the upper rear. (Those figures do not include implants that anchor a full set of artificial teeth, which put less stress on the devices.) Highly experienced practitioners have reported somewhat better results than those figures. But there are virtually no data for the many inexperienced practitioners, who undoubtedly do worse.

- **Implants are hard to maintain.** While implants won't constantly remind you that you're wearing false teeth, you can't just forget about them, either. The gum does not hug the artificial tooth as tightly as it hugs a healthy natural tooth, so the chance of local inflammation is greater than normal You need to clean the implant more carefully than you would a natural tooth, in many cases using a special implement, since parts of the device may be hard to reach with an ordinary toothbrush and floss. And you need to see your dentist for a checkup and cleaning more often than the usual twice a year. If you have trouble keeping your teeth clean, a common cause of tooth loss in the first place, dental implants may not be for you.

- **Implants cost plenty.** The bill can range from about $1500 to $3000 for a single tooth to as much as $25,000 for an entire jaw. Implants cost two to three times as much as fixed bridgework, four to eight times as much as a partial denture, and 10 to 15 times as much as a full-jaw denture.

  And you'll probably have to foot the entire bill yourself. Most dental insurance plans cover dentures and bridges but refuse to pay for implants.

  You could probably get the work done much more cheaply— say, at half the price—at a dental school, where closely supervised graduate students perform the procedure. But in this new field, there's no guarantee that even the faculty members are expert implanters. Note that there's often a long waiting list for dental-school treatment, and that students work more slowly than practicing dentists.

Finding the Right Dentist

Despite those formidable drawbacks, implants may make sense for some people, particularly those who can't adjust to dentures or just don't want to try. A second opinion can help you determine whether you are a good candidate for implants. If you do choose implants, be prepared to choose a practitioner carefully—especially if you will need particularly difficult work, such as multiple or upper-rear implants.

While the American Dental Association does not recognize implantology as a specialty, the American Academy of Implant Dentistry (AAID) does. The AAID certifies dentists who have had extensive training and experience and passed an examination. It also grants the titles of fellow and associate fellow, which have somewhat less rigorous requirements than full certification, particularly for associate fellow. Call the Academy at (312) 335-1550 to see whether any AAID-endorsed dentists practice in your area.

Since the AAID may not have approved a dentist in your area, you may have to ask your own dentist or periodontist to recommend an implanter. Periodontists can be especially useful for referrals; as specialists in saving teeth from gum disease, they often see the work of various implanters, and can evaluate it.

Dental specialists (oral surgeons, periodontists, and prosthodontists) are trained in many of the general skills required for implantation, and are often the best practitioners to do the procedure. However, the most important factor is training and experience specifically in implantation. Any dentist can do implantation well if he or she has studied the procedure thoroughly and done it on many patients.

Whether you choose a specialist or generalist, you'll have a better chance of success if the practitioner has these qualifications:

- **Training:** At least one course in implant technique lasting six months or more, or many shorter courses.

- **Experience:** At least three to five years doing implants, including a minimum of 50 cases overall and 10 to 15 cases similar to yours.

- **Success:** Three- to five-year success rates comparable to the rates cited above for survival of the implant in different parts of the mouth.

- **Flexibility:** Experience with at least two or three different implant devices.

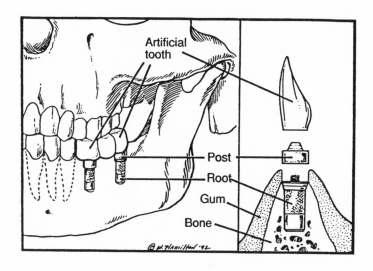

Figure 51.1. *At the right, the three components of a dental implant: root, post, and tooth, each usually installed in a separate procedure. At left is a typical result, with two roots and posts anchoring a set of three artificial teeth.*

Checking Out the Implant

It's important to find out about the implant as well as the implanter. The Food and Drug Administration has not yet established standards for implants, and manufacturers are rushing new devices onto the market, sometimes without extensive testing. Inferior devices may attract bacteria, be difficult to clean, or trigger inflammatory reactions in the tissues of the mouth. Worse still, the implants may fail to bond firmly with the bone, or may even bend or break under the pressure of chewing.

Fortunately, the American Dental Association (ADA) now evaluates these devices. The ADA deems a device fully acceptable after the manufacturer submits five-year data demonstrating its safety and effectiveness. Three-year results can earn provisional acceptance. So ask your dentist whether the ADA has at least provisionally accepted the device he or she plans to use, or write:

American Dental Association
Department of Public Information and Education
211 E. Chicago Ave.
Chicago, IL 60611

Chapter 52

Implant Dentistry: Where Are We Now?

Dental implants can dramatically change a patient's self-esteem and quality of life. But too few people receive implants because of the cost and lack of education in this growing field. More training, systems standardization and practice guidelines will improve implant treatment availability.

Implant dentistry has emerged as a major component of dental practice in response to the more than 125 million Americans who are missing some or all of their teeth. Today, dental implants are an acceptable alternative capable of providing bone-anchored fixed prostheses for improved quality of life and self-esteem for many of these patients. Implant dentistry, however, is still not practiced uniformly throughout the profession.

Implant treatment will become a routine part of everyday dentistry when general dentists have a key role in providing comprehensive implant dentistry services.

Implant Uses and Classification

Dental implants reduce the need to prepare healthy teeth; eliminate maintenance of teeth with questionable prognoses; provide retention for partial and complete over-dentures; and provide abutment support for single-tooth, partial and complete arch fixed restorations.

The many implant modalities currently available are classified in three ways according to their relationship to bone:

- **Endosseous implants** are placed into the bone. Their overall shape of cylindrical cones and thin plates (blades) is designed to engage the endocortex for fixation. They can be used in all areas of the mouth.

- **Subperiosteal implants** are custom-cast frames that rest on the bone. They can be used for complete and partial arch restoration in both jaws, usually when there is inadequate bone in which to place endosseous implants.

- **Transosteal implants** combine a subperiosteal plate component with an endosseous component that passes through the bone. They are used only in the anterior mandible primarily as partial support for tissue-borne over-dentures.

The cylindrical endosseous implants are, by far, most commonly used. These implant systems consist of three parts: the fixture, the transmucosal abutment and the prosthesis retainer. The fixture surface can be threaded, grooved, perforated or textured to engage the cortex and to provide immediate and long-term bone anchorage.

The transmucosal abutment can be connected to the fixture by screws, cement or swaging in place. Often the abutment engages an internal or external hexagon at the occlusal aspect of the fixture for anti-rotation of single crowns and registration during transfer procedures. The prosthesis is attached to the abutment with screws, cement or precision attachments.

Longevity

It is difficult to draw specific conclusions on longevity of implant treatment because criteria for success vary. Most research is based on case series studies. There is, however, a large body of experiential data accumulating that demonstrates implants function regularly for 10 years or more. The original Branemark research showed five-year implant survival rates of 90 percent in the anterior mandible and 82 percent in the anterior maxilla for totally edentulous patients. Fixed prosthesis survival in these studies was higher, 100 percent in the mandible and 89 percent in the maxilla.

We see that every implant is not needed for reconstructive success and that there is about a 10 percent difference in survival rates between the maxilla and mandible. As more partially edentulous patients are being treated, implants are needed for all areas. In these applications, the prognosis for osseointegration—absence of clinical mobility—and long-term success varies from more than 95 percent in the anterior mandible to 72 percent in the posterior maxilla.

Implant survival relates directly to cortical and trabecular density of available bone. Density is greatest in the anterior mandible. This region is followed in descending order by the anterior maxilla (because of the cancellous bone and thinner cortex); the posterior mandible (because of its hollow nature and the location of the mandibular nerve); and the posterior maxilla, which contains the hollow sinus bordered by eggshell-thin cortex.

Patient Selection

From the psychological point of view, the ideal candidate has a strong desire for fixed rather than removable dentures, realizes that the state of the art is still evolving and is willing to work with the dentist to achieve his or her goal. In general, there are few medical conditions in which implants cannot be used if the patient's general health is adequate to withstand the required surgical and reconstructive procedures. Specific medical conditions representing poor risks for implant therapy are uncontrolled diabetes, addiction to alcohol, blood dyscrasias, the effects of high doses of corticosteroid or immunosuppressive drug therapy and high doses of radiation therapy to the jaws.

Sequence of Implant Treatment

Implant treatment is usually performed in five phases: pre-surgical planning, fixture installation, healing abutment placement, final abutment connection and prosthesis fabrication, and follow-up and maintenance.

Pre-surgical planning is imperative since the implant position and type of abutment connection determine the final prosthesis. The first treatment procedure consists of fabricating the diagnostic prosthesis to determine the final restoration's emergence profile, arch form, vertical dimension and occlusal plane. A transparent duplicate of this prosthesis becomes a surgical template that guides the placement of the implants into the optimum position for tooth support. The diagnostic prosthesis becomes the provisional restoration that the patient will use during the different stages of implant treatment.

Implant Placement

The implant site is precisely prepared using traumatic techniques of slow-speed bone drilling with burs of sequentially increasing diameter, and copious irrigation. Implants are seated by gently tapping press-fit implants or screwing threaded implants into place. All implant procedures are done under sterile conditions to prevent infection and contamination of the highly specialized biomedical surface, which allows osseointegration to occur. Tissues are sutured over or around the implant to allow a stress-free healing period during which the implant is osseointegrating. This takes about four months in the mandible and six months in the maxilla.

In a second surgical procedure, after osseointegration is confirmed by the absence of mobility, a transmucosal healing abutment is attached to the fixture. The provisional prosthesis is then modified to fit over these interim abutments.

Although the process of final restoration can begin at any time, a healing period during which the gingival tissue matures to its final position often helps to obtain the best final abutment height. At this point, the procedures followed depend on the patient's specific treatment plan and personal requirements. Final impressions will transfer either the occlusal aspect of the fixture for custom abutment fabrication or the occlusal aspect of a prefabricated abutment that has replaced the healing abutment.

Once the final prosthetic teeth are in place, the patient follows an individualized maintenance program. In most cases, the patient is asked to return every three months for a close watch on implants and final restoration. Bacteria and plaque are removed, and the screws or attachments that maintain the prostheses are checked for tightness.

Restorative Challenges

Decisions on the type and number of implants to be used are dictated by residual bone structure and the presence of teeth. When periodontally compromised teeth occupy potentially good implant supportive bone anterior to the maxillary sinus and neurovascular bundle, it is preferable to sacrifice them in favor of more predictable anterior implant therapy.

Since cortical bone dictates fixture position, and arch form, vertical dimension and occlusal plane dictate crown position, the restorative challenge is to bridge the gap between the occlusal aspect of the fixture and the apical aspect of the restoration. Many patients suffering from edentulism have significant residual ridge resorption to the lingual and palatal aspects of the normal arch form. This dictates fixture placement to the lingual or palatal aspect of the existing arch form and opposing dentition.

In restoring function and esthetics, the restoration must be cantilevered buccally to create the desired occlusal scheme. Implant prostheses often do not duplicate natural root position or gingival anatomy and have some space between the teeth and the tissue. This is generally not an esthetic problem since the lips cover these areas.

Lingually placed or angled implants in patients with high lip lines may expose the gingival margins of the final restoration. This situation requires an implant system including abutments that allow restorations to emerge directly from the implant. The crown will then meet the gingival tissues in an aesthetically pleasing fashion. In some fully edentulous patients, resorption, resulting in lingual placement, of implants that support fixed restorations may require removable prosthetic gingiva.

In fully edentulous patients, implants are usually placed anterior to the mental foramina and maxillary sinus. The prosthesis is cantilevered posteriorly as much a 20 millimeters in the mandible and 10 mm in the maxilla This allows reconstruction with fixed restorations to first molar occlusion. Occlusal forces are minimized by distributing implants evenly over the widest possible area and connecting them with an implant bridge as rigid and passively fitting as possible.

Implant placement is limited by existing residual bone, proximity of adjacent teeth and opposing dentition. With tooth loss, the residual ridge resorbs lingually or palatally. To align the restoration with remaining adjacent and opposing dentition, angulation of the implants or angled abutments, or both, are often necessary.

Frequently, the restoration will need to be cantilevered buccally to create the desired occlusal scheme and arch form. Abutments retained by screws are difficult or impossible to angle. Furthermore, unlike multiple abutment bridges, the crown retained by a single screw may loosen and rotate on its abutment. Cemented abutments are more difficult to use but can avoid this problem. Screw attachments can be retrieved, but access holes require maintenance, may compromise occlusion and are not attractive.

Because of the difference in their attachments to bone, there's no consensus whether osseointegrated implants can or should be bridged directly to natural teeth. When natural teeth are mobile, cantilevering forces to the implant result. Forces can be stress-broken with interlocks or by seating retainers on the implant without cement while cementing them to natural teeth.

Horizontal and vertical displacement of integrated implants is about one-tenth as much as healthy natural teeth. Integrated implant movement is a function of the elastic property of bone. If an implant-supported restoration is adjusted for the partially edentulous patient with conventional prosthetic guidelines, more force will be placed on the implants than the natural dentition To overcome this discontinuity, the implant-supported restoration should be adjusted 50 to 100 microns in infra-occlusion to account for the compression of the periodontal ligament. This can be achieved with multiple strips of occlusal foil.

Occlusion should allow for equal force transfer between the implants and the natural abutments and reduce the effect of angulation and prematurities. The occlusal technique for partially edentulous patients is to develop a long centric occlusion. The implant-supported restoration is adjusted to eliminate protrusive and lateral prematurities and to be in lighter centric contact than natural teeth. Whenever possible, disclusion is achieved on natural dentition. Implants are most susceptible to the detrimental effects of premature occlusal forces in the maxilla where cancellous bone and minimal cortex are present.

Relationship of the Implant

Natural tooth reconstruction requires special attention because of the difference in the support mechanisms of implants by bone and teeth by periodontal ligament. When natural teeth are mobile, there will be cantilevering forces to the implants. As a result of direct attachment of implant restorations to natural teeth, the following problems have been observed: implant fracture, loosening of attachment screws and crown cement failure resulting in decay.

Implant systems are available with flexible polymer elements between the implant and its abutment. Proponents of these systems claim that the elements simulate natural tooth movement during function, thereby damping or stress-breaking the effects of occlusal and lateral forces. Others claim these elements require frequent changes, don't really offer advantages over rigid elements and complicate the restorative and maintenance process.

When possible, tooth implant-borne restorations should be avoided in favor of totally implant-supported restorations. When this is not possible, interlocks in implant tooth restorations are recommended to allow for any difference in support mechanisms. If interlocks are used, they should be placed closer to the implant than the natural teeth to reduce the cantilever effect on the implant caused by tooth movement.

When natural abutment support must be incorporated into the reconstruction, the prosthesis should be a one-piece frame cemented over copings or cemented to natural teeth with hard cement and to the implant abutment with soft cement. If the hard cement fails, the prosthesis is easily removed from the implant for recementing.

Looking to the Future

As implant dentistry approaches the turn of the century, the key factors of public awareness and demand, insurance, research, regulation and education will influence its advancement.

Demand

While demand for implant services is steadily increasing, the current estimate of 300,000 implants each year is well below potential need, when we consider the more than 40 million totally edentulous and many more partially edentulous patients who could benefit from implants. With this increasing demand, greater numbers of complex cases will emerge and increase the need for implant systems designed for specific anatomic conditions.

There is great demand for insurance coverage but traditionally, insurance carriers do not provide benefits for this type of care. Some dental insurers provide minimal benefits for the prosthetic aspect and related treatment. Some major medical insurance may cover a portion of the cost of the surgical procedure, but this frequently relates to the type of procedure and whether it is performed in the hospital. As insurance coverage becomes available, more patients will seek implant treatment.

In the midst of rapid expansion, providers of implant services are being faced with the question of professional liability coverage.

Unfortunately, today's underwriting decisions are based on negligence claims for implants inserted several years ago when technology was not as well developed and dentists were not as well informed. As guidelines for practice and standards of education are instituted, this trend should be reversed.

Device guidelines have been established by the American Dental Association, but compliance with the Association's acceptance program is voluntary. Some manufacturers have applied and received full acceptance (Nobelpharma and IMZ, fully and partially edentulous arches of two or more units; Oratronics, one-stage blade partially edentulous arches) or provisional acceptance (Core-Vent, Integral, ITI and Steri-Oss systems; and Nobelpharma single-tooth replacement). This endorsement will become more important as patients begin to request credible information on the devices they are receiving.

Research

Research in basic biology, materials and methodology will be critical to growth and development. Many leading-edge questions are now being addressed:

- the management of biomaterials-based infection
- efficacy of hydroxylapatite and other coatings for improved support and healing
- guided tissue regeneration to eliminate bone defects and increase implant-supporting bone, and
- bone augmentation to improve available bone and esthetic appearance.

Procedures for lateral mandibular nerve repositioning during fixture placement and sinus augmentation and grafting using various combinations of autogenous, freeze-dried bone and hydroxylapatite promise increased implant application in the future.

Methods of shortening the healing period through the addition of growth factors and evaluation of efficacy of placement of implants into fresh extraction vs. healed sites, and into immediate function, are also being studied.

Studies on the biomechanics of implant design are evaluating the effects of stress on implant devices and bone attachment mechanisms in both free-standing and combined tooth-bone/implant prostheses. Luting agents, stress-breaking mechanisms and simpler abutments for overcoming angulation difficulties are being developed. Researchers are working on prosthesis design for improved esthetics, strength, comfort and ease of fabrication.

Other factors, such as cost-effectiveness and relative value of alternative treatments, in terms of patient outcome, are under evaluation. There are efforts to simplify case management through standardized treatment plans and diagnostic guidelines, using decision sciences research methodology.

412

As a collaborative effort, the National Dental Implant Registry was initiated by the Department of Veterans Affairs, with initial support from the American Academy of Implant Dentistry. More recently it has been expanded to include the American Academy of Periodontology, the American College of Prosthodontists, the Academy of Osseointegration, the American Association of Oral and Maxillofacial Surgeons, the U.S. Army, the Agency for Health Policy and Research and the National Institute of Dental Research.

This registry will give practitioners and researchers access to a large body of scientific data on implants, heretofore unavailable. In another government/industry collaboration, a Dental Implant Clinical Research Group has been formed to conduct an extensive, multicentered, randomized, controlled, clinical trial jointly funded by the VA and Core-Vent Corp. The study, which began in January 1991, will follow more than 680 patients at 30 VA medical centers for six years.

Further Food and Drug Administration regulations can be expected to lead to an increase in efficacy research. Endosseous dental implants are currently classified as Class III devices. This classification requires manufacturers to conduct clinical trials demonstrating that their devices are safe and effective in order to market them. In response, a group of manufacturers formed the Dental Implant Manufacturers Association, which petitioned the FDA to reclassify endosseous dental implants to Class II, claiming this research is unnecessary based on the long history of the use of endosseous implants. The FDA is expected to make its decision in the first quarter of 1993. The cost of this research is staggering and will strain manufacturers, but the challenge is to support regulation without stifling new development.

Education

Implant education varies widely for practicing dentists, postdoctoral students and pre-doctoral students. There is a pressing need for national educational standards. Currently, most education is provided by implant manufacturers in short weekend courses. These programs can be expected only to orient the practitioner to a particular system rather than to the discipline of oral implantology.

There are many categories of patients and a wide range of treatment difficulty. Many problems are emerging because of the recent widespread increase in implant application. It is becoming increasingly important for the practicing dentist to acquire basic implant education in a comprehensive program lasting at least several months.

It is also becoming apparent that the profession needs implant specialists who focus exclusively on advancing implant dentistry through research, education and treatment of complex cases. This will shift basic implant surgical and restorative services to trained and qualified general dentists.

While educational institutions are aware of the need and are striving to provide broad training in implantology, most are just beginning to introduce implant training into their curricula. Limited funds and unavailability of trained professors, coupled with overcrowded curricula and a natural resistance to change must be overcome. Undoubtedly, the October 1992 ADA House of Delegates' resolution (89RC) will stimulate predoctoral education in the diagnosis, placement and restoration of oral implants. This resolution urges the Council on Dental Education to work with the American Association of Dental Schools to develop appropriate standards in these areas.

If the profession is to meet the public's demand for high-quality and cost-effective care, comprehensive clinical implant training in the pre-doctoral dental curriculum must provide the general dentist with the same fundamental training in implant dentistry as for other dental disciplines. If this is not done, some young dentists may get their education only from manufacturers.

Conclusion

The implant field is in a state of exciting flux that promises to change the way we practice. The advantages of the implant solution can dramatically change a person's self-esteem and quality of life. Today, however, the cost of implant treatment places it beyond the reach of many who could reap its benefits. As practitioners are trained, implant systems standardized and practice guidelines established, implant treatment will evolve into a routine part of general practice.

The opinions expressed are those of the author and do not necessarily reflect the opinion or official policies of the American Dental Association. Dr. Schnitman is in private practice limited to implant dentistry; director, Boston Seminars in Implant Dentistry; immediate past president, American Academy of Implant Dentistry; and founder and former head, Department of Implant Dentistry, Harvard School of Dental Medicine.

— by Paul A Schnitman, D.D.S., M.S.D.

Chapter 53

Dental Implant Care: Should It Be a Specialty?

The ADA's Council on Dental Education and the House of Delegates Have Twice, in 1985 and 1987, denied the American Academy of Implant Dentistry's application for specialty recognition of dental implantology. The specialty application committee of AAID plans to continue efforts toward attaining specialty recognition.[1,2]

This issue points out a valuable attribute of our profession—a willingness to address changing trends through formal channels like the ADA Council on Dental Education and the ADA House of Delegates.

An objective overview of the dental implant specialty recognition issue might lend insight to the subject.

Discussion

There are six criteria that must be met to receive the ADA's recognition as a specialty.[1] In its application, AAID has failed to meet the third, fourth and sixth criteria. The third and sixth criteria deal with education. The new specialty shall not be coincident with other recognized specialties (criteria 3), and there must be formal advanced education programs of at least two years (postdoctoral) capable of educating and training qualified individuals for the specialty (criteria 6). The fourth criterion requires a determination that current dentists and specialists are unable to meet the public demand and need for implant care. This will be discussed later.

©1993 *Journal of American Dental Association* (JADA Vol 124, April 1993). Reprinted with permission.

Dental implants definitely are an integral component of the formal education programs for oral and maxillofacial surgeons, periodontists; and prosthodontists.[1] At issue is the argument that existing dental programs cannot adequately cover the scope of dental implants or give a "unique emphasis" that an implant specialist program could.[3,4]

Currently, there are or will be requirements at the in-depth and proficiency level for advanced education in dental implants for oral and maxillofacial surgery, periodontics and prosthodontics that provide a standardized means of assuring appropriate implant education.[5-7] This is the basis for the team approach to implant dental care.[8] It offers a broad multitalented knowledge base of shared expertise.

The cooperative team approach also provides a corrective mechanism for specialty bias or "specialty myopia"—treatments viewed only through a particular specialty.[9] The team coordinator is usually a general dentist, implant-educated general dentist or prosthodontist.[3] There is no question that for the general dentist to assume the team leadership role, he or she needs standardized education to ensure basic knowledge of dental implants. But it is debatable whether this person needs to possess in-depth knowledge and demonstrated proficiency in all phases of dental implants.

The requirements at the predoctoral level currently do not go beyond the familiarity and understanding level of instruction and will probably require future upgrades.[10,11] Postdoctoral curriculum guidelines for general practice residency and advanced education in general dentistry are written for the understanding level with highly desirable recommendations that the postdoctoral student demonstrate competency in diagnosis, treatment planning and maintenance procedures.[12]

Most U.S. dental schools provide required lectures and elective courses on dental implants. A few schools provide pre-doctoral patient care experiences with surgical and restorative phases.[3,13] In addition, four institutions provide postdoctoral dental implant programs for general dentists and specialists.

Dental implantology is a clinical method available to solve oral deficiencies. It shares a multidisciplinary approach with craniomandibular disorders and dental occlusion. All of these rely on basic research in areas such as biomechanics, bioengineering, biomaterials, physiology and interdisciplinary team efforts in terms of diagnosis, treatment planning and treatment methodologies.

Although there are orofacial pain clinics, postdoctoral programs and departments of occlusion and craniomandibular disorders in dental schools, specialty status has not been a prominent agenda item for these disciplines. Dental implantology has probably been thrust into the profession's conscience because the resurgence of dental implants as a treatment method can be traced to basic animal and clinical studies that provided a long-term, predictable treatment option not previously available.[14]

Despite great strides, implantology remains just one of several treatment options available to patients. It is an excellent treatment option, and many documented articles deal with patient satisfaction.[15-16] Realistically, though, many patients cannot afford the cost, and some cannot deal with the time and commitment required. Some are unwilling to undergo the surgical phases required for implant placement. Dental implants are still prostheses placed in a variable and dynamic environment subject to the limitations that govern all of our treatment modalities. It is not a 100 percent fail-safe method. Some of the limitations identified with other prosthodontic options also influence the treatment outcomes for patients selecting dental implant care.[21-25]

If we look to our medical colleagues for a similar example of a clinical procedure evolving into a specialty, we are unable to find a comparison. Implants do not fall under one discipline or specialty, nor is there a specialty of implantology in medicine.

The sixth criterion for ADA specialty recognition requires documentation that current dentists and specialists are unable to meet the public need and demand for implant care. Predictions for increased demand are evident, and more and more implants are being placed.[3,26-28]

There is a definite U.S. population of employed adults and seniors with one or both edentulous arches who may be seeking dental implant care as a treatment option.[29] A 1985-86 National Survey of Oral Health conducted by the National Institute of Dental Research revealed 50 percent of U.S. seniors 65 years and older are completely edentulous. Employed adults aged 45 to 64 make up the largest group who have mandibular bilateral or unilateral edentulism.[29]

Patients with bilateral or unilateral edentulism require surgical implant placement in a zone of the mouth with higher risk factors and only a developing documentation of longevity.[30] Between 1986 and 1990, there was a decreasing proportion of general dentists and an increasing proportion of specialists placing implants.[27] This may be the result of risk management issues and proposed curriculum changes to advanced education programs that mandate in-depth dental implant education, for example, in periodontics.[31]

Despite some compelling contentions, there is no indication the dental profession is not currently meeting the public demand and needs for dental implant care.[9] As with all changing trends, however, dentistry must continually monitor these changes and modify its educational programs accordingly.

Our goal as health professionals is to provide the most effective therapies to our patients.[30] Unfortunately, dental care—particularly dental implant care—is reaching only a select socioeconomic population.[15-17] Dental care often is viewed by the public as a discretionary expense with some consumers feeling they get poor value for their money.[26,32]

High-technology equipment and procedures have clouded our view of some basic issues. Our society has not determined what level of primary medical care everyone should be entitled to, nor have we in the dental profession addressed the same question as it applies to dentistry.[33]

Conclusion

There is a growing demand and need for dental implant care as a treatment option for selected patient populations. The current team approach to this care is accommodating this demand and need. Not only must we closely monitor this need and modify our education programs accordingly, but we must also explore avenues to make this treatment option available to a broader patient population.

As standards of patient care are being developed, they must include dental implant therapy. As dentists become more involved in such high technology as esthetic computer imaging, preventive education and primary care should be directed toward specific patient populations that are still becoming partially or totally edentulous.

The opinions expressed or implied in this article are strictly those of the author and do not necessarily reflect the opinion or official policies of the American Dental Association or Omnigraphics.

—by Lee M. Jameson, DDS., M.S.

References

1. McCann D. Implantology—does it merit specialty status? JADA 1990;121(3): 322-8.
2. Evasic R. Statement of the American Academy of Implant Dentistry. J Dent Educ 1988;52(12):765-6.
3. Misch C. Dental education: meeting the demands of implant dentistry. JADA 1990;121(3):334-8.
4. Schnitman P. Education in implant dentistry. JADA 1990;121(3): 330-2

5. Commission on Dental Accreditation. The standards for advanced specialty education programs in oral and maxillofacial surgery. Chicago: American Dental Association, 1991.
6. Commission on Dental Accreditation. Draft revision document. The standards for advanced specialty education programs in periodontics. Chicago: American Dental Association, February 2-5, 1991.
7. Commission on Dental Accreditation. The standards for advanced Specialty education programs in prosthodontics. Chicago: American Dental Association, 1992.
8. Laney W. Team communication. Int J Oral Implantol 1990; 5(1):3.
9. Misch C. Implantology seeks specialty recognition. Dentistry Today 1993;12(2):36-9.
10. Curriculum guidelines for fixed prosthodontics. J Dent Educ 1993,57(1): 49-55.
11. Curriculum guidelines for predoctoral implant dentistry. J Dent Educ 1991;55(11):751-3.
12. Curriculum guidelines in implant dentistry for general practice residency and advanced education in general dentistry programs. J Dent Educ 1993;57(1):56-8
13. Bavitz J. Dental implantology in U.S. dental schools. J Dent Educ 1990;54(3):205-6.
14. Zarb G. Implants for complete denture therapy. J Dent Educ 1988;52(12):721-4.
15. Nihill P. Expectations and satisfaction with implants (Masters thesis). Chicago: Northwestern University Dental School;1991.
16. Tavares M, Branch L, Shulman L. Dental implant patients and their satisfaction with treatment. J Dent Educ 1990; 54(11) 670-9.
17. Kiyak H, Beach B, Worthington P Taylor T, Bolender C, Evans J. The psychological impact of osseointegrated dental implants. Int J Oral Maxillofac Implants 1990;5(1)619.
18. Grogano A, Lancaster D, Finger I Dental implants: A survey of patients' attitudes. J Prosthet Dent 1989;62(5) 573-6.
19. Brecker S. Clinical procedures in occlusal rehabilitation. 2nd ed. Philadelphia: Saunders 1966:449-47.
20. Fenton A. The roll of dental implants in the future. JADA 1992,123(1):37.
21. Langer A, Michman J, Seifert I. Factors influencing satisfaction with complete denture in geriatric patients. J Prosthet Dent 1961;11(6):1019-31.

22. Van Waas M. The influence of clinical variables on patient's satisfaction with complete dentures. J Prosthet Dent 1990; 63(5):307-10.
23. Newton A The difficult denture patient. Br Dent J 1975;138(3) 93-7.
24. Friedman N, Landesman H, Wexler M. The influences of fear, anxiety and depression on the patient's adaptive responses to complete dentures. Part II. J Prosthet Dent 1988;59(1):45-8.
25. Davis E, Albino J, Tedesco L, Portenoy B. Expectations and satisfaction of denture patients in a university clinic. J Prosthet Dent 1986;55(1):59-43.
26. McCann D. The dental work force: meeting the public's and the profession's needs JADA 1989-118(4):423.
27. Stillman N. The developing market for dental implants. JADA 1993;124(4):514.
28. Worthington P: Current implant usage. J Dent Educ 1988; 52(12) 692-5.
29. Meskin L, Brown L Prevalence and patterns of tooth loss in US. employed adult and senior populations, 1985-86. J Dent Educ 1988;52(12):686-91.
30. Zarb G, Zarb F, Schmitt A. Osseointegrated implants for partially edentulous patients. Dent Clin North Am 1987;31(3):457-72.
31. O'Leary D. New priorities for quality of care evaluation. JADA 1988;117(1):147.
32. Howard T. Good deal or rip-off? Consumers value basics. Chicago Tribune 1993;Feb 16:1,2.
33. Loucks V Jr. Health care: A test of leadership: Chicago Tribune 1992;Nov 18:23.

Chapter 54

Children at Risk from Not Using Head & Mouth Gear During Sports

Dental experts are reminding parents that children risk broken teeth and other dental and facial injuries if they are not wearing protective face and mouth gear on the playing field. The reminder comes after the release of the first national data that shows children do not consistently wear mouthguards and headgear during organized sports. The information was contained in a paper by NIDR researchers, published in the current issue of Public Health Reports. "Even though protective devices for the face and mouth have been around for decades and have been shown to prevent injury, we found that their use is spotty and varied except in football," said NIDR's Ruth Nowjack-Raymer, RDH, MPH, the report's lead author. The findings further suggest that although there are differences in use of protective equipment by race, grade level, and socioeconomic status, the differences are not consistent across all sports and are therefore not predictive of use. Injuries to the face and mouth include facial bone fractures, broken and knocked out teeth, jaw joint injuries, concussion, blinding eye injuries, permanent brain injury, and in rare cases, trauma that can result in death. Experts have not determined exactly how many sports-related orofacial injuries occur each year, but it is estimated that almost one-third of all dental injuries are due to sports-related accidents.

Survey Results

The data on children and protective gear were extracted from the 1991 National Health Interview Survey (NHIS) conducted by the

National Institute of Dental Research. http://www.nidr.nih.gov

National Center for Health Statistics. NIDR researchers analyzed the answers of parents or guardians of 9,630 children aged 7 to 17 responding to questions about their children and sports. Data on the sample population were used to estimate how many of the approximately 38 million school-aged children in the U.S. play certain sports and whether the youngsters wear protective headgear and mouthguards. Included in the survey were questions about baseball and softball, soccer, football, field or ice hockey, wrestling, lacrosse, rugby, boxing, and karate or judo.

An estimated 14 million schoolchildren play at least one of the listed organized sports, with over one-fourth of that group involved in two or more sports activities, according to the authors. Baseball and softball are the most popular organized children's sports in the U.S. The researchers reported that almost a quarter of school-aged children play some form of the national pastime.

Differences among Sports

Among the youngsters who play baseball or softball, 35 percent wear headgear and 7 percent wear mouthguards all or most of the time. Children at or below the poverty level wore headgear less often than their more affluent peers. Mouthguard use in baseball differed by race, with African American youngsters wearing protective mouthguards more often than white children. High school students were more likely to wear mouthguards than kids in elementary school during baseball or softball. Almost 5 million youngsters play soccer, the second most popular sport among school-aged children, according to the survey. Only 4 percent of soccer players wore headgear and 7 percent wore mouthguards all or most of the time. Mouthguards were worn more often by high school athletes than by elementary schoolchildren playing soccer.

In football, the third most popular sport played by youngsters, nearly three-fourths of children wore protective headgear and mouthguards all or most of the time. "Part of the reason for the use of protective equipment in football is rules established in the early 1960s requiring use of mouthguards and headgear," said Nowjack-Raymer. "Before that time, half of all football injuries were to the mouth and face. Now, facial and dental injuries account for less than 2 percent of injuries in football."

High school players wore both headgear and mouthguards more often than younger players during football. Youngsters who lived above the poverty level and those whose parents had more education were more likely than other children to wear headgear.

Need for Rules and Education

Based on the findings, the authors say that enforcing rules and regulations already on the books could help decrease sports injuries. In football, where rules are enforced, kids are more likely to wear protective equipment than in baseball, where not all teams or leagues require use of safety equipment or only selected player positions are covered by rules. During soccer, a sport in which rules for wearing protective mouthguards are virtually nonexistent, children are much less likely to wear them than youngsters playing football or baseball.

The researchers also suggested advising parents and coaches of the potential for injury during sports and the importance of head and mouth protection. Educating coaches is particularly important, Nowjack-Raymer said, since research has shown that they greatly influence the behavior of their student-athletes.

Another consideration in attempting to increase the use of protective gear is product design. Mouthguards, for example, must be engineered to be comfortable, functional, and able to accommodate growing children's mouths and orthodontic appliances, the researchers noted.

The NIDR paper, "Use of Mouthguards and Headgear in Organized Sports by School-aged Children," appears in the January-February issue of *Public Health Reports*.

Chapter 55

Bridges and Dentures: Many Ways to Replace Missing Teeth

Bridges and Dentures

Almost everyone missing a front tooth wants it replaced, but is it necessary to replace missing posterior teeth? The answer depends on how many teeth are missing and whether or not the empty space presents a problem. It also depends on the patient's finances and, more often than not, whether there is dental insurance to defray at least 50 percent of the cost. Insurance may be the decisive factor, often accounting for treatment that otherwise would be considered nonessential.

The Economics of Bridges and Dentures

Replacement of missing teeth is very expensive and provides a major source of income to dentists. Because people are conditioned to pay for appliances and mechanical devices, it is customary to charge fees for prostheses that generate higher hourly income than for fillings. To be sure, crowns, bridges, and dentures are expensive because of the time involved and the added cost of laboratory construction, including the labor of the technician and the costs of materials. Nonetheless, when these costs are deducted from the total fee for the appliance, dentists earn more per hour for this kind of work than for most other services.

Because fees vary, reflecting the competitive dental marketplace, it is not a bad idea to obtain a few estimates whenever a lot of expensive bridgework is required. But price should never be the only determinant. As John Ruskin is quoted on the nineteenth-century marketplace: There is hardly anything in this world that one man cannot make worse and sell for less. The person who considers price only is this man's lawful prey.

One way to "make worse and sell for less" is to rush through treatment. Good dental technique requires careful attention to details, which takes more time and, not infrequently, repetition of a procedure or an impression until the correct result is achieved. The less time a dentist spends on a procedure for which a fee has been established, the higher the hourly income; therefore, the lowest-priced dentist may be less able to resist the temptation to cut corners. On the other hand, there is no guarantee that a high-priced dentist will be more conscientious. The goal, then, is to locate a dentist who is competent in technique and reasonable in his or her charges. This requires that the consumer have at least a basic understanding of the basis for treatment.

Preference for Fixed Bridges Is Natural

Fixed bridges are virtually indistinguishable from the natural teeth, in contrast to a partial denture that is bulkier and must be removed to clean around the metal-plastic base and clasps. Yet if the larger expenditure of multiple fixed bridges is beyond one's means, a well-designed partial denture can be as comfortable as fixed bridges.

If nothing is known of a dentist's skills, a removable bridge is the safest way to replace missing teeth. After all, if the fit is poor, it can always be thrown away. Not so with a fixed bridge that is cemented onto adjacent teeth that have been cut down for artificial crowns to which the missing teeth are attached. If the crowns are poorly done, the bridge will be lost in a few years along with the teeth.

How Permanent Are Bridges?

A good fixed bridge will last a decade or longer. When a bridge fails within a few years of placement, the reason is almost always poor dentistry, not patient neglect. Much less expensive removable bridges—partial dentures—last as long as good fixed bridges if they are properly constructed and cared for. Patients who have resisted persuasive arguments to replace well-functioning partial dentures with fixed bridges have been known to wear the same appliance for 15 or 20 more years. An experienced dentist knows not to tinker with success and does not recommend replacements in the absence of obvious need. Some fixed bridges, however, rival the Golden Gate in span, stretching from a back molar on one side to the last molar on the other side with too few supporting teeth in between. An "ear to ear" or "roundhouse" bridge costs thousands of dollars more than a removable bridge and seldom lasts longer. Too often these great bridges are monuments to the ambitions of the dentists but end up as disasters to their patients when they come loose and have to be removed along with the teeth that have decayed extensively underneath. Nevertheless, if enough strong teeth remain, if good oral hygiene is maintained, and if the dentist is experienced and conscientious, fixed bridges, large and small, are well worth the effort and the money.

Restorations seem to last longer when there is no dental insurance to pay for replacement. Willing patients and those with insurance may be receptive to suggestions that they replace crowns and bridges even when all that is required is a small gum line filling to repair a decayed margin. Most insurance plans limit coverage for crowns, bridges, and dentures to once in five years. This seems like an arbitrary limitation, but it does help prevent the worst abuses.

There Needs to Be a Problem

Most often the decision to replace teeth should be made on a sense of felt need for improvement of appearance or function, though account should be taken of the future consequences of leaving things as they are. The dentist's responsibility the condition of the remaining teeth and the patient's ability to chew and otherwise function effectively. The dentist should also predict for the patient what will likely occur if the missing teeth are not replaced. But because dentists are trained to think in terms of restoring every mouth to an ideal state, patients cannot rely solely on professional recommendations. Before going ahead with bridgework, you should be convinced that there really is a problem that needs correction, not just an empty space that offends the dentist's sensibilities.

Reasons for Replacing Missing Teeth

In addition to restoring function and appearance, replacement of missing teeth prevents other teeth from moving into the empty spaces, which in turn prevents periodontal breakdown and possible loss of other teeth. But teeth are not stacked in the mouth like a row of dominoes. Extraction of one or a few teeth does not necessarily lead to loss of other teeth. Except for appearance, functional reasons for replacing every lost tooth are often exaggerated. Nevertheless, there are good reasons for replacements, such as the missing front tooth that discourages smiling or where insufficient back teeth remain for adequate mastication, causing the front teeth to be overworked and eventually to be broken down.

Early Loss of a Six-year Molar: the Case for a Second Extraction

The permanent teeth that are most frequently lost in childhood are the first molars. If the child's second molars have not yet erupted, they can be an excellent replacement. For example, if a child's 6-year molar is extracted because of gross decay before the eruption of the second permanent or 12-year molar, the developing second molar will drift forward into the space of the first molar. But the opposing first molar will move up or down into the empty space, depending on which tooth was lost, upsetting the position of all the molars in that arch. To prevent super-eruption of the opposing molar, it should be extracted at the same time, thereby allowing the upper and lower second molars a chance to replace the first molars. This also provides room for the third molars to erupt without difficulty. Even if the second molars do not replace the first molars perfectly, the condition will still be better than if only one first molar is extracted.

Not All Teeth Super-erupt

Teeth do not always extrude into open spaces. In a young person, there is a high probability of tooth movement into spaces vacated by extracted teeth. The older the patient, the less likely it is to occur, and then it is not always harmful. There is the example of a patient in his mid-fifties who had all his upper teeth and a lower partial denture replacing a few lost molars. It fit well but was a constant annoyance because he could not stop tongue-doodling with the appliance. Having been warned by his former dentist of the dire consequence of super-eruption of the unopposed molars without the partial denture, he continued to wear it despite the constant annoyance. When he explained his inability to adjust, a more sympathetic dentist suggested that he try doing without the partial since he had enough teeth to chew with. Twenty years later he is still grateful for the suggestion. The other teeth have held up, and his unopposed upper molars have stabilized in bone, not extruded downward.

This kind of non-treatment is very successful because it does no harm and relieves the patient of discomfort, but it is not very popular among dentists because it provides them little professional or economic satisfaction.

When to Replace a Missing Tooth

Assuming all the first and second molars are in normal occlusion and the lower first molar is extracted sometime during adolescence, the second molar frequently drifts and tilts forward into the space. The bicuspid in front of the space is less likely to drift backward because it is held in place by occluding with the upper teeth. At this early age, the upper first molar super-erupts slightly down into the space below until further movement is prevented by contact with the shifting lower teeth in adjacent spaces. Quite often the teeth stabilize at this point, but it is not uncommon for small spaces to remain, which collect food particles and plaque, causing further tooth decay and periodontal breakdown. Thus, it is desirable to prevent shifting of other teeth by replacing the missing tooth soon after extraction. But there should be at least a two-month delay to allow the tooth socket to heal so that the artificial tooth (pontic) will fit snugly against the gum ridge. If the tooth is replaced immediately after extraction, the gum is likely to shrink away from the pontic, creating a food trap that is a constant annoyance.

What if the extraction was many years ago, and the teeth have already shifted so that the space is small and the situation has stabilized? What if the adjacent teeth are sound, with only small fillings or perhaps no filling at all? What if the bone support is strong and there is no periodontal breakdown around these teeth? What if you do not miss the tooth until your dentist reminds you of the small space and recommends a fixed bridge? Listen to what your dentist has to say, but before consenting to any new bridge, make sure that the case for not leaving well enough alone is truly persuasive. If you face the circumstances outlined above, a bridge will probably be recommended.

Restoring Chewing Surfaces

Many dentists insist that a full complement of teeth is necessary for proper mastication, a conclusion that is unrelated to reality. If many posterior teeth are missing, replacement with fixed or removable bridges is generally advisable to balance the chewing table even though the need for replacement may not be felt. Otherwise there is a tendency to chew more on the front teeth, which can be very damaging since the incisors are designed for cutting food, not grinding. However, two-thirds of the natural teeth in occlusion is sufficient for adequate mastication. If chewing contact is present from the first molar on one side to the second bicuspid on the other side, replacement of missing teeth is not essential. In fact, many people get along very well with only bicuspids to chew on following loss of all their molars.

For the Sake of Appearance

Almost everyone wants to replace a missing front tooth. Not so the old man who ran a cheap restaurant near a dental school in New York City. His missing upper central incisor provided a space that was just the right width to hold an ever-present cigarette. He could talk, smile, and chew gum without missing a puff. Since the cigarette was part of his face, replacing the tooth would serve no purpose.

We cannot be faulted for wanting to look our best, and that includes the appearance of our teeth, but we can be faulted for accepting or insisting on cosmetic treatment that has no cosmetic value. As an example, dentists often place a porcelain-covered metal crown on an upper second molar instead of an unbreakable full metal crown. The only way another person can see such a tooth is if the patient does a headstand with his or her mouth wide open and the other person kneels with a flashlight. It is just as foolish to have porcelain-covered metal crowns on lower second molars. The same can usually be said for the lower first molars since they are not visible in normal speaking and smiling. The best restoration for a molar, assuming filling is not possible, is a gold onlay or a three-quarter or full gold crown.

Small spaces may be the result of an extraction at a young age or may simply be related to the fact that the circumference of the jaw is too large for all the teeth to be held in contact. In the absence of functional or esthetic problems, grinding down healthy teeth at the risk of nerve injury to place a small bridge is potentially more harmful than ignoring the space. It is even more foolish if to see the space you have to hold a mirror six inches in front of your face and then grimace to lower the lower lip. This is quite different from the normal movements of the lips, which draw back over the lower front and side teeth when one smiles, rendering them even less visible than in normal speech. But there are some people whose teeth are visible back to the lower first molars. For them, replacement of missing teeth even where the space is small or covering first molar crowns with porcelain veneers makes esthetic sense.

Types of Bridges and Dentures

Fixed bridges. Fixed bridges are usually constructed of crowns on either side of missing teeth that are cemented to natural teeth, called abutments, and pontics or artificial teeth suspended between the crowns. Abutment teeth are reshaped to remove bulges so that the artificial crowns can fit over them to hold the bridge in place.

Fixed bridges usually replace one or two teeth. If three or more teeth are to be replaced, the abutments must have long and strong roots, or else they will be loosened by the additional stress. Long-span bridges sometimes require double abutments at one or both ends to share the load, particularly when the abutment teeth are short. But if the crowns and the roots are short, the patient is well advised to consider a removable rather than a long, overloaded fixed bridge.

When the space is small, five or six millimeters in width as in the case of a lateral incisor or small bicuspid, only one abutment or attachment tooth is necessary from which the pontic is cantilevered. The attachment teeth are usually covered by full crowns for maximum retention. By retention is meant the resistance of the bridge to loosening. If the crown is not made properly, the cement bond will not be strong enough to hold the bridge in place. The skill of the dentist and the design of the bridge—not the strength of the cement—determines success or failure. For this reason, bridges generally should be made with crowns on the abutments, rather than inlays or onlays, because the latter lack sufficient retentive strength. An exception would be a very small bridges in which case strong onlays, or three-quarter crowns on large teeth, are satisfactory.

Most fixed bridges are made by fusing porcelain to a semiprecious or nonprecious metal base. Semiprecious metal avoids the risk of a hypersensitivity reaction to the nickel in nonprecious metal, without significantly increasing cost. Since a porcelain veneer can chip or fracture, the chewing surfaces of the bridge should be made entirely of metal. Also, porcelain on an occlusal surface acts like a millstone, grinding away the enamel of opposing natural teeth.

An alternative to conventional bridges. The Maryland bridge, named after the university dental school where it was developed in the 1970s, is an alternative to a small conventional fixed bridge. It has the distinct advantage of requiring only minor modification of abutment teeth. Instead of grinding off all the enamel and some dentin, small metal wings are bonded to the inside enamel of the natural crown on either side of the pontic to hold it in place. Success is dependent on careful case selection, design, and bonding. The Maryland bridge is not suitable for replacement of more than one molar or a few anterior teeth. Too long a span results in torquing and breaking of the bond. But if only one or two small teeth are involved, and if the abutment teeth would not otherwise benefit from artificial crowns, the Maryland bridge is an ideal choice.

Defective bridges. As with any restoration, the bite of a bridge must be correct. All the teeth should come together evenly and without interference or "tripping" over opposing teeth in lateral movements. There should be no high spots or sense of imbalance. Patients should never tell a dentist that they can get used to the bridge if the bite feels even slightly off center or high. A good dentist continues to adjust the bite until it feels just right.

If a fixed bridge comes loose in a few years, the cause is usually faulty design and poor abutment tooth preparation. Most often the crowns are not long enough and the attachment teeth are overtapered. Or in the case of the Maryland bridge, the attachment arms are too small or the bonding was defective. Sometimes a bridge can be recemented or rebonded. If it comes loose more than once, it should be remade.

Gum line sensitivity following cementation is due to a crown that does not completely cover the surfaces of the tooth that were ground off or to an open margin. When a cavity develops in two or three years, the cause is most likely poor construction of the crown with a deficient margin at the gum line. This is especially true, if the cavity is on the inaccessible proximal surface between teeth. A deficient bridge should be remade at no charge. A small gum line defect on the outside buccal or the lingual surface of a crowned tooth can be corrected satisfactorily with a filling.

Patients are often blamed for causing the cavity by eating too many sweets and not keeping the bridge clean. Since many people do not brush thoroughly, such accusations have a ring of truth to them. But it is the rare person who through neglect develops a gum line cavity around a fixed bridge so soon after placement. When such a cavity occurs, the dentist should not make the patient a scapegoat. If poor dental treatment is suspected, an independent examination (second opinion) should be obtained. Although dentists are reluctant to criticize colleagues, a good dentist will at least describe the problem and let the patient draw his or her own conclusion.

Removable Bridges—Partial Dentures. The removable partial denture is best suited to the replacement of a number of teeth that are missing all around the arch. It is the only choice where there are no posterior teeth to which a fixed bridge can be attached. (For exceptions, see the section in this chapter on implants.) They also provide less chance of injury to the nerves of sound teeth because none have to be ground down for crowns.

A partial denture consists of saddles to hold artificial teeth, the underside literally saddling toothless ridges, a base or bar connected to the saddles in different parts of the mouth, and retainers or clasps to grip abutment teeth and hold the partial denture in place. Rests or small extensions of clasps sit on the occlusal or chewing surfaces of the abutments to prevent the partial from sinking into the tissue.

The base is customarily cast in a stainless-steel alloy. This alloy has great strength, allowing the framework and clasps to be kept thin. Before the price of gold became too high, many partial dentures were constructed of gold. Prior to 1950, gold was a superior material because in those days the stainless steel was too brittle. The modern dental chrome alloy is not only stronger than gold but also flexible so that clasps can be adjusted and tightened from time to time. Gold no longer has any advantages in the construction of removable partial dentures unless one has an allergy to stainless steel.

Artificial teeth used on partial dentures are the same as for full dentures. Made of plastic or porcelain, the denture teeth are attached to the saddle base with pink denture plastic—acrylic—to resemble the gum tissue. The underside of the saddle, which fits on the ridge of the jaw, is also lined with acrylic. Since the ridge changes over time, this design permits periodic relining of the saddle to maintain a close fit.

Before constructing a bridge or partial denture, dentists are likely to grind off an extruded tooth to realign it with the other teeth, sometimes to the extent that root canal therapy and crown coverage become necessary. However, these teeth can be shortened slightly without inflicting nerve damage. The partial denture can also be designed with an irregular line of occlusion to accommodate extruded teeth. While it may be desirable to have an even occlusal plane, in practice the mouth really does not know the difference. If extreme extrusion has occurred in the back of the mouth, the partial can be designed with a thin metal chewing plate to restore function without having to crown or extract any of the natural teeth to make space for artificial teeth.

When to crown a clasped tooth. Some dentists recommend crowning abutment teeth that will be clasped in order to reshape their contours and to help prevent future decay. Unless a tooth requires a crown for other reasons, such as extensive decay or fracture, the added expense is unnecessary. With few exceptions, clasps can be designed to fit attachment teeth even if tilted or out of normal position. Teeth can also be reshaped without crowning by selective reduction of excessive bulges to permit easy placement and removal of the partial denture as well as to brace the teeth securely. Decay of supporting teeth is minimized by proper design and good daily oral hygiene, including cleansing of the denture base and clasps, preferably after each meal.

Clasps usually can be designed so that they are not visible, even when smiling, but sometimes the clasps come so far forward or the patient's smile is so broad that the clasps are truly unsightly. In such cases, crowns can be designed to completely hide a clasp. The very expensive precision attachments used years ago have been replaced by a dowel and dimple design that is less expensive and just as effective. The dowel is part of the partial denture and fits into a groove in the crown of the abutment tooth. A half-clasp with a pimple on the end encircles the inner surface of the crown where it is invisible. The pimple snaps into a small dimple or corresponding concavity on the inside surface of the crown to hold the partial in place. Since only visible teeth benefit from dowel and dimple design, conventional clasps can be used on all the other support teeth.

Single-tooth removable bridge. The unilateral removable bridge, also called a Nesbit after the name of the dentist who promoted it decades ago, is frowned upon by most dentists. Since only one tooth—occasionally two—is replaced, it is not uncommon for a patient to leave it out of the mouth from time to time. If it is left out a few days, the adjacent teeth sometimes shift slightly so that the bridge no longer fits. Although unlikely, the danger of swallowing a small removable bridge if it dislodges while eating is something to be considered. Since the clasps are like little hooks, surgery is necessary if it gets caught in the stomach or intestines. Poorly fitted crowns and onlays also come loose and not infrequently are swallowed. Fortunately, these things usually pass through the body without harm.

Despite these disadvantages, a person who cannot afford a fixed bridge may be well served by a Nesbit until finances permit a fixed restoration. Sometimes it is a logical choice to solve a special problem, as in the case of a patient who had to lose part of an extensive bridge that had been made years before. Since he was recovering from a stroke, extensive treatment to remake the entire bridge was inadvisable. As he was partially paralyzed, there was some doubt about his ability to remove and replace the little bridge, but he was well motivated and the Nesbit functioned successfully until his death almost a decade later.

Even though fixed bridges are customarily recommended by dentists, many patients are satisfied with unilateral removable bridges. Thus, it is not inappropriate to question the wisdom of grinding down perfectly healthy teeth to place a one-tooth posterior permanent bridge—which, if poorly done, will last only a few years. A Nesbit might serve as well, provided that the clasped teeth and the appliance are kept clean.

Proper fit. Maintaining a close fit is particularly important when the partial denture has a free-end saddle. This saddle is partly tissue supported because there is no posterior tooth to hold a clasp. Occlusal forces have to be distributed evenly over the teeth and gums. If the saddle does not fit properly, chewing forces the free end to sink down into the ridge rather than be supported by it. If the clasps are too tight or are improperly designed, the partial rotates and loosens the abutment teeth, eventually causing their loss. Partial dentures should be checked once a year by the dentist, or whenever they become bothersome, and adjusted and relined as necessary to maintain a balanced fit.

As with fixed bridges, poorly constructed removable bridges do more harm than good. If the clasps are put in the wrong position, they act as levers to loosen the teeth. A properly designed clasp that is too tight has the same effect. Thus, a removable partial denture should not snap into position. It should seat gently and be held in place without any sense of pressure. Likewise, its removal should require no more than gentle pressure and no moving of the support teeth. The saddles should be extensive and tight enough to keep all but the smallest particles of food from getting underneath.

If the bite is incorrect or the base or connecting bars press too hard against the mucosa, sore teeth and tissue sores develop. Occasional discomfort is no cause for alarm since the bite or the area of the denture irritating the gum can be relieved easily by the dentist's grinding away an insignificant amount of material. If frequent sores occur, the partial denture needs relining or replacement. A sore should heal completely within two weeks after denture adjustment. If it does not, further adjustment is necessary. To avoid shifting of abutment teeth, a partial denture should not be left out of the mouth for more than a day while waiting for an adjustment or for a sore to heal. Once the teeth shift, no matter how slightly, the partial may never fit again.

Full Dentures

Many people expect to lose all their teeth eventually because their parents ended up with dentures. They think all their dental problems will be over with false plates. Such is not the case. Among the big sales items in drugstores are denture adhesives and do-it-yourself reliners, proving that denture wearers are constantly troubled with loose fits and sore gums.

The number of edentulous (toothless) persons in the United States is decreasing. Among the reasons are the reduction of tooth decay and consequent tooth loss and the increasing availability of dental insurance to pay, at least in part, for expensive restorative treatment rather than extractions. With proper dental care, few people should lose all their teeth. Nevertheless, by age 65, over 40 percent of the population is edentulous, and nearly 50 percent by age 80. When all the permanent teeth are lost in the same arch (upper or lower), a full denture—also called false teeth or a plate—is necessary to restore function and appearance.

Some patients ask for dentures as a deliverance from the unpleasantness of dental care. Good dentists will persuade their patients to keep at least a few strategic teeth that can be clasped for support of a removable partial denture. They will not extract sound teeth. Extracting healthy teeth at the request of a patient is essentially mutilation by consensus.

Immediate dentures. If the remaining teeth cannot be saved, it is customary to have an immediate denture placed at the same time that the front teeth are extracted. The back molars and bicuspids will have been removed at least a month earlier to allow healing and better control over the construction of the new denture. Since the underlying bone and gums continue to shrink following extractions, an immediate denture gradually loosens and has to be relined. The permanent relining should be delayed for at least six months to allow complete ridge healing. During the interim, the denture can be tightened with a soft, gel-like lining material called tissue conditioner. Tissue conditioner can last several months and may also be used as a semipermanent reliner by a denture wearer who otherwise never gets a satisfactory fit.

Dentures have a way of breaking on Saturday night just before going out to dinner or when one is about to leave for work. Therefore, if the cost is not prohibitive, the immediate denture should be replaced by a new one and the immediate denture kept as a spare. A completely new denture allows improvement of the bite, of the overall fit of the denture base, and of the appearance of the artificial teeth.

An immediate denture does not have to be replaced if the fit is satisfactory after the gums have healed and the base has been relined. A duplicate denture can be made of inexpensive base and tooth acrylic by the dental laboratory at a fraction of the cost of a new denture. It can be worn for a short time while the regular denture is being repaired

Overdentures. When a tooth is extracted, the top part of the bone that surrounded the root is resorbed while the lower part of the tooth socket fills in with new bone. In other words, there is a leveling process that reduces the crest or height of the alveolar ridge. When many teeth are extracted because of advanced periodontal bone loss, the entire ridge flattens out, making denture retention and stability very difficult. This is more likely to occur in the lower jaw where the entire alveolar ridge is resorbed, leaving a thin, horseshoe-shaped jawbone termed an atrophied mandible. The only way to achieve any degree of stability on an atrophied mandible is to build up the ridge artificially with a graft or by inserting an implant with posts to support the denture base. (See the discussion of grafts and implants in this chapter.)

As long as roots are present, resorption of the alveolar bone is slowed if not completely prevented. Even where teeth are too weak to support a denture, it is sometimes possible to save a few roots, ideally the cuspids. The top parts of the roots may be left above the gum for direct support of the denture—now called an overdenture—or they may be cut off to the level of the bone and covered over by the gum. Either way, the roots remain, giving support not only to the denture above but also to the alveolar ridge bone. Although this principle applies to both arches, it is particularly relevant to the lower arch, or mandible, since that is the location of most denture problems.

More positive retention is obtained by inserting special attachments (connectors) into these roots that stick out above the gum and snap into the overdenture base. The attachments should be designed to allow minor movement of the base caused by chewing without torquing and loosening the roots. Another concern is decay of the exposed roots. All surfaces must be kept clean and free of plaque to prevent root decay.

The main disadvantage of an overdenture is the expense of root canal therapy and connectors. If connectors are not used, the opening to the root canal can be filled with amalgam, avoiding the cost of a gold cap that some dentists place over the stump, ostensibly to prevent decay. But the stump, capped or not, will decay if meticulous oral hygiene is not maintained. Application of fluoride gels and rinses will also inhibit decay.

Some patients report a better sense of "feel" with an overdenture, more like chewing on natural teeth, but there is no certainty that an overdenture will be significantly more satisfactory: Many people never adjust completely to any type of denture. Nonetheless, there is little to lose and perhaps much to gain, provided initial costs are kept to a minimum. Cutting off the crown at the level of the bone, filling the root canal, closing the canal with amalgam, and then suturing over the gum tissue sounds complex, but it is actually quite simple. It costs about as much as an extraction, a single root canal filling, and a small amalgam filling—about $275 in 1990 dollars. Connectors increase the cost per root by another $100. If more than two roots are to be retained, the dentist should be asked to reduce the charges for the additional roots. After all, it does not take four times as long to do four teeth or twice as long to do two teeth when all are done at once.

If a partial denture is supported by too few natural teeth, the teeth may eventually loosen. Anticipating their loss, which is by no means certain, some dentists recommend an overdenture so that at least the roots will be preserved to support the underlying ridge bone. Good, strong cuspids (canines or eyeteeth) are sometimes cut in half to make an overdenture when they could have been retained to support a partial denture. If the remaining teeth are strong enough to avoid a full denture, neither extraction nor removal of the crown of the tooth for root retention should be done. If only two lower cuspids remain, neither one wiggles on finger pressure, and the X-ray film shows close to 50 percent of bone remaining about the roots, a conventional partial denture is the treatment of choice.

The Natural look. Dentures are made of an acrylic base and porcelain or plastic artificial teeth. Artificial teeth come in a variety of shapes and colors to match real teeth. Denture teeth look unreal if set too straight. They can be set into the base with slight irregularities that impart a more natural look. Some patients, anticipating a new denture, ask for bright white teeth, regardless of the shade of their natural teeth and skin tones. Teeth that are too light look flashy instead of blending into the color of the face. Healthy teeth have a yellow hue, becoming slightly more yellow with age.

The color of the denture base should also be natural. Denture acrylic is usually light to medium pink, but it can be tinted darker to match a patient's gums. An extra charge for tinting a denture base is unwarranted since it costs no more to produce in the laboratory. There is no sense paying extra for a clear plastic palate on the upper denture. The palate is not visible, and if it could be seen, the clear acrylic would look more unreal than the pink of the denture base. However, characterized front teeth that simulate stained enamel fracture lines or slight mottling or a gold inlay effectively disguise a denture look. The additional charge should be nominal since characterized teeth cost about $25 more than a regular set of denture teeth; the laboratory cost of an inlay in a denture tooth is about $50.

Advice to senior denture wearers. If a denture is comfortable but requires replacement because the teeth are badly worn and chipped or the base has cracked and been repaired a number of times, it should be duplicated as closely as possible. If you are 60 years old, the teeth should not be set as though you were still 20. Don't expect the dentist to eliminate all the wrinkles around your mouth by making the teeth and the denture bases longer—what dentists call "opening the bite." The bite should be opened only if the previous dentures are so short that your mouth overcloses, making you look prematurely older. Even so, there are limits to how much the bite can be opened to lengthen your profile and smooth out your wrinkles. Improvement can often be obtained by thickening the peripheral borders of the dentures to plump out lips and cheeks that appear to have fallen in, but the wrinkles of age cannot be so easily erased.

Denture Problems

Movement in action. The upper denture with a full palatal base is more easily tolerated than the lower horseshoe-shaped denture. It fits on the broader, more solid base of the hard palate, whereas the lower ridge is narrower, and the gum tissue is thinner and more fragile. The lower denture seldom seals like the upper denture, so that it is easily displaced by action of the tongue, cheeks, and lips along the borders of the denture base.

Although the upper denture feels more secure and almost always fits tighter, both upper and lower dentures actually move and rock during chewing, swallowing, and talking. In a sense, there is no such thing as a tight denture. All are simply better or worse than others. The success of dentures is as much due to the ability of the patient to adapt as to the skill of the dentist. Even a properly fitted denture may not be successful, and sometimes a poorly constructed one is completely satisfactory to the patient. But the risk of failure is always greater if the bite is incorrect or the denture base is undersize.

Denture adhesives. Denture adhesives provide a little more security but should not substitute for a proper fit. A well-fitting upper denture rarely needs an adhesive. Since a comparable fit is seldom achieved with a lower denture, an adhesive can help for a few hours. There is no general advantage of one type of adhesive over another. Some people prefer powders, others pastes. Whatever works best is best.

Many people, especially the elderly, wear their dentures only for appearance, removing them to eat. Without teeth to chew, the pleasure of eating is severely diminished. If food is not cut into small pieces, attempting to swallow it whole is dangerous. Death from suffocation has happened all too often when a large piece of steak lodged in the throat, cutting off the airway. But the more common complaints deal with the misery of being unable to chew without pain or to laugh and smile and speak without a denture coming loose, and of the distaste for the gobs of adhesive powders and pastes that literally gum up the works.

Diminished taste and gagging. New denture wearers occasionally complain about the lack of feeling when the palate is completely covered, but they soon get used to it. Some patients complain of loss of taste, since 25 percent of taste buds are located on the hard and soft palate. However, this complaint is rare because most taste buds are located on the tongue. Then there are the gaggers, people who simply cannot tolerate the denture extending onto the soft palate, the postdam area, which provides the suction-like seal of the upper denture. A few people cannot even tolerate the plate covering the center of the hard palate. While it is preferable to cover the entire hard palate for maximum stability, with extension of the postdam two or three millimeters onto the soft palate, it is possible to make a horseshoe-shaped upper plate that leaves the palate bare. A horseshoe palate decreases retention ability, but it may be the only solution for an otherwise uncontrollable gagger.

The inaccuracy of articulation. Some dentists claim that to make the best dentures and bridges requires a special device, an expensive

440

anatomical articulator set to the measurements of the patient's natural jaw movements. This adds hundreds or even thousands of dollars to the cost. Any additional accuracy obtained by special measurements transferred to complex articulators is lost in the imprecision of the fabricating process. In addition, the slight movement of every denture on the viscous oral tissue renders such accuracy meaningless. There is no reason to pay the extra cost of anatomical articulation. The same result is obtained by any skilled dentist using a simple laboratory articulator.

Functional artificial teeth. It makes no difference what kind of teeth or base materials are used. Only the front denture teeth need to look exactly like natural teeth. The bicuspids and molars also have to look natural on the visible sides but not on the occlusal or chewing surfaces. Chewing surfaces should not have high cusps that lock in the bite and limit the free movement of dentures from side to side. Patients have less trouble if chewing surfaces are flat, albeit with special grooves to assist cutting, shearing, and grinding food. Even these grooves are not too important since teeth just barely touch on chewing. It is more the pressure of the teeth that tears and grinds food particles, not the cutting edges. Some artificial posterior teeth are designed as cutting bars to improve chewing efficiency. Magnets in reverse, or repelling, position can be set in opposite dentures so that the dentures seat more tightly as they come together. Nevertheless, none of these devices provide reliable solutions for some denture wearers, no matter how good the device seems in theory. To some problems there simply are no easy solutions.

Relines and Remakes

How long should dentures last? Some people have worn the same dentures for decades without needing relines. They are the exceptions. Most denture wearers benefit from refitting every few years as the jaw ridges continue to shrink. The inside of the old denture is ground out and relined with new acrylic plastic that bonds perfectly to the outside base. On average, a denture should last five years or longer. Regardless of its age, a denture that satisfies a patient should not be changed. New dentures, like new shoes, never fit the same. One can seldom go back to the old denture with the same comfort if it has been out of the mouth for weeks or months and the new denture has somehow changed the tissue adaptation. By the same token, do not blame your dentist for a new denture that does not fit the way you remember the old denture fitting years ago. You and your mouth are no longer the same.

Soft tissue relines. Because the hard denture base rubs on the soft tissue or skin of the mouth, denture wearers are likely to develop occasional sores. The dentist provides relief by grinding away a small amount of the denture base to reduce the pressure over the sore spot. If sores occur frequently, the denture can be relined periodically with a plastic that is semisoft or rubbery in consistency. The material gradually hardens. It is also more porous than hard acrylic and may retain unpleasant odors. But a soft reline can provide relief for months at a time.

For some denture wearers there are no permanent solutions, not even when permanency is measured in months or a year. They are the purchasers of the do-it-yourself reline pads available at drugstores. These replaceable cushions help some individuals, but they generally fit poorly and may accelerate the shrinkage of the underlying bone. A better solution is to have a dentist place a soft tissue conditioner as an inexpensive temporary liner in the denture. The material is mixed to a creamy consistency and spread on the underside of the denture, where it sets like foam rubber.

The tissue conditioner provides immediate relief from painful sores and markedly improves retention of the denture. It may be comfortable for only a few weeks or months as the material gradually hardens, and then the denture loosens again and new sores develop. Instead of looking for a permanent reline, patients with this kind of recurrent problem should have the tissue conditioner replaced as needed by the dentist or a trained assistant. Think of it as going to the hairdresser every month or having a car serviced every two or three months. Patients can also be taught to apply the material themselves at home, with periodic checkups by the dentist to assure the oral tissues are healthy. Both patients and dentists have to get over the idea that there is anything permanent about a denture base.

Because soft liners are porous, microorganisms settle into the material increasing the risk of yeast infections. This can be prevented by soaking the dentures daily for 15 minutes in a disinfectant solution.

Care of dentures. Denture materials are essentially the same as plastic and porcelain dinnerware. Soap and water clean them as well as commercial denture cleansers. Commercial denture cleansers or household chlorine bleach diluted one to 10 parts of water are convenient for overnight soaking and disinfection. Do not use harsh abrasives such as scouring powder that scratch the surface, nor full-strength bleaches that leach the color out of the plastic. The denture should be cleaned often, preferably after each meal. Small round brushes are handy for cleaning the inside of partial denture clasps, and larger denture brushes are available to reach inside the denture base. Some dentists recommend leaving dentures out of the mouth at night to give the gums a chance to recuperate, but there is no clear evidence that doing so makes any difference. Most important, dentures should always be kept in water when not worn. If the base dries out, the acrylic shrinks and distorts, affecting the fit adversely. The base also becomes more brittle.

Annual tissue examination. Even though dentures fit all right and there are no apparent problems, denture wearers should still have an annual dental examination. It takes a dentist only a few minutes to examine the oral tissues for changes and for sores that might become cancerous. Denture wearers should be particularly wary of a painless sore in the mouth. Of course, if it does not hurt, how is one to know it is there? This is one of the reasons that periodic dental examinations are recommended. It is also a reason why a denture wearer should regularly feel around his or her mouth, particularly under the tongue, to detect breaks in the tissue or painless "ulcers."

Ordinary sores caused by the pressure and movement of dentures heal in 10 to 14 days after adjustment of the denture by the dentist. If a sore persists despite repeated relief of the denture base, the problem is more serious. The constant irritation of a denture, particularly around the underside of the tongue, can cause cancer. Though uncommon, oral cancer represents about 4 percent of all cancers and 2.2 percent of cancer deaths. Suspicious areas should be examined by an oral pathologist or an oral surgeon with a biopsy for microscopic examination of the tissue. Delay could be catastrophic.

Dental Implants

The ideal implant attaches to the jawbone like the root of a tooth. It supports the crown of an individual tooth or serves as an abutment for a fixed bridge. Implants can be inserted into the jawbone to hold a full denture. While there has been significant improvement in the design of dental implants, they lack two essential features, which eventually leads to failure: an elastic attachment membrane similar to the periodontal ligament, and an epithelial attachment. The elastic membrane cushions the shock of chewing, grinding, and clenching forces applied to the root, and the epithelial attachment seals the tooth where it extrudes through the gum to prevent bacterial invasion and infection. Careful design and placement minimizes adverse forces on the "root" of the implant. Frequent professional prophylaxis and meticulous home care are essential to keep the tissue tight around the attachment post, although the implant seal will never be as complete as a true epithelial attachment.

An implant inserted into the bone is firm at first, with new bone growing into the irregularities of its design. In time, the supporting bone begins to resorb, and the implant loosens to the point where it must be removed. The problem is not simply that the material is basically incompatible with bone. The same resorption and loosening takes place with an inherently compatible implant, one's own tooth that has been knocked out and replanted. The problem is the 150 or more pounds per square inch of biting force, which inevitably breaks down both the rigid, nonelastic attachment of an artificial implant and a reimplanted natural tooth. Newer materials and improved surgical techniques have increased the success rate of implants significantly, but the five-year failure rate may still be as high as 25 percent.

Types of Implants

Osseous-integrated (bone) implants. The osseous-integrated implant is the current rage in dental implantology, representing a major advance over older methods. Success is critically dependent on careful patient selection and technical surgical performance. The implant consists of a small perforated titanium cylinder that is placed into a hole drilled in the jawbone. The gum tissue is sutured back over the implant, where it remains undisturbed for three to six months as new bone grows into and around the cylinder. After the implant has become firmly fixed in the bone, a post is screwed into the cylinder. The post sticks up through the gum for attachment of the bridge or denture.

Multiple implants are necessary for large fixed bridges and dentures. Since there are two surgical procedures, first to place—the implants, second to uncover them and insert the posts, the cost for the surgery and implants ranges from a few thousand to over $10,000. Then there is the added cost of the bridge or denture.

Blade implants. Not too long ago, blade implants were the "in" procedure, touted by enthusiasts then claiming the same high rate of success as advocates of osseous-integrated implants claim today.

Long-term outcome proved less than promised. Yet many blade implants have successfully supported fixed bridges for 10 or more years even though the five-year failure rate is over 25 percent.

One type of blade implant resembles a crescent, one end of which is driven into the vertical jawbone behind the lower third molar area, and the other end a post extruding through the gum to support the back part of a fixed bridge. Another type of blade, shaped like mother's old hand-operated chopper, is placed directly into the body of the mandible.

Subperiosteal implants. The periosteum is the tough fibrous membrane that covers bone. A subperiosteal implant is a thin metal framework that is placed under the periosteum next to the bone. While the periosteum is usually strong enough to hold the implant in place, the frame is sometimes stapled to the jawbone by long pins. The procedure requires two fairly extensive operations. In the first, the underlying jawbone is uncovered for an accurate impression. The implant is constructed in the laboratory and then inserted during the second operation.

The subperiosteal implant is used almost exclusively for denture wearers with atrophied mandibles where the ridge has worn completely flat. Four posts stick out of the gum and fit into the base of the denture to stabilize and retain it. The main cause of failure is the inflammation and infection that set in-around the posts and gradually extend to loosen the entire implant. The implant also loosens under the heavy pressure of the denture, but it can provide substantial improvement if not complete satisfaction for a few years to persons otherwise described as "denture cripples."

Implants Are Not Forever

Advocates of implants promise an end to partial and full denture miseries. Newspapers, senior citizen magazines, radio and television present advertisements by dentists claiming to be experts in dental implantology. Unfortunately, the reader of such ads too seldom tries to confirm the training and certification of these experts. But even the best dentists working on the best patients will have implant failures; dental implants are foreign objects, and the body is prone to reject them.

Success and failure are relative terms. If life with a lower denture is miserable and the price is affordable, a subperiosteal or osseous-integrated implant is a success even if it provides only a few years of improved comfort. Is it worth thousands of dollars for temporary implants to hold one or two teeth that a patient could probably do without? If only money were at risk, the answer would be relatively simple. The patient can either afford it or not. But there is also the risk of nerve or sinus injury, or extensive bone degeneration around the implants as they loosen, destroying even more of the base bone and leaving the patient with more of a problem than before. While the improvements in dental implants have been impressive, the potential for harm should not be underestimated. Implants should not be undertaken unless more conventional and less risky alternatives have been unsuccessful.

Such caveats are unlikely to deter the true dental cripple, the totally frustrated denture wearer who cannot imagine things being worse than they are. Before embarking on an implant, however, you should investigate the dentists' qualifications. Ask about their training. Find out how many implants they have done and over what period of time. Ask to see checkup X rays on their patients' implants. If they claim a success rate close to 100 percent, it is because they have performed too few or have only just begun to do them. It is 5- and 10-year success rates that indicate whether or not a dentist is sufficiently qualified to deserve your confidence.

Grafts for Dentures

Prior to implants, the only way to increase the underlying support for dentures was to build up the ridge, using either bone or skin grafts. More recently, an artificial bone graft procedure called ridge augmentation has been introduced. These types of grafts continue to have limited effectiveness, as evidenced by ongoing efforts to develop better remedies.

The bone graft serves two functions. It improves denture retention and reinforces a lower jaw that has been weakened by complete resorption of the dental ridge, leaving only a narrow, thin mandible that can fracture from the slightest blow. The graft is formed from a section of a rib or hipbone (iliac crest) that is shaped in the form of a U to replace the ridge. Hospital surgery is required to obtain the graft and then to insert it beneath the gum.

The skin graft is a roll of skin taken from the abdomen or thigh that is sutured in place over either the upper or the lower jawbone, forming a ridge to support a denture. Although not as hard or firm as a bone graft, skin grafts also improve denture retention.

Artificial bone grafts are composed of a special material, commonly hydroxylapatite to those who enjoy tongue twisters, that is placed beneath the periosteum, the tough fibrous membrane enveloping bone. The surgery is relatively simple compared to bone or skin grafts, both of which require hospitalization. Artificial bone grafts or ridge augmentation can be done in the private dental office. The procedure consists of making a minor incision through the gum tissue and separating the periosteum from the bone by tunneling an instrument along the length of the dental ridge area, thereby creating a space into which the artificial bone is injected. The material sets hard in a few weeks, during which time fibrous tissue grows into it, intertwining with the graft to stabilize it.

The relative ease of placement and the lower cost give artificial grafts a distinct advantage over bone and skin grafts. The value of any graft remains sharply limited, however, because it does not provide the positive retention of an implant. The most one can hope for is some support from the built-up ridge, some increased stability for an intrinsically movable denture.

Natural and artificial bone grafts can be combined with implants to significantly improve denture retention, as long as the grafts and implants are not rejected. To the edentulous person with severely atrophied jaws, any improvement is a godsend. If the graft implant permits wearing of an otherwise unwearable denture, if it strengthens the jawbone to reduce the risk of fracture, if it prevents a lower denture from impinging on nerves that can trigger shooting pains or create facial numbness, clearly it has value beyond the measure of dollars.

Part Seven

Special Needs and Concerns

Chapter 56

Dental Health in Children with Phenylketonuria (PKU) and Other Inborn Errors of Amino Acid Metabolism Managed by Diet

Introduction

This chapter has been prepared to inform medical and dental professionals about the dental health needs of children with PKU and similar inborn errors of amino acid metabolism. Many of these children are managed on specifically formulated diets which are high in free sugar content. Professionals have been concerned that this diet might place these children at increased risk for dental caries.

Phenylketonuria or PKU is an inherited deficiency of phenylalanine hydroxylase, the enzyme which converts phenylalanine to tyrosine. As a result of this enzyme deficiency, phenylalanine builds up to excessive levels in the blood. There is a relative deficiency of tyrosine, and there is increased excretion of phenylalanine and its organic acid metabolites, the phenylketones in the urine. Without early recognition and treatment, the child with PKU will develop moderate to severe mental retardation. However, with early diagnosis, institution of a specifically formulated dietary regime in the first month of life, and careful management of this diet, normal intellectual development is expected. Because of the need for early recognition and treatment, PKU was the first inborn error of metabolism targeted by mass newborn screening. While PKU remains the prototype inherited disorder of amino acid metabolism, many other related inherited deficiency states are now recognized and can be managed with nutritional therapies designed individually for each disorder.

U.S. Department of Health and Human Services. Publication No. HRS-D-MC 84-1.

451

The management of these inborn errors of amino acid metabolism involves restriction of a specific amino acid such as phenylalanine in the child with PKU, or restriction of a group of amino acids such as the branched-chain amino acids (leucine, isoleucine and valine) in Maple Syrup Urine Disease. There may be supplementation by an amino acid product of the blocked reaction, such as tyrosine in the child with PKU, or cysteine, in the child with homocystinuria. While a single amino acid, or a small group of amino acids is restricted, these nutritional therapies do not result in protein restriction. Through specifically designed formulae and supplemental foods, these individuals receive well over the minimum daily requirement of protein (2 grams/kg/day) with intakes usually in the range of 3-4 grams/kg/day of protein. Since other protein-containing foods are very carefully restricted in these diets, supplemental calories to meet energy needs are frequently provided by foods and drinks which are high in free sugar and/or other carbohydrates.

Parents and professionals have long been concerned about the potential for dental caries resulting from a diet which emphasizes foods high in free sugar. The data in this area are limited primarily to studies of children with PKU, and the results have been somewhat mixed. However, well-controlled studies of non-institutionalized children with PKU suggest that they do not have an increased frequency or severity of dental caries. However, just like other children in the general population, their dental health can be improved, and their dietary management requires specific prophylaxis and management for optimal dental health.

Dental Health and Amino Acid Disorders: What Is Known

Phenylketonuria (PKU) is the most studied of the amino acid inborn metabolic errors, yet findings related to oral health remain equivocal, due to limited clinical studies in this area. Four major areas of dental health have been investigated, including dental caries, malocclusion, oral hygiene, and hypoplastic or developmental defects of teeth.[1-7]

The rarity of most amino acid disorders makes generalization of oral findings difficult. None have been studied to the extent of PKU. It is worth noting that persons with amino acid disorders are subject to the same dental problems as the general population, including the extremes of disease brought on by lack of attention to good oral hygiene and regular care.

Dental Caries

Perhaps the most consistent finding in the dental studies of PKU is the caries rate (dental decay) or these patients.[2-5,7] The rate of dental caries in PKU children and adults has been found to be similar to, or in some cases less than, the general population or other comparison groups, such as siblings or institutionalized groups. Attempts to explain the caries rate have included:

- closer attention to diet and health by families of children in active PKU treatment, and

- patient oral hygiene levels equivalent to or better than comparison groups.

No adequate explanation has been found. Despite a diet that may involve frequent ingestion of carbohydrate and, for many PKU children, consumption of carbohydrate in forms adherent to teeth, PKU patients do not as a group appear to experience an increased rate of dental decay.

Dental Development and Orthodontic Problems

Available data suggest that PKU children do not experience significant alterations in tooth eruption, orthodontic problems, or malocclusion. One would have to conclude that for the person with PKU, the same factors leading to malocclusion—primarily genetic influences or premature and untreated loss of primary teeth—are important.

Oral Hygiene

Because oral hygiene care (removal of plaque and food particles by brushing and flossing) reflects numerous social and environmental variables, its study is complicated. In the few studies available, no differences in plaque accumulations between PKU children and comparison groups were noted.[4,7] Institutionalized adults with PKU may have poorer hygiene than PKU individuals who live at home, due to lack of attention to oral health in some large institutions. This difference is related to PKU only in that the institutional environment may not provide adequate care. The difference may also be related to mental retardation and behavioral problems in institutionalized untreated PKU patients.

No data are available on periodontal health in PKU patients. Oral hygiene is sometimes an indication of periodontal health, but the lack of scientific information on PKU patients makes generalization difficult.

Hypoplasia and Developmental Defects of Teeth

An area of controversy is the prevalence of congenital defects—pits, grooves, discolored areas of enamel—on both primary and permanent teeth in PKU patients. Some studies suggest an increased incidence of these abnormalities in PKU patients[1], while others do not.[4,5,7] Untreated rather than treated PKU patients appear to be at risk. Study design, however, has been inconsistent, often comparing untreated PKU patients to other mentally retarded persons, many of whom have craniofacial and other syndromal abnormalities.

DISORDER	POSSIBLE ORAL MANIFESTATIONS
Alkaptonuria	brownish tint to buccal mucosa reported intrinsic discoloration of teeth
Homocystinuria	tendency toward high-arched palate crowding and irregular alignment of teeth
Hydroxykynureninuria	stomatitis ulcerated gingiva gingivitis
Hyperlysinemia	protruding tongue and habitual open mouth high arched palate high wide maxilla
Cystinosis	stomatitis delayed eruption of primary and permanent teeth interdental bone loss bell-shaped roots enlarged pulp chambers periapical radiolucencies absence of lamina dura

Table 56.1. *Amino Acid Disorders and Possible Oral Findings*

Other Amino Acid Disorders

Hyperlysinemia and homocystinuria[8] have been associated with high arched palate and a wide maxilla. The Marfan-like appearance of homocystinuria also may include crowding of teeth.[9] Persons with cystinosis can have numerous abnormal oral findings, including stomatitis, delayed calcification and eruption of both primary and permanent teeth, and assorted morphological aberrations in teeth and bones. The stomatitis reported to be associated with cystinosis may be painful and lead to eating problems. Table 56.1 is a list summarizing available data on various amino acid disorders and assorted oral abnormalities.

Dental Disease Process

This section deals mainly with dental caries and diet in the child with PKU. The principles developed will generally apply to other disorders of amino acid metabolism treated with restricted amino acid intake. The two other major dental diseases active in humans are periodontal disease and malocclusion, each of which will be covered briefly in this section.

Dental Caries

Dental caries is believed to be an infectious disease involving bacteria such as *Streptococcus mutans* and a susceptible individual. A third necessary element is an energy source or substrate for bacterial metabolism, most commonly, the fermentable carbohydrate found in the diet. Some dental researchers would include a fourth element, time, because carious lesions develop over months, in contrast to other infectious diseases which may develop in a few days.

When all four factors are present in the oral cavity, dental caries begins. Cariogenic bacteria, which are a part of the normal oral flora, metabolize fermentable carbohydrate to produce mucopolysaccharide chains, which form dental plaque. When plaque matures, in about a day, acid is produced in sufficient concentration to decalcify the enamel surface of a susceptible tooth. If the bacterial plaque is not removed, it continues to produce both plaque and acid. The decay process, which is an acid dissolution of tooth structure, continues until one of the three main factors—bacteria, tooth susceptibility, or fermentable carbohydrate—is eliminated.

Periodontal Disease

Periodontal disease is also considered an infection involving bacteria, food, and a susceptible individual. Bacteria use carbohydrate and other nutrients to produce a toxin which attacks the soft tissue or gingiva, as well as the ligaments supporting teeth in the bones of the jaw. The toxic attack continues until the bacteria are removed. Unlike the caries process in which diet and tooth susceptibility are controllable, periodontal disease remains a disease prevented mainly by good oral hygiene. Extremes in diet such as lack of vitamins B and C can also aggravate periodontal disease, as can systemic illness such as leukemia or diabetes. Minimal and transient deficiencies in diet do not appear to have a major effect on the progress of periodontal disease.

The beginning stage of periodontal disease (gingivitis) is reversible. With adequate oral hygiene, the infection can be eliminated and health of soft tissues restored. Failure to eliminate the infection leads to periodontitis. By definition, periodontitis involves destruction of the alveolar bone which supports the teeth. The destruction progresses from the clinically visible gingival surface, down through the sulcular space between tooth and gingival tissue into the periodontal ligament and bone. The damage at this point cannot be repaired. Surgical treatment used for periodontitis is not a cure, but a reconstructive technique to minimize the progress of the disease.

Current research is directed at non-surgical management using chemotherapeutic methods to prevent disease. These agents include peroxide and tetracycline, both aimed at altering destructive oral flora, and slowing or eliminating the infection.

No data are available on periodontal disease in persons with PKU. In the absence of data, we must approach periodontal disease in PKU as with the general population, noting that the person with PKU can benefit from oral hygiene.

Malocclusion

Malocclusion includes a range of orthodontic problems, many of which require treatment. The person with PKU appears to be no more prone to having a malocclusion than anyone else. The etiology of most malocclusion is complex, and most often inherited via poorly understood polygenic mechanisms. Malocclusion of this type is unpredictable and unpreventable. In the pre-fluoride era, and still in some non-fluoridated areas or indigent populations, malocclusion can be the result of premature primary tooth loss from decay. The loss of the space-holding primary tooth results in crowding and malocclusion.

The child or adult with PKU who has a malocclusion may be treated with orthodontic therapy. Any child or adult with healthy bone support for teeth can be a candidate for orthodontic treatment, and PKU children can benefit from early intervention. To date, no special contraindications to orthodontic treatment exist for the child with PKU. Mental deficiency in PKU patients or persons with other amino acid disorders who are untreated or inadequately treated may make compliance with orthodontic treatment difficult, and for this reason an orthodontist may recommend a delay or discontinuance of treatment.

Dental Caries, Fluoride, Dietary Carbohydrates and Other Dietary Factors

Historical Perspectives

Until recently, the incidence of dental caries was considered directly related to the amount of sugar in the diet. More specifically, a direct relationship was hypothesized between the total amount of dietary sucrose consumption and caries incidence. In addition, a food was considered deleterious solely on its carbohydrate content. The logical extension of this simplistic view was a preventive approach to dietary management that

- minimized sucrose in the diet, often with disregard for individual energy needs and overall diet, and

- substituted dentally sound, but potentially unhealthful foods such as artificial sweeteners, high fat and high sodium foods, and foods with a low nutrient-to-energy ratio.

Current Concepts

Within the last decade, review of available human and animal research suggested a more complex view of the role of dietary carbohydrate is caries development. The re-examination focused on differing design elements of accepted studies with a view toward factors other than the presence of sucrose or the amount of sucrose in the diet. Dentistry today recognizes the following statements to characterize the role of fermentable carbohydrates in the initiation of dental caries:

Fermentable carbohydrates are related to dental caries. Sufficient data exist to implicate carbohydrates in the caries process. Diets free of carbohydrates or comprised of non-fermentable carbohydrate do not support dental decay.

Carbohydrate-containing foods are not equally destructive of teeth. The concept of good and bad foods based on carbohydrate content is no longer an accepted one. Foods of varying carbohydrate content, when used in animal studies, often produced unexpected results, because of the role of factors other than concentration.

No direct proportional relationship exists between concentration of fermentable carbohydrates and the extent or frequency of dental caries. Diets rich in fermentable carbohydrate need not be associated with a high caries rate, especially if control of other cariogenic factors is maintained.

Frequency of eating is at least as important as the total amount of carbohydrate consumed. In retrospect, it is easy to see how frequency and amount were confused in interpretation of research studies. Animals often were not restricted in frequency of feeding, yet the quantification of consumption of carbohydrate in those designs simply looked at amount of carbohydrate consumed rather than how often it was consumed. Today we know that if carbohydrate is consumed in bulk, and at lower frequency, much of it can pass through the oral cavity unused by bacteria. If the same amount of carbohydrate is consumed in many smaller increments, the oral cariogenic bacteria have more opportunities to use it for acid production. The teeth are subject to acid attack more often in a given time period.

Food retention is an important factor in caries generation. Food retention and clearance from the oral cavity go hand in hand. Liquid carbohydrate tends to be less cariogenic than highly retentive solid carbohydrate because it is cleared from the mouth more rapidly. In many animal studies, liquid sucrose diets using high concentrations proved to be less cariogenic than solid diets of lower sucrose concentration. The difference was in retention of food on the teeth. This retention permits bacteria access to food and thus the tooth is subjected to bacteria for longer periods of time. Saliva cannot dilute solid retentive foods as quickly.

Food properties such as acid buffering can influence cariogenic potential. Foods that have buffering capacity act to prevent a sharp drop in pH and to make the drop of shorter duration, thus subjecting the tooth to a shorter, less serious acid attack. Chocolate bars may be less cariogenic than granola bars because of the fat and cocoa content, both of which act as caries retardants.

It is difficult, if not impossible, to measure the cariogenic potential of an individual food in the diet. Although some methods are available to measure acid production, none can account for the host of factors involved in dietary cariogenesis. The most common method used to "predict" cariogenicity of a food is to measure oral acid production for a time period after consumption. Other methods use enamel dissolution by acid produced or retentiveness on teeth after eating a particular food. It should be apparent that one food within the entire diet, even if deemed cariogenic, is of little consequence. Another complicating factor in measuring cariogenicity is that many foods are eaten together, yet cariogenicity is measured in the laboratory on single foods. Two foods, in fact, may not be as dangerous to teeth when eaten simultaneously. Table 56.2 shows the varying cariogenicities of foods using various measures.

Other Dietary Factors Relating to the Development of Caries-Resistant or Caries-Susceptible Teeth

- Animal studies suggest adequate iron during tooth development imparts some resistance to decay. No human studies are available in this area.

- Protein deficiency during development can also markedly affect the quality of the dentition and, to some degree, its caries resistance (based on animal data).

- The role of trace elements such as manganese, selenium, and tin in tooth development and subsequent caries susceptibility remains equivocal.

- Extremes of deficiencies of vitamins such as vitamins C, A and D can lead to abnormal development and increased susceptibility to decay.

Unfortunately, human data describing the relationship between minor nutritional deficiencies and dental decay are minimal. The most

Table 56.2. *Cariogenicity of Various Foods by Various Measures (pH Depression, Retentiveness)*

FOOD (ALPHABETICAL ORDER)	RETENTIVENESS[1] (mg CHO)	FOOD pH	pH DEPRESSION[2]	FERMENTATION ACID[3] (ml 0.05M Na OH)	ENAMEL[4] DISSOLVED (mg)
Angel Food Cake	11.39	5.15	4.48	---	---
Chocolate Cake	10.63	8.20	3.66	1.96	0.56
Chocolate Graham Cracker	3.43	7.13	3.66	1.64	0.31
Coca Cola®	3.56	2.65	3.20	0.16	0.90
Jelly Candy	---	5.04	4.45	0.37	0.29
Milk	3.66	6.6	0.75	0.17	0.35
Peanuts	3.29	6.55	0.09	---	---
Sucker (Fruit)*	3.60	2.92	4.30	0.00	7.11
Sugarless Gum	2.00	5.8	0.46	---	---
White Bread	10.12	---	---	1.35	0.74

1. *Retentiveness* measured by carbohydrate retained in mouth after eating food where samples are collected from expectorated oral fluid after 15 minutes.

2. *pH Depression* measured as the sum of pH depressions for 30 minutes.

3. *Fermentation Acid* is measured by acid production by salivary bacteria.

4. *Enamel Dissolved* is measured by the amount of enamel dissolved by acid produced by salivary bacteria using 2% sucrose = 1 as a control value.

*Various flavors combined.

460

sensible and accepted control of development of a caries-resistant dentition is a well-balanced diet during tooth development.

Fluoride and Dental Caries

Fluoride (F⁻) is undeniably the single most safe, most effective and economic caries-preventive measure available. Fluoride is considered both a nutritional and a therapeutic anti-caries measure.

A nutritional perspective emerging in dentistry is the concept of fluoride as an essential nutrient rather than a supplement to manage the problem of caries. The term fluoride-deficient describes anyone whose intake of fluoride is below optimal levels. Optimal intake has been determined to be 0.05 mg/kg/day.

During tooth development, ingested fluoride can be incorporated into the enamel; post-eruptive fluoride maintains the tooth's resistance to decay, mainly by its topical effect as it passes through the oral cavity.

The mechanism of fluoride action is still under study. The long-held yet simplistic theory that fluoride incorporated into enamel during development imparts resistance to decay still holds true. In addition, the current belief is that fluoride imparts caries protection by inhibiting bacterial metabolism. A third theory currently under evaluation is that fluoride facilitates the remineralization of teeth. Remineralization is a newly recognized homeostatic mechanism in which minerals in saliva replace those lost in the acid dissolution of the tooth surface enamel. The mechanism is not entirely understood, but recent experimental evidence suggests that this process is active in the oral cavity and that fluoride acts to shift the equilibrium from tooth dissolution to tooth remineralization. Remineralization is essentially a healing process for very small beginning carious lesions. This mechanism, as well as the action of fluoride on bacterial metabolism, may account for post-eruptive fluoride caries resistance from topical action in communal water supplies, rinse programs, and fluoride dentifrices.

Dietary Management of PKU and Amino Acid Disorders with Concern for Dental Health Problems

Although the few studies available seem to indicate that persons with PKU do not have a higher caries rate than the general population, some patients can still experience extremes in dental caries. Until more data are available, it is reasonable to assume that the person with PKU or an amino acid disorder is at risk for developing dental decay. The special potential risk factors for these patients related to diet may include the following:

Special Diet High in Carbohydrate

The diet for PKU contains sufficient carbohydrate to present more than the usual potential for dental decay. Current knowledge on the role of carbohydrate in dental caries initiation provides optimism that the carbohydrate concentration can be overcome by attention to other characteristics of foods, as well as to fluoride intake and oral hygiene care. Enough evidence exists from studies of isolated populations world-wide with similar high carbohydrate diets and low caries rates to suggest that high carbohydrate intake alone may not be very significant. Dietary management of PKU that relies on a carbohydrate-rich diet needn't be in conflict with dental health.

Management: Wise choice of foods, appropriate tooth cleaning, and adequate fluoride intake make goals for dental health compatible with those for recommended PKU management.

Frequent or Prolonged Bottle Use

A common problem in bottle-fed infants is nursing bottle caries, an early and insidious decaying of primary teeth from prolonged and frequent daily or night-long bottle feeding. The disease process involves a fermentable carbohydrate such as milk (lactose), formula, juice (fructose) or sugared soft drinks (sucrose), normal oral bacteria, and a susceptible dentition exposed to these fluids for extended periods. The most common pattern is for the child to use a bottle throughout the night or during naps for several months. The child falls asleep and stops actively feeding, but the sugar-containing liquid continues to bathe the teeth and is metabolized to acid by oral bacteria. Saliva flow is slowed during sleep, minimizing its protective effects such as dilution. Frequent bottle feedings during the day for the purpose of insuring adequate calorie intake or pacifying the child can also lead to nursing bottle caries. Several anecdotal reports in the dental literature have even implicated breast feeding when the child has unlimited access to the breast, or when the child sleeps with mother, nursing throughout the night.

Clinically, children with nursing bottle caries have badly decayed or chalky, decalcified upper front teeth. The lower front teeth may be paradoxically free of caries, often attributed to the protective feeding position of the tongue and cleansing action of saliva from sublingual salivary glands. Advanced decay often leaves the teeth so weak that the crowns fracture at the gum line, giving the impression the teeth have exfoliated. Abscesses also can develop and endanger the permanent tooth buds.

Management: Management of nursing bottle caries involves providing parents with alternatives. The first option is not letting the child sleep with the bottle or use it for a pacifier during the day. A second choice, as effective, is to substitute water in the bottle. Still another effective technique is to use a pacifier (without sweetening the nipple) instead of a bottle, if behavior is the problem. Weaning to a glass as soon as advisable can also help. Sips from a cup can be started as early as six months of age. Oral hygiene with a toothbrush and adequate fluoride via an oral-topical route are good adjunctive, even as early as the eruption of the first tooth. Education of parents to recognize the signs of nursing bottle decay can provide secondary prevention via early treatment, as can early visits to a dentist.

Frequent Feedings and Snacking

Frequency of carbohydrate consumption is now believed to be as significant as the total amount of carbohydrate eaten. Improved knowledge about the *in vivo* decay process at the level of the tooth surface suggests that each carbohydrate challenge is potentially dangerous.

A beneficial concept for understanding the impact of frequency is pH depression of dental plaque after carbohydrate consumption. A pH of 5.5 is thought to be needed for tooth decay to begin, although the duration of pH depression needed to support decay is unknown. Oral ingestion of fermentable carbohydrate in the presence of mature plaque (about a day old) usually depresses the pH for up to an hour (Figure 56.1). Carbohydrate in liquid, fibrous, or other non-retentive forms tend to depress the pH for shorter periods of time.

If a day's required intake of carbohydrate involves many feedings, the number of risk periods when pH may drop into caries-supporting range is increased. In addition, carbohydrate clearance depends largely on dilution by stimulated saliva, so the total time the oral cavity is in pH depression is also increased. Figure 56.2 shows graphically a hypothetical situation for an average day in the life of a 22-month-old on a low phenylalanine diet. The shaded areas depict the time the child's oral cavity is in pH depression and, therefore is at risk for decay.

Management: Frequency of feeding may not be manipulated as easily as alteration in food consistency or oral hygiene habits. The following steps can be used to minimize the risk of frequent carbohydrate challenges:

- Maintain good oral hygiene to prevent plaque from maturing to the point at which it can support decay. Figure 56.1 suggests that a clean mouth resists significant pH depression. Brushing after meals is ideal. At the very minimum, once-daily brushing, and for older children, once-daily flossing is recommended.

- Attempt to use carbohydrate in liquid form when possible to encourage oral clearance. Although plaque uses liquid carbohydrate more readily, liquids are cleared far more rapidly than solid and retentive foods. The pH also returns to dentally safe levels more readily when the carbohydrate challenge is in liquid form.

- Follow ingestion of retentive carbohydrates with tooth cleaning or rinsing with water when possible. Another alternative is to follow retentive foods with fibrous ones to effect some food removal. A liquid such as milk, liquid formula, or water can be used to follow a carbohydrate challenge to dilute the sugar and minimize the length of pH depression.

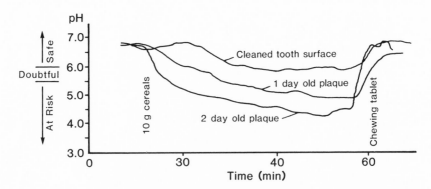

(Modified from: Bibby, B.: Food Relationships to Caries, In: Hefferren, J.J. and Koehler, H.M.: Foods, Nutrition, and Dental Health, Park Forest South (Illinois): Pathotox Publishers, 1981.)

Figure 56.1. *The pH of interdental plaque after eating a breakfast cereal of three subsequent days (telemetric recording), showing pH depression into caries-initiating areas.*

- If possible, snacking and other carbohydrate intake should be controlled. The control of meals and snacking in overall PKU diet management, as well as the attention to detail on food amounts, would seem to fit well into a low frequency carbohydrate exposure program for dental health. This attention to detail in diet programs has already been suggested as a possible reason for the low caries rates seen in studies of PKU.

- Finally, explanation to parents about the role of frequency of carbohydrate consumption and the effect of extremes such as nursing bottle caries or uncontrolled access to candy helps focus their efforts. It is important to develop an overall concept of carbohydrate in the diet as relates to PKU management and dental health.

Formula Use Encouraging Retention on Teeth

As a child grows, the need for increasing caloric intake requires modification of diet. A common practice in PKU management is to modify formula consistency by decreasing the amount of water in the mixture, and thus obtain a higher calorie-to-volume ratio. In some cases, the formula mixture may take on the consistency of pudding. Formula may also be eaten dry or as a paste. The thicker the formula the more retentive the carbohydrate, and the more resistant it becomes to clearance. The pH depression persists for a prolonged period.

Management: Some management techniques directed at frequency also work for problems with retention caused by formula thickening. Good oral hygiene care to eliminate plaque is an important first step. Introduction of fibrous foods as well as liquids to encourage clearance helps. In some cases, it may be preferable to include other types of carbohydrate when possible. Increased frequency of a thinner mix may need to be balanced against fewer challenges with a thicker retentive carbohydrate. A decision on management of frequent intake of highly retentive carbohydrates should include:

- Overall caloric needs of the child
- Adequacy of oral hygiene
- Options for substitution of foods of lower retentive consistency
- Sequencing and choice of foods to encourage oral clearance
- Current oral health status of the child

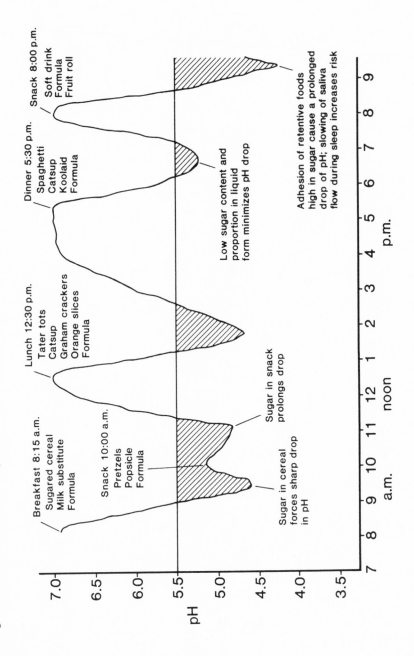

Figure 56.2. Diagrammatic Depiction of a day's Diet for a 22-Month-Old Child with PKU, Showing pH Depression in the Danger Area When Mature Plaque is Present on the Teeth.

Free Foods High in Carbohydrate

Supplementation with free foods, many of which are high in readily available sugars, must be recognized as a potential dental health problem for the child with PKU. With appropriate management, the high carbohydrate concentration need not be a problem. Animal and some human data suggest that the concentration of sugar and caries rate need not have a linear relationship. The evidence available indicates that once a certain threshold concentration of sucrose or other sugar is reached, dental caries incidence does not increase appreciably. When sugar concentrations in diet drop below the threshold, roughly about 15 percent, dental caries begin to decrease with concentration. The dependence of this very general threshold concept on other diet factors such as consistency, frequency and sequencing of carbohydrate, as well as non-diet factors within these research studies, should caution against eliminating foods solely based on sugar content.

Management: Although it is difficult, if not impossible, to make specific recommendations on an individual's free food management, several general guidelines may help in minimizing potential negative effects of free food sugars on individual diets:

* Retention and frequency are as important as sugar content.

* Clearance from the oral cavity, whether by sequencing fluid intake, consumption of liquid free food, or by oral hygiene, is a major preventive measure.

* Cultural and food-specific eating styles can play a role in cariogenicity. For example, hard candy and lollipops are most commonly kept in the oral cavity for prolonged periods. The clearance factor of these foods is high, but plaque exposure is prolonged because of the way the food is consumed.

* Fruit and so-called natural sugars are potentially as cariogenic as refined sugars. Fruit juices, granola products, and honey are all excellent substrates for cariogenic bacteria. No appreciable benefit would be obtained by replacing refined sugar with honey. However, substitution of fruit in place of more retentive forms of refined sugar may help.

467

Fluoride Deficiency

The child with PKU can benefit significantly from optimal fluoride intake. Potential for fluoride deficiency (which is considered less than optimal intake of 0.05 mg/kg/day) exists from:

- lack of communal water fluoridation at 60 percent of optimal levels (optimal levels are defined as 0.7 to 1.2 ppm);

- sole reliance on human or cow's milk, estimated to have approximately 0.10 mg F-/L for formula supplementation.

Fluoride intake also comes via ingestion of natural and processed foods. Fluoride content in natural sources can vary greatly, depending on food type and growing area. Processed foods, even those of a common brand name, can have varying fluoride levels. The variability in community water fluoridation, especially in urban centers where food is processed, has made fluoride estimation in diet a more difficult task. Children can also ingest fluoride in dentifrice used for brushing, if it is swallowed accidentally. Because of wide individual variation of fluoride intake and the difficulty in estimating the fluoride content of each food on a day-to-day basis, standard tables and general rules based on population norms are used to determine fluoride needs. The following guidelines are considered when determining adequacy of fluoride intake:

	F⁻ CONC. (PPM)		
AGE	<0.3	0.3 to 0.7	>0.7
2 wks. to 2 yrs.	0.25	0	not needed
2 yrs. to 3 yrs.	0.50	0.25	not needed
3 yrs. to 14 yrs.	1.00	0.50	not needed

Table 56.3. *Recommended Fluoride (F⁻) Supplementation (MG/Day). Table shows amount of fluoride supplementation needed for various age ranges and drinking water concentrations of fluoride. American Academy of Pediatrics, Committee on Nutrition:* Pediatrics *63:150, 1979.*

- Human and cow's milk are considered poor sources of fluoride.

- Water fluoridation should be optimal; a sample showing less than 60 percent of optimal is considered the point at which supplementation is considered. Table 56.3 provides specific dose increments based on water levels.

- Fluoride estimation is usually done independently of food fluoride content; a patient's community water source is the baseline for determination of fluoride intake.

- The fluoride provided in water and food is mainly a systemic benefit. The ingestion via mouth provides some topical effect, but calculations are directed toward systemic intake.

- The concern with excess fluoride is enamel fluorosis, which occurs when fluoride levels are above optimal doses. Fluorosis includes a range of permanent enamel defects. Minor fluorosis is usually seen as white spotting on teeth. Moderate to severe fluorosis can appear as brown areas and, in some cases, pits and other disfiguring defects on the enamel. Unfortunately, fluorosis is difficult to predict. The tables used for fluoride supplementation are designed to minimize the possibility of fluorosis in most children. Tables used to calculate fluoride intake are based on average weights of children. Table 56.4 shows optimal fluoride intake based on child's weight and age.

- Infant formulas and low phenylalanine preparations have little or no fluoride. Fluoride in mixtures made from these is assumed to come mainly from added water.

- Systemic supplementation is usually continued until age 14 when all permanent teeth except third molars have erupted.

Management: Tabulation and the use of group norms have made systemic fluoride supplementation simpler. The steps in the process are as follows:

- Determine the fluoride available to the child via water supply (drinking water). Community fluoridation levels should be available from the department of health. Rural water supplies from wells can be analyzed by the department of health and private laboratories or university health centers.

- Identify age of the child.

- Find the intersection of age and fluoride concentration of drinking water on Table 56.3 to identify the supplement needed for a particular child. This is the amount needed to be added to diet.

- Determine with parents the best vehicle for fluoride supplementation, such as tablets, drops, or if indicated, a fluoride-vitamin combination.

- Discuss with parents administration of fluoride within the overall diet to determine how best to insure compliance.

- Reevaluate every six months to adjust for growth and dietary changes. Figure 56.3 shows a sample calculation for a 2-1/2 year-old child.

AGE	AVERAGE BODY WEIGHT (kg)	OPTIMUM F⁻ INTAKE (mg F/day)
1 mo	4.4	0.22
3 mo	5.6	0.28
6 mo	7.2	0.36
1 yr	9.5	0.475
1½ yr	11.0	0.55
2 yr	12.3	0.615
2½ yr	13.4	0.67
3 yr	14.4	0.72
4 yr	16.5	0.825
5 yr	18.6	0.96
6 yr	21.1	1.06

Table 56.4. Optimal fluoride intake based on 0.05 mg F/kg body weight/ day. From Wei, S.H.Y.: Fluoride Supplementation, In: Stewart, R.E., et al: Pediatric Dentistry, Scientific Foundations and Clinical Practice, St.Louis: C.V. Mosby, 1982, p. 741.

Figure 56.3. Sample Fluoride Calculation for 2-1/2 Year-Old Child

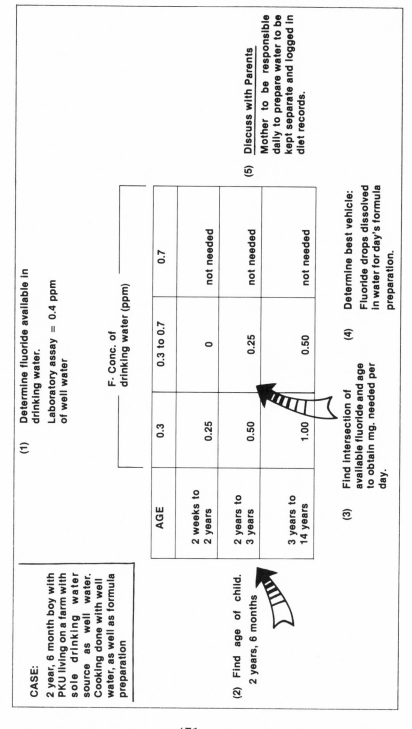

CASE:

2 year, 6 month boy with PKU living on a farm with sole drinking water source as well water. Cooking done with well water, as well as formula preparation

(1) Determine fluoride available in drinking water.

Laboratory assay = 0.4 ppm of well water

F. Conc. of drinking water (ppm)

AGE	0.3	0.3 to 0.7	0.7
2 weeks to 2 years	0.25	0	not needed
2 years to 3 years	0.50	0.25	not needed
3 years to 14 years	1.00	0.50	not needed

(2) Find age of child.
2 years, 6 months

(3) Find intersection of available fluoride and age to obtain mg. needed per day.

(4) Determine best vehicle: Fluoride drops dissolved in water for day's formula preparation.

(5) **Discuss with Parents**

Mother to be responsible daily to prepare water to be kept separate and logged in diet records.

471

A Summary of Recommendations about Diets and Dental Health for Parents of Children with PKU

1. Despite a special diet high in carbohydrates, children with PKU and other amino acid disorders can enjoy good dental health.

2. A child sleeping with a bottle of formula or any sugar-containing liquid can develop nursing caries. Try substituting water or even better, eliminate the practice of sleeping with a bottle.

3. Good daily oral hygiene removes plaque and prevents decay and gum disease. Brushing after eating is best.

4. Sugar in non-retentive forms such as liquids is better than forms which stick to teeth.

5. Frequent ingestion of carbohydrate such as sugar can be as important in dental decay as the amount of carbohydrate eaten. Try to limit the number of times carbohydrates are consumed.

6. Eating sweets at mealtime may help to minimize their influence on dental decay.

7. Following sweets with a liquid to cleanse the mouth can help clear sticky foods.

8. Fluoride protection is the simplest, least expensive preventive measure to combat tooth decay. Be sure your child is getting enough fluoride.

9. See a dentist as soon as your child has a tooth. This first visit can provide a wealth of information and prevent problems from developing.

10. Good overall nutrition with attention to both general and dental health is the best thing one can do from a dietary standpoint to control dental diseases.

Additional Reading on Nutrition and Dental Health

Nizel, A.D.: *Nutrition in Preventive Dentistry, Science and Practice.* 2nd Edition, Philadelphia: W.B. Saunders Company, 1981.

Hefferren, J.J. and Koehler, H.M.: *Foods, Nutrition, and Dental Health.* Park Forest South (Illinois): Pathotox Publishers, Inc., 1981.

The Food That Stays. New York, Medcom, Inc., 1977.

Changing Perspectives in Nutrition and Caries Research. New York, Medcom, Inc., 1979.

Wei, S.H.Y. (Ed.): *National Symposium on Dental Nutrition.* Iowa City, Iowa: University of Iowa Press, 1979.

—*by Paul S. Casamassimo, D.D.S., M.S. Beverly Entwistle, R.D.H., M.P.H., Arlene Ernest, M.A., Edward McCabe, M.D., Ph.D.*

Chapter 57

Diabetes and Periodontal Disease: A Guide for Patients

A Guide for Patients

If you have diabetes, you know the disease can harm your eyes, nerves, kidneys, heart and other important systems in the body. Did you know it can also cause problems in your mouth? People with diabetes have a higher than normal risk of periodontal diseases.

Periodontal diseases are infections of the gum and bone that hold the teeth in place. In advanced stages, they lead to painful chewing problems and even tooth loss. Like any infection, gum disease can make it hard to keep your blood sugar under control.

What Is the Link Between Diabetes and Periodontal Disease?

Diabetic Control. Like other complications of diabetes, gum disease is linked to diabetic control. People with poor blood sugar control get gum disease more often and more severely, and they lose more teeth than do persons with good control. In fact, people whose diabetes is well controlled have no more periodontal disease than persons without diabetes. Children with IDDM (insulin-dependent diabetes mellitus) are also at risk for gum problems. Good diabetic control is the best protection against periodontal disease.

Studies show that controlling blood sugar levels lowers the risk of some complications of diabetes, such as eye and heart disease and

NIH Publication No. 94-2946.

nerve damage. Scientists believe many complications, including gum disease, can be prevented with good diabetic control.

Blood Vessel Changes. Thickening of blood vessels is a complication of diabetes that may increase risk for gum disease. Blood vessels deliver oxygen and nourishment to body tissues, including the mouth, and carry away the tissues' waste products. Diabetes causes blood vessels to thicken, which slows the flow of nutrients and the removal of harmful wastes. This can weaken the resistance of gum and bone tissue to infection.

Bacteria. Many kinds of bacteria (germs) thrive on sugars, including glucose, the sugar linked to diabetes. When diabetes is poorly controlled, high glucose levels in mouth fluids may help germs grow and set the stage for gum disease.

Smoking. The harmful effects of smoking, particularly heart disease and cancer, are well known. Studies show that smoking also increases the chances of developing gum disease. In fact, smokers are five times more likely than nonsmokers to have gum disease. For smokers with diabetes, the risk is even greater. If you are a smoker with diabetes, age 45 or older, you are 20 times more likely than a person without these risk factors to get severe gum disease.

How Does Periodontal Disease Develop?

Gingivitis. Poor brushing and flossing habits allow dental plaque, a sticky film of germs, to build up on teeth. Some of these germs cause gum disease. The gums can become red and swollen and may bleed during tooth-brushing or flossing. This is called gingivitis, the first stage of periodontal disease.

Gingivitis can usually be reversed with daily brushing and flossing and regular cleanings by the dentist. If it is not stopped, gingivitis could lead to a more serious type of gum disease called periodontitis.

Periodontitis. Periodontitis is an infection of the tissues that hold the teeth in place. In periodontitis, plaque builds and hardens under the gums. The gums pull away from the teeth, forming "pockets" of infection. The infection leads to loss of the bone that holds the tooth in its socket and might lead to tooth loss.

There are often no warning signs of early periodontitis. Pain, abscess, and loosening of the teeth do not occur until the disease is advanced. Since periodontitis affects more than just the gums, it cannot be controlled with regular brushing and flossing. Periodontitis should be treated by a periodontist (a gum disease specialist) or by a general dentist who has special training in treating gum diseases.

As plaque builds up, the gums become inflamed and, in time, affected teeth may loosen and could be lost.

How Is Periodontal Disease Treated?

Plaque Removal. Treatment of periodontitis depends on how much damage the disease has caused. In the early stages, the dentist or periodontist will use deep cleaning to remove hardened plaque and infected tissue under the gum and smooth the damaged root surfaces of teeth. This allows the gum to re-attach to the teeth. A special mouthrinse or an antibiotic might also be prescribed to help control the infection.

Deep cleaning is successful only if the patient regularly brushes and flosses to keep the plaque from building up again.

Periodontal Surgery. Gum surgery is needed when periodontitis is very advanced and tissues that hold a tooth in place are destroyed. The dentist or periodontist will clean out the infected area under the gum, then reshape or replace the damaged tooth-supporting tissues. These treatments increase the chances of saving the tooth.

If You Have Diabetes . . .

- It's important for you to know how well your diabetes is controlled and to tell your dentist this information at each visit.

- See your doctor before scheduling treatment for periodontal disease. Ask your doctor to talk to the dentist or periodontist about your overall medical condition before treatment begins.

- You may need to change your meal schedule and the timing and dosage of your insulin if oral surgery is planned.

- Postpone non-emergency dental procedures if your blood sugar is not in good control. However, acute infections, such as abscesses, should be treated right away.

- For the person with controlled diabetes, periodontal or oral surgery can usually be done in the dentist's office. Because of diabetes, healing may take more time. But with good medical and dental care, problems after surgery are no more likely than for someone without diabetes. Once the periodontal infection is successfully treated, it is often easier to control blood sugar levels.

Are Other Oral Problems Linked to Diabetes?

Dental Cavities. Young people with IDDM have no more tooth decay than do nondiabetic children. In fact, youngsters with IDDM who are careful about their diet and take good care of their teeth often have fewer cavities than other children because they don't eat many foods that contain sugar.

Thrush. Thrush is an infection caused by a fungus that grows in the mouth. People with diabetes are at risk for thrush because the fungus thrives on high glucose levels in saliva. Smoking and wearing dentures (especially when they are worn constantly) can also lead to fungal infection. Medication is available to treat this infection. Good diabetic control, no smoking, and removing and cleaning dentures daily can help prevent thrush.

Dry Mouth. Dry mouth is often a symptom of undetected diabetes and can cause more than just an uncomfortable feeling in your mouth. Dry mouth can cause soreness, ulcers, infections, and tooth decay.

The dryness means that you don't have enough saliva, the mouth's natural protective fluid. Saliva helps control the growth of germs that cause tooth decay and other oral infections. Saliva washes away sticky foods that help form plaque and strengthens teeth with minerals.

One of the major causes of dry mouth is medication. More than 400 over-the-counter and prescription drugs, including medicines for colds, high blood pressure or depression, can cause dry mouth. If you are taking medications, tell your doctor or dentist if your mouth feels dry. You may be able to try a different drug or use an "artificial saliva" to keep your mouth moist. Good blood glucose control can help prevent or relieve dry mouth caused by diabetes.

Keep Your Teeth

Serious periodontal disease not only can cause tooth loss, but can also cause changes in the shape of bone and gum tissue. The gum becomes uneven, and dentures may not fit well. People with diabetes often have sore gums from dentures.

If chewing with dentures is painful, you might choose foods that are easier to chew but not right for your diet. Eating the wrong foods can upset blood sugar control. The best way to avoid these problems is to keep your natural teeth and gums healthy.

How Can You Protect Your Teeth and Gums?

Harmful germs attack the teeth and gums when plaque builds up. You can stop plaque build-up and prevent gum disease by brushing and flossing carefully every day.

- Use a piece of dental floss about 18 inches long.
- Using a sawing motion, gently bring the floss through the tight spaces between the teeth.
- Do not snap the floss against the gums.
- Curve the floss around each tooth and gently scrape from below the gum to the top of the tooth several times.
- Rinse your mouth after flossing.
- Gently brush teeth twice a day with a soft nylon brush with rounded ends on the bristles.
- Avoid hard back-and-forth scrubbing.
- Use small circlular motions and short back-and-forth motions.
- Gently brush your tongue, which can trap germs.
- Use a fluoride toothpaste to protect teeth from decay.

Check Your Work. Dental plaque is hard to see unless it is stained. Plaque can be stained by chewing red "disclosing tablets" sold at grocery stores and drug stores or by using a cotton swab to smear green food coloring on the teeth. The color left on the teeth shows where there is still plaque. Extra flossing and brushing will remove this plaque.

Dental Check-ups. People with diabetes should have dental check-ups at least every six months, or more often if recommended by their dentist. Be sure to tell your dentist you have diabetes. Frequent dental check-ups are needed to find problems early when treatment is most effective. See your dentist as soon as possible if you have any problem with your teeth or mouth.

Preventing or controlling gum disease depends on teamwork. The best defense against this complication of diabetes is good blood sugar control, combined with daily brushing and flossing and regular dental check-ups.

Dental Tips for Diabetics

- Controlling your blood glucose is the most important step you can take to prevent tooth and gum problems. People with diabetes, especially those whose blood glucose levels are poorly controlled, are more likely to get gum infections than non-diabetics.

A severe gum infection can also make it more difficult to control your diabetes. Once such an infection starts in a person with diabetes, it takes longer to heal. If the infection lasts for a long time, the diabetic person may lose teeth.

- Much of what you eat requires good teeth for chewing, so it is extremely important to try to preserve your teeth. Because the bone surrounding the teeth may sometimes be damaged by infection, dentures may not always fit properly and may not be perfect substitutes for your natural teeth.

- Taking good care of your gums and teeth is another important measure. Use a soft-bristle brush between the gums and the teeth in a vibrating motion. Place the rubber tip on the toothbrush between the teeth and move it in a circle.

- If you notice that your gums bleed while you are eating or brushing your teeth, see a dentist to determine if you have a beginning infection. You should also notify your dentist if you notice other abnormal changes in your mouth, such as patches of whitish-colored skin.

Have a dental checkup every six months. Be sure to tell your dentist that you have diabetes and ask him or her to demonstrate procedures that will help you maintain healthy teeth and gums.

Chapter 58

Dental Care for Adults with Heart Disease

Prepared by the Committee on Rheumatic Fever and Infective Endocarditis of the American Heart Association's Council on Cardiovascular Disease in the Young.

The information contained in this chapter based on the brochure entitled "Dental Care for Adults with Heart Disease" is considered by the American Dental Association to be in accord with current scientific knowledge, (1987 and still current in 1997).

If you have heart disease, you need special consideration when you get dental treatment. Physicians and dentists know this, but this may be news to you. And that's why this chapter was written: to tell you and your family about the special steps required to avoid complications of heart disease arising from dental treatment.

As someone with heart disease, you have three responsibilities. First, you need to establish and maintain a healthy mouth. That means practicing good oral hygiene and visiting your dentist regularly. Second, you need to make sure your dentist knows you have a heart problem. Finally, you must carefully follow your physician's and dentist's instructions when they prescribe special medications such as antibiotics.

Your dentist wants to be sure that dental care won't complicate your heart problem. Therefore, he or she will ask you about the nature of your heart problem and what, if any, medications you're taking for it. Be prepared to provide this information. Also, be prepared to give your dentist:

1. your physician's name and address and
2. your permission to consult your physician about your heart problem.

Several heart problems require you and your dentist to take special precautions. These include:

Heart Attack

Until a person has completely recovered from a heart attack, only emergency dental care should be performed. The reason is that in rare instances the stress of a dental procedure and exposure to local anesthetics can complicate the early recovery from a heart attack.

Irregular Heartbeat

Minor irregularities of the heartbeat ordinarily aren't affected by dental treatment. Certain serious heartbeat irregularities treated by drugs or a pacemaker may be affected by dental procedures or by drugs used in dental treatment, however. Check with your physician about the specifics of your condition.

Heart Failure

If you're taking medication for heart failure, it's especially important to maintain good dental health. Dental infection associated with severe pain or high fever can seriously increase your heart's workload and interfere with the beneficial effects of these medications. If you have trouble breathing when lying flat on your back, tell your dentist. That way he or she will know not to tilt you back any more than is absolutely necessary to work in your mouth.

Angina Pectoris

If you're subject to angina (chest pain or discomfort due to narrowing of arteries to the heart), tell your dentist what's likely to trigger an attack. If you can control the attacks with medication, be sure to tell your dentist what medications you use. And carry a fresh supply of nitroglycerine or other comparable medicine to your dental appointment. If the stress of a dental procedure causes an attack of angina, postpone the procedure until a later date if possible.

Heart Murmur

A heart murmur may or may not be important. Some innocent murmurs don't signify structural abnormalities in the heart and are nothing to worry about. But another group of murmurs (significant murmurs) are the result of structural abnormalities in the heart.

Most structural abnormalities in the heart make the valves or lining of the heart more susceptible to serious infection (infective or bacterial endocarditis) when bacteria enter the bloodstream. And bacteria can enter the bloodstream from any dental procedure that causes bleeding. Consequently, if you have a significant murmur, special precautions during your dental treatment will be required. Antibiotics may be used to prevent infection. (For more information refer to the section "Antibiotics to Prevent Bacterial Endocarditis.")

Artificial Heart Valve

Artificial heart valves are especially susceptible to infections. If you have an artificial heart valve, your dentist will probably give you an injection of antibiotics before treatment. That way you'll have maximum protection. (For more information refer to the section "Antibiotics to Prevent Bacterial Endocarditis.") If you're taking an anticoagulant (drug to thin the blood), be sure to tell your dentist.

Heart Pacemaker

Individuals with pacemakers have a very low risk of heart infection from dental procedures. Consequently, if you have a pacemaker it's unlikely your dentist or physician will administer antibiotics if the dental treatment is routine and your mouth is healthy. Of course if you have an infection in your mouth, you should have it treated immediately.

Some electrical devices used in dental offices may interfere with pacemakers. An electrical pulp tester and an electrical surgical device are two such examples. Both have non-electrical alternatives that can be used, so be sure to tell your dentist if you wear a pacemaker.

Bypass Surgery

If you've had a coronary artery bypass graft, you won't need any special precautions during dental treatment unless you also have another heart problem. If you're taking aspirin or persantin, be sure to tell your dentist.

Vascular Surgery

If part of one of your arteries has been replaced by a synthetic device or material, or if a device (such as a shunt for renal dialysis) has been implanted in a vessel, antibiotic protection may be advisable during dental procedures that cause bleeding. If you've had vascular surgery, ask your physician or dentist if you need to take antibiotics during specific dental procedures.

Antibiotics to Prevent Bacterial Endocarditis

Bacterial endocarditis is a serious infection of the heart valves or the tissues lining the heart. It occurs rarely, but it's a real threat to people with structural abnormalities of the heart or artificial heart valves, or to individuals who have had certain types of vascular surgery. The American Heart Association (AHA) and the American Dental Association (ADA) specifically recommend to dentists and physicians that they give antibiotics before performing dental procedures on these patients. The reason is that the antibiotics prevent infection of the heart by destroying bacteria that get into the bloodstream. The AHA and ADA currently recommend only a short period of antibiotic administration, typically one dose before and after a dental procedure. In many instances antibiotics can be given by mouth, but for maximum protection injecting antibiotics may be necessary.

Heart Medications

It's very important for your dentist to know the names and the doses of all medicines you take. Your dentist needs this information to avoid interfering with your medicine's effects. This is especially important for people taking blood-thinning drugs (anticoagulants).

Dental Care at Home

If you have heart disease, ask your dentist about precautions to take in caring for your mouth. And be sure to follow your dentist's instructions when using dental floss to minimize injury to your gums. Some home procedures, such as water irrigation devices, can force bacteria into the bloodstream and may cause endocarditis. Accordingly, if you have a valve or other structural abnormality of the heart, avoid these procedures. All heart patients should maintain a healthy mouth by practicing good oral hygiene at home and visiting their dentist frequently. That way, they can avoid most dental problems that complicate heart disease. If you have questions about dental care and your heart problem, don't hesitate to ask your dentist or physician.

Chapter 59

Chemotherapy and Oral Health

Why do I need to see a dentist?

If you are going to receive chemotherapy, it is important that you have a complete oral examination before you begin treatment. Many patients may not realize that chemotherapy can cause oral and dental side effects. But if dental care is started early, you can prevent or minimize these problems.

Your cancer physicians should coordinate your treatment with a dental team. If possible, any dental work you need should be performed before chemotherapy begins. Later, problems in your mouth may be more complicated and harder to treat. Tooth decay, for example, can become a serious problem, and removing a tooth will require special care. It is also important that you learn how to maintain a healthy mouth to avoid future oral problems. Even if you wear dentures, you need to be evaluated by a dentist. Research shows that preventive dental care can reduce the oral complications of cancer treatment.

What should a dental evaluation include?

The initial appointment with a dentist should include examination of the mouth and teeth and dental x-rays. This examination allows the dentist to diagnose conditions that require treatment. In consultation with your physician, the dentist will plan dental treatment to meet your individual needs.

NIH Publication No. 93-3583.

Treatment may include filling decayed teeth or removing infected or badly decayed teeth.

Dental staff should clean your teeth and show you how to control the plaque in your mouth that can cause tooth decay and gum disease. This includes careful daily brushing and flossing. To prevent tooth decay, your dentist may also recommend that you use a prescription-strength fluoride gel that you apply daily in custom-made trays. Good self-care is essential for maintaining a healthy mouth.

What oral problems can result from chemotherapy?

Chemotherapy is likely to affect the mouth and teeth to some degree. People respond differently to treatment; you may have all, or none, of the problems associated with chemotherapy. Some problems last only a short time, while others continue longer.

Certain chemotherapy drugs cause mouth sores to develop during treatment. The soft tissues of the mouth may become sensitive and irritated. The lips may crack and peel. Your dentist and physician can assist you in making your mouth more comfortable by providing mouthrinses and pain relievers. Changes in the mouth are usually at their worst shortly after you receive chemotherapy. They can be expected to heal during the recovery period.

At times during the chemotherapy cycle, you may undergo temporary periods when your resistance to infection is reduced and the ability of your blood to clot is decreased. During these times, your physician may tell you to stop brushing and flossing. Special mouthrinses to reduce plaque may be prescribed instead.

Other problems caused by chemotherapy include dry mouth, tooth development changes, and jaw or tooth pain. You may notice a change in the consistency of your saliva and your mouth may feel dry. Taking small bites, chewing slowly, and sipping liquids with your meal will make eating more comfortable. Dry mouth due to chemotherapy is usually temporary. In young people, exposure to chemotherapy drugs may lead to abnormal development of teeth that are still in the formative stages. Tooth or jaw pain may develop for no apparent reason and may be a result of nerve changes. These pains should be evaluated by your dentist.

How should I care for my mouth and teeth after chemotherapy?

You should continue regular dental checkups and good personal dental care after chemotherapy is completed. Be sure your dentist is familiar with your health. Your dentist, or physician, will need to initially check your blood counts, to be certain that your ability to fight infection and your blood's ability to clot have returned to normal. Continue with the routine you learned for cleaning and caring for your teeth and mouth. Excellent oral hygiene is the key to preventing future mouth problems.

Chapter 60

Radiation Therapy and Oral Health

Why do I need to see a dentist?

If you are going to receive radiation therapy to the head or neck area, it is important that you have a complete oral examination before you begin treatment. Many patients may not realize that radiation therapy can cause oral and dental side effects. But if dental care is started early, you can prevent or minimize these problems.

Your cancer physicians should coordinate your treatment with a dental team. If possible, any dental work you may need should be performed before you receive radiation therapy. After radiation, oral problems may be more complicated and harder to treat. Tooth decay, for example, can become a serious problem, and removing a tooth will require special care. It is also important that you learn to maintain a healthy mouth to avoid future oral problems. Even if you wear dentures, you should be evaluated by a dentist. Research shows that preventive dental care can reduce the oral complications of cancer treatment.

What should a dental evaluation include?

The initial appointment with a dentist should include examination of the mouth and teeth and dental x-rays. This examination allows the dentist to diagnose conditions that require treatment. In consultation with your physician, the dentist will plan dental treatment to

NIH Publication No. 93-3584.

491

meet your individual needs. Treatment may include filling decayed teeth or removing infected or badly decayed teeth.

Dental staff should clean your teeth and show you how to control the plaque in your mouth that can cause tooth decay and gum disease. This includes careful daily brushing and flossing. To prevent tooth decay, your dentist may also recommend that you use a prescription strength fluoride gel that you apply daily in custom-made trays. Good self-care is essential for maintaining a healthy mouth.

What oral problems can result from radiation therapy?

Radiation therapy to the head or neck area is likely to affect the mouth and teeth to some degree. People respond differently to treatment; you may have all, or none, of the problems associated with radiation therapy. Some problems last only a short time, while others are permanent.

Your mouth may become dry because of reduced saliva production. Dry mouth or thick saliva is often noticed during the first weeks of radiation. Some dryness persists after radiation therapy is completed. Having too little saliva may make chewing and swallowing difficult. Taking small bites, chewing slowly, and sipping liquids with your meal will make eating more comfortable. Reduced saliva may lead to severe tooth decay, so it is essential that you follow instructions given to you about oral hygiene and fluoride use.

Some patients experience a partial loss of taste during radiation therapy. Foods that were previously enjoyable may become unpleasant. Fortunately, these taste changes are usually temporary. Most people recover their ability to taste several months after completing treatment.

Mouth sores may develop during radiation therapy. The soft tissues of the mouth may become sensitive, irritated, and sometimes bleed. The lips may crack and peel. Your dentist and physician can assist you in making your mouth more comfortable by providing mouthrinses and pain relievers. Mouth sores are usually at their worst during radiation therapy. They generally heal during the weeks after radiation is completed.

Other problems may include muscle stiffness, tooth development abnormalities, and jaw bone changes. The muscles involved in opening the mouth and chewing may become stiff during radiation. To help maintain a full range of motion, your dentist may prescribe special jaw exercises. In young people, exposure to radiation may lead to abnormal development of teeth that are still in the formative stages.

Radiation therapy also can affect the ability of jaw bone to heal. If you need to have a tooth extracted after radiation therapy is completed, special precautions must be taken to avoid complications such as infection.

How should I care for my mouth and teeth after radiation therapy?

You should continue regular dental checkups and good personal dental care after you complete your radiation therapy. Be sure your dentist is familiar with your health. Your dentist will need to know what area was irradiated and what dose was used. If you have dry mouth, you should see your dentist three times a year. You should continue with the routine you learned for cleaning and caring for your teeth and mouth, including daily applications of fluoride. *Excellent oral hygiene* is the key to preventing future oral problems.

Chapter 61

Recommended Practices for Infection Control in Dentistry

Summary

This document updates previously published CDC recommendations for infection-control practices in dentistry to reflect new data, materials, technology, and equipment. When implemented, these recommendations should reduce the risk of disease transmission in the dental environment, from patient to dental health-care worker (DHCW), from DHCW to patient, and from patient to patient.

Based on principles of infection control, the document delineates specific recommendations related to vaccination of DHCWs; protective attire and barrier techniques; handwashing and care of hands; the use and care of sharp instruments and needles; sterilization or disinfection of instruments; cleaning and disinfection of the dental unit and environmental surfaces; disinfection and the dental laboratory; use and care of handpieces, antiretraction valves, and other intraoral dental devices attached to air and water lines of dental units; single-use disposable instruments; the handling of biopsy specimens; use of extracted teeth in dental educational settings; disposal of waste materials; and implementation of recommendations.

Introduction

This document updates previously published CDC recommendations for infection-control practices for dentistry (13) and offers guidance for

May 28, 1993 Centers for Disease Control and Prevention. Recommended infection-control practices for dentistry, 1993. MMWR 1993; 42(No. RR-8): 1-12.

reducing the risks of disease transmission among dental health-care workers (DHCWs) and their patients.

Although the principles of infection control remain unchanged, new technologies, materials, equipment, and data require continuous evaluation of current infection-control practices. The unique nature of most dental procedures, instrumentation, and patient-care settings also may require specific strategies directed to the prevention of transmission of pathogens among DHCWs and their patients. Recommended infection-control practices are applicable to all settings in which dental treatment is provided. These recommended practices should be observed in addition to the practices and procedures for worker protection required by the Occupational Safety and Health Administration (OSHA) final rule on Occupational Exposure to Bloodborne Pathogens (29 CFR 1910.1030), which was published in the Federal Register on December 6, 1991 (4).

Dental patients and DHCWs may be exposed to a variety of microorganisms via blood or oral or respiratory secretions. These microorganisms may include cytomegalovirus, hepatitis B virus (HBV), hepatitis C virus (HCV), herpes simplex virus types 1 and 2, human immunodeficiency virus (HIV), Mycobacterium tuberculosis, staphylococci, streptococci, and other viruses and bacteria specifically, those that infect the upper respiratory tract. Infections may be transmitted in the dental operatory through several routes, including direct contact with blood, oral fluids, or other secretions; indirect contact with contaminated instruments, operatory equipment, or environmental surfaces; or contact with airborne contaminants present in either droplet spatter or aerosols of oral and respiratory fluids. Infection via any of these routes requires that all three of the following conditions be present (commonly referred to as the chain of infection): a susceptible host; a pathogen with sufficient infectivity and numbers to cause infection; and a portal through which the pathogen may enter the host. Effective infection-control strategies are intended to break one or more of these links in the chain, thereby preventing infection.

A set of infection-control strategies common to all health-care delivery settings should reduce the risk of transmission of infectious diseases caused by bloodborne pathogens such as HBV and HIV (2,5-10). Because all infected patients cannot be identified by medical history, physical examination, or laboratory tests, CDC recommends that blood and body fluid precautions be used consistently for all patients (2,5). This extension of blood and body fluid precautions, referred to as universal precautions, must be observed routinely in the care of all dental patients (2). In addition, specific actions have been recommended to reduce the risk of tuberculosis transmission in dental and other ambulatory health-care facilities (11).

Confirmed Transmission of HBV and HIV in Dentistry

Although the possibility of transmission of bloodborne infections from DHCWs to patients is considered to be small (12-15), precise risks have not been quantified in the dental setting by carefully designed epidemiologic studies. Reports published from 1970 through 1987 indicate nine clusters in which patients were infected with HBV associated with treatment by an infected DHCW (16-25). In addition, transmission of HIV to six patients of a dentist with acquired immunodeficiency syndrome has been reported (26,27). Transmission of HBV from dentists to patients has not been reported since 1987, possibly reflecting such factors as incomplete ascertainment and reporting, increased adherence to universal precautions including routine glove use by dentists and increased levels of immunity due to use of hepatitis B vaccine.

However, isolated sporadic cases of infection are more difficult to link with a healthcare worker than are outbreaks involving multiple patients. For both HBV and HIV, the precise event or events resulting in transmission of infection in the dental setting have not been determined; epidemiologic and laboratory data indicate that these infections probably were transmitted from the DHCWs to patients, rather than from one patient to another (26,28). Patient-to-patient transmission of bloodborne pathogens has been reported, however, in several medical settings (29-31).

Vaccines for Dental Health-Care Workers

Although HBV infection is uncommon among adults in the United States (1 to 2 percent), serologic surveys have indicated that 10 to 30 percent of health-care or dental workers show evidence of past or present HBV infection (6,32). The OSHA bloodborne pathogens final rule requires that employers make hepatitis B vaccinations available without cost to their employees who may be exposed to blood or other infectious materials (4). In addition, CDC recommends that all workers, including DHCWs, who might be exposed to blood or blood-contaminated substances in an occupational setting be vaccinated for HBV (68). DHCWs also are at risk for exposure to and possible transmission of other vaccine-preventable diseases (33); accordingly, vaccination against influenza, measles, mumps, rubella, and tetanus may be appropriate for DHCWs.

Protective Attire and Barrier Techniques

For protection of personnel and patients in dental-care settings, medical gloves (latex or vinyl) always must be worn by DHCWs when there is potential for contacting blood, blood-contaminated saliva, or mucous membranes (1,2,46). Non-sterile gloves are appropriate for examinations and other nonsurgical procedures (5); sterile gloves should be used for surgical procedures. Before treatment of each patient, DHCWs should wash their hands and put on new gloves; after treatment of each patient or before leaving the dental operatory, DHCWs should remove and discard gloves, then wash their hands. DHCWs always should wash their hands and reglove between patients. Surgical or examination gloves should not be washed before use; nor should they be washed, disinfected, or sterilized for reuse. Washing of gloves may cause wicking (penetration of liquids through undetected holes in the gloves) and is not recommended (5). Deterioration of gloves may be caused by disinfecting agents, oils, certain oil-based lotions, and heat treatments, such as autoclaving.

Chin-length plastic face shields or surgical masks and protective eyewear should be worn when splashing or spattering of blood or other body fluids is likely, as is common in dentistry (2,5,6,34,35). When a mask is used, it should be changed between patients or during patient treatment if it becomes wet or moist. Face shields or protective eyewear should be washed with an appropriate cleaning agent and, when visibly soiled, disinfected between patients.

Protective clothing such as reusable or disposable gowns, laboratory coats, or uniforms should be worn when clothing is likely to be soiled with blood or other body fluids (2,5,6). Reusable protective clothing should be washed, using a normal laundry cycle, according to the instructions of detergent and machine manufacturers. Protective clothing should be changed at least daily or as soon as it becomes visibly soiled (9). Protective garments and devices (including gloves, masks, and eye and face protection) should be removed before personnel exit areas of the dental office used for laboratory or patient-care activities.

Impervious-backed paper, aluminum foil, or plastic covers should be used to protect items and surfaces (e.g., light handles or x-ray unit heads) that may become contaminated by blood or saliva during use and that are difficult or impossible to clean and disinfect. Between patients, the coverings should be removed (while DHCWs are gloved), discarded, and replaced (after ungloving and washing of hands) with clean material.

Appropriate use of rubber dams, high-velocity air evacuation, and proper patient positioning should minimize the formation of droplets, spatter, and aerosols during patient treatment. In addition, splash shields should be used in the dental laboratory.

Handwashing and Care of Hands

DHCWs should wash their hands before and after treating each patient (i.e., before glove placement and after glove removal) and after barehanded touching of inanimate objects likely to be contaminated by blood, saliva, or respiratory secretions (2,5,6,9).

Hands should be washed after removal of gloves because gloves may become perforated during use, and DHCWs hands may become contaminated through contact with patient material. Soap and water will remove transient microorganisms acquired directly or indirectly from patient contact (9); therefore, for many routine dental procedures, such as examinations and nonsurgical techniques, handwashing with plain soap is adequate. For surgical procedures, an antimicrobial surgical handscrub should be used (10).

When gloves are torn, cut, or punctured, they should be removed as soon as patient safety permits. DHCWs then should wash their hands thoroughly and reglove to complete the dental procedure. DHCWs who have exudative lesions or weeping dermatitis, particularly on the hands, should refrain from all direct patient care and from handling dental patient-care equipment until the condition resolves (12). Guidelines addressing management of occupational exposures to blood and other fluids to which universal precautions apply have been published previously (68,36).

Use and Care of Sharp Instruments and Needles

Sharp items (e.g., needles, scalpel blades, wires) contaminated with patient blood and saliva should be considered as potentially infective and handled with care to prevent injuries (2,5,6).

Used needles should never be recapped or otherwise manipulated utilizing both hands, or any other technique that involves directing the point of a needle toward any part of the body (2,5,6). Either a one-handed scoop technique or a mechanical device designed for holding the needle sheath should be employed. Used disposable syringes and needles, scalpel blades, and other sharp items should be placed in appropriate puncture-resistant containers located as close as is practical to the area in which the items were used (2,5,6). Bending or breaking of needles before disposal requires unnecessary manipulation and thus is not recommended.

Before attempting to remove needles from non-disposable aspirating syringes, DHCWs should recap them to prevent injuries. Either of the two acceptable techniques may be used. For procedures involving multiple injections with a single needle, the unsheathed needle should be placed in a location where it will not become contaminated or contribute to unintentional needle sticks between injections. If the decision is made to recap a needle between injections, a one-handed scoop technique or a mechanical device designed to hold the needle sheath is recommended.

Sterilization or Disinfection of Instruments

Indications for Sterilization or Disinfection of Dental Instruments

As with other medical and surgical instruments, dental instruments are classified into three categories critical, semi-critical, or noncritical depending on their risk of transmitting infection and the need to sterilize them between uses (9,37-40). Each dental practice should classify all instruments as follows:

- **Critical.** Surgical and other instruments used to penetrate soft tissue or bone are classified as critical and should be sterilized after each use. These devices include forceps, scalpels, bone chisels, scalers, and burs.

- **Semi-critical.** Instruments such as mirrors and amalgam condensers that do not penetrate soft tissues or bone but contact oral tissues are classified as semi-critical. These devices should be sterilized after each use. If, however, sterilization is not feasible because the instrument will be damaged by heat, the instrument should receive, at a minimum, high-level disinfection.

- **Non-critical.** Instruments or medical devices such as external components of x-ray heads that come into contact only with intact skin are classified as non-critical. Because these noncritical surfaces have a relatively low risk of transmitting infection, they may be reprocessed between patients with intermediate-level or low-level disinfection (see Cleaning and Disinfection of Dental Unit and Environmental Surfaces) or detergent and water washing, depending on the nature of the surface and the degree and nature of the contamination (9,38).

Methods of Sterilization or Disinfection of Dental Instruments

Before sterilization or high-level disinfection, instruments should be cleaned thoroughly to remove debris. Persons involved in cleaning and reprocessing instruments should wear heavy-duty (reusable utility) gloves to lessen the risk of hand injuries.

Placing instruments into a container of water or disinfectant/ detergent as soon as possible after use will prevent drying of patient material and make cleaning easier and more efficient. Cleaning may be accomplished by thorough scrubbing with soap and water or a detergent solution, or with a mechanical device (e.g., an ultrasonic cleaner).

The use of covered ultrasonic cleaners, when possible, is recommended to increase efficiency of cleaning and to reduce handling of sharp instruments.

All critical and semi-critical dental instruments that are heat stable should be sterilized routinely between uses by steam under pressure (autoclaving), dry heat, or chemical vapor, following the instructions of the manufacturers of the instruments and the sterilizers. Critical and semi-critical instruments that will not be used immediately should be packaged before sterilization.

Proper functioning of sterilization cycles should be verified by the periodic use (at least weekly) of biologic indicators (i.e., spore tests) (3,9). Heat-sensitive chemical indicators (e.g., those that change color after exposure to heat) alone do not ensure adequacy of a sterilization cycle but may be used on the outside of each pack to identify packs that have been processed through the heating cycle. A simple and inexpensive method to confirm heat penetration to all instruments during each cycle is the use of a chemical indicator inside and in the center of either a load of unwrapped instruments or in each multiple instrument pack (41); this procedure is recommended for use in all dental practices. Instructions provided by the manufacturers of medical/dental instruments and sterilization devices should be followed closely.

In all dental and other health-care settings, indications for the use of liquid chemical germicides to sterilize instruments (i.e., cold sterilization) are limited. For heat-sensitive instruments, this procedure may require up to 10 hours of exposure to a liquid chemical agent registered with the U.S. Environmental Protection Agency (EPA) as a sterilant/disinfectant. This sterilization process should be followed by aseptic rinsing with sterile water, drying, and, if the instrument is not used immediately, placement in a sterile container.

EPA-registered sterilant/disinfectant chemicals are used to attain high-level disinfection of heat-sensitive semi-critical medical and dental instruments. The product manufacturers directions regarding appropriate concentration and exposure time should be followed closely. The EPA classification of the liquid chemical agent (i.e., sterilant/disinfectant) will be shown on the chemical label. Liquid chemical agents that are less potent than the sterilant/disinfectant category are not appropriate for reprocessing critical or semi-critical dental instruments.

Cleaning and Disinfection of Dental Unit and Environmental Surfaces

After treatment of each patient and at the completion of daily work activities, countertops and dental unit surfaces that may have become contaminated with patient material should be cleaned with disposable toweling, using an appropriate cleaning agent and water as necessary. Surfaces then should be disinfected with a suitable chemical germicide.

A chemical germicide registered with the EPA as a hospital disinfectant and labeled for tuberculocidal (i.e., mycobactericidal) activity is recommended for disinfecting surfaces that have been soiled with patient material. These intermediate-level disinfectants include phenolics, iodophors, and chlorine-containing compounds.

Because mycobacteria are among the most resistant groups of microorganisms, germicides effective against mycobacteria should be effective against many other bacterial and viral pathogens (9,38-40,42). A fresh solution of sodium hypochlorite (household bleach) prepared daily is an inexpensive and effective intermediate-level germicide. Concentrations ranging from 500 to 800 ppm of chlorine (a 1:100 dilution of bleach and tap water or 1/4 cup of bleach to 1 gallon of water) are effective on environmental surfaces that have been cleaned of visible contamination. Caution should be exercised, since chlorine solutions are corrosive to metals, especially aluminum.

Low-level disinfectants EPA-registered hospital disinfectants that are not labeled for tuberculocidal activity (e.g., quaternary ammonium compounds) are appropriate for general housekeeping purposes such as cleaning floors, walls, and other housekeeping surfaces. Intermediate- and low-level disinfectants are not recommended for reprocessing critical or semi-critical dental instruments.

Disinfection and the Dental Laboratory

Laboratory materials and other items that have been used in the mouth (e.g., impressions, bite registrations, fixed and removable prostheses, orthodontic appliances) should be cleaned and disinfected before being manipulated in the laboratory, whether an on-site or remote location (43). These items also should be cleaned and disinfected after being manipulated in the dental laboratory and before placement in the patients mouth (2). Because of the increasing variety of dental materials used intraorally, DHCWs are advised to consult with manufacturers regarding the stability of specific materials relative to disinfection procedures. A chemical germicide having at least an intermediate level of activity (i.e., tuberculocidal hospital disinfectant) is appropriate for such disinfection. Communication between dental office and dental laboratory personnel regarding the handling and decontamination of supplies and materials is important.

Use and Care of Handpieces, Antiretraction Valves, and Other Intraoral Dental Devices Attached to Air and Water Lines of Dental Units

Routine between-patient use of a heating process capable of sterilization (i.e., steam under pressure [autoclaving], dry heat, or heat/chemical vapor) is recommended for all high-speed dental handpieces, low-speed handpiece components used intraorally, and reusable prophylaxis angles. Manufacturers instructions for cleaning, lubrication, and sterilization procedures should be followed closely to ensure both the effectiveness of the sterilization process and the longevity of these instruments. According to manufacturers, virtually all high-speed and low-speed handpieces in production today are heat tolerant, and most heat-sensitive models manufactured earlier can be retrofitted with heat-stable components.

Internal surfaces of high-speed handpieces, low-speed handpiece components, and prophylaxis angles may become contaminated with patient material during use.

This retained patient material then may be expelled intraorally during subsequent uses (44-46). Restricted physical access particularly to internal surfaces of these instruments limits cleaning and disinfection or sterilization with liquid chemical germicides. Surface disinfection by wiping or soaking in liquid chemical germicides is not an acceptable method for reprocessing high-speed handpieces, low-speed handpiece components used intraorally, or reusable prophylaxis angles.

Because retraction valves in dental unit water lines may cause aspiration of patient material back into the handpiece and water lines, antiretraction valves (one-way flow check valves) should be installed to prevent fluid aspiration and to reduce the risk of transfer of potentially infective material (47). Routine maintenance of antiretraction valves is necessary to ensure effectiveness; the dental unit manufacturer should be consulted to establish an appropriate maintenance routine.

High-speed handpieces should be run to discharge water and air for a minimum of 2030 seconds after use on each patient. This procedure is intended to aid in physically flushing out patient material that may have entered the turbine and air or water lines (46). Use of an enclosed container or high-velocity evacuation should be considered to minimize the spread of spray, spatter, and aerosols generated during discharge procedures. Additionally, there is evidence that overnight or weekend microbial accumulation in water lines can be reduced substantially by removing the handpiece and allowing water lines to run and to discharge water for several minutes at the beginning of each clinic day (48). Sterile saline or sterile water should be used as a coolant/irrigator when surgical procedures involving the cutting of bone are performed.

Other reusable intraoral instruments attached to, but removable from, the dental unit air or water lines such as ultrasonic scaler tips and component parts and air/water syringe tips should be cleaned and sterilized after treatment of each patient in the same manner as handpieces, which was described previously.

Manufacturers directions for reprocessing should be followed to ensure effectiveness of the process as well as longevity of the instruments.

Some dental instruments have components that are heat sensitive or are permanently attached to dental unit water lines. Some items may not enter the patient's oral cavity, but are likely to become contaminated with oral fluids during treatment procedures, including, for example, handles or dental unit attachments of saliva ejectors, high-speed air evacuators, and air/water syringes. These components should be covered with impervious barriers that are changed after each use or, if the surface permits, carefully cleaned and then treated with a chemical germicide having at least an intermediate level of activity. As with high-speed dental handpieces, water lines to all instruments should be flushed thoroughly after the treatment of each patient; flushing at the beginning of each clinic day also is recommended.

Single-Use Disposable Instruments

Single-use disposable instruments (e.g., prophylaxis angles; prophylaxis cups and brushes; tips for high-speed air evacuators, saliva ejectors, and air/water syringes) should be used for one patient only and discarded appropriately. These items are neither designed nor intended to be cleaned, disinfected, or sterilized for reuse.

Handling of Biopsy Specimens

In general, each biopsy specimen should be put in a sturdy container with a secure lid to prevent leaking during transport. Care should be taken when collecting specimens to avoid contamination of the outside of the container. If the outside of the container is visibly contaminated, it should be cleaned and disinfected or placed in an impervious bag (49).

Use of Extracted Teeth in Dental Educational Settings

Extracted teeth used for the education of DHCWs should be considered infective and classified as clinical specimens because they contain blood. All persons who collect, transport, or manipulate extracted teeth should handle them with the same precautions as a specimen for biopsy (2). Universal precautions should be adhered to whenever extracted teeth are handled; because preclinical educational exercises simulate clinical experiences, students enrolled in dental educational programs should adhere to universal precautions in both preclinical and clinical settings. In addition, all persons who handle extracted teeth in dental educational settings should receive hepatitis B vaccine (68).

Before extracted teeth are manipulated in dental educational exercises, the teeth first should be cleaned of adherent patient material by scrubbing with detergent and water or by using an ultrasonic cleaner. Teeth should then be stored, immersed in a fresh solution of sodium hypochlorite (household bleach diluted 1:10 with tap water) or any liquid chemical germicide suitable for clinical specimen fixation (50).

Persons handling extracted teeth should wear gloves. Gloves should be disposed of properly and hands washed after completion of work activities. Additional personal protective equipment (e.g., face shield or surgical mask and protective eyewear) should be worn if mucous membrane contact with debris or spatter is anticipated when the specimen is handled, cleaned, or manipulated. Work surfaces and equipment should be cleaned and decontaminated with an appropriate liquid chemical germicide after completion of work activities (37,38,40,51). The handling of extracted teeth used in dental educational settings differs from giving patients their own extracted teeth. Several states allow patients to keep such teeth, because these teeth are not considered to be regulated (pathologic) waste (52) or because the removed body part (tooth) becomes the property of the patient and does not enter the waste system (53).

Disposal of Waste Materials

Blood, suctioned fluids, or other liquid waste may be poured carefully into a drain connected to a sanitary sewer system. Disposable needles, scalpels, or other sharp items should be placed intact into puncture-resistant containers before disposal. Solid waste contaminated with blood or other body fluids should be placed in sealed, sturdy impervious bags to prevent leakage of the contained items. All contained solid waste should then be disposed of according to requirements established by local, state, or federal environmental regulatory agencies and published recommendations (9,49).

Implementation of Recommended Infection-control Practices for Dentistry

Emphasis should be placed on consistent adherence to recommended infection-control strategies, including the use of protective barriers and appropriate methods of sterilizing or disinfecting instruments and environmental surfaces. Each dental facility should develop a written protocol for instrument reprocessing, operatory cleanup, and management of injuries (3). Training of all DHCWs in proper infection-control practices should begin in professional and vocational schools and be updated with continuing education.

Additional Needs in Dentistry

Additional information is needed for accurate assessment of factors that may increase the risk for transmission of bloodborne pathogens and other infectious agents in a dental setting. Studies should address the nature, frequency, and circumstances of occupational exposures. Such information may lead to the development and evaluation of improved designs for dental instruments, equipment, and personal protective devices. In addition, more efficient reprocessing techniques should be considered in the design of future dental instruments and equipment. Efforts to protect both patients and DHCWs should include improved surveillance, risk assessment, evaluation of measures to prevent exposure, and studies of post-exposure prophylaxis. Such efforts may lead to development of safer and more effective medical devices, work practices, and personal protective equipment that are acceptable to DHCWs, are practical and economical, and do not adversely affect patient care (54,55).

Use of trade names is for identification only and does not imply endorsement by the Public Health Service, the U.S. Department of Health and Human Services, or Omnigraphics.

References

1. CDC. Recommended infection-control practices for dentistry. MMWR 1986;35:237-42.

2. CDC. Recommendations for prevention of HIV in health-care settings. MMWR 1987;36:(No.2S).

3. US Department of Health and Human Services. Infection control file: practical infection control in the dental office. Atlanta, GA/Rockville, MD:CDC/FDA, 1989. (Available through the US Government Printing Office, Washington, DC, or the National Technical Information Services, Springfield, VA.)

4. Department of Labor, Occupational Safety and Health Administration. 29 CFR Part 1910.1030, occupational exposure to bloodborne pathogens; final rule. Federal Register 56(235):64004-182, 1991.

5. CDC. Update: universal precautions for prevention of transmission of human immunodeficiency virus, hepatitis B virus, and other bloodborne pathogens in health-care settings. MMWR 1988;37:37782,387-8.

6. CDC. Guidelines for prevention of transmission of human immunodeficiency virus and hepatitis B virus to health-care and public-safety workers. MMWR 1989;38(suppl. No. S-6):1-37.

7. CDC. Protection against viral hepatitis: recommendations of the Immunization Practices Advisory Committee (ACIP). MMWR 1990;39(No. RR-2).

8. CDC. Hepatitis B virus: a comprehensive strategy for eliminating transmission in the United States through universal childhood vaccination. MMWR 1991;40(No. RR-13).

9. Garner JS, Favero MS. Guideline for handwashing and hospital environmental control, 1985. Atlanta: CDC, 1985; publication no. 99-1117.

10. Garner JS. Guideline for prevention of surgical wound infections, 1985. Atlanta: CDC, 1985; publication no. 99-2381.

11. CDC. Guidelines for preventing the transmission of tuberculosis in health-care settings, with special focus on HIV-related issues. MMWR 1990;39(No. RR-17).

12. CDC. Recommendations for preventing transmission of human immunodeficiency virus and hepatitis B virus during exposure-prone invasive procedures. MMWR 1991;40(No. RR-8).

13. CDC. Update: investigations of patients who have been treated by HIV-infected health-care workers. MMWR 1992;41:344-6.

14. Chamberland ME, Bell DM. HIV transmission from health care worker to patient: what is the risk? Ann Intern Med 1992;116:871-3.

15. Siew C, Chang B, Gruninger SE, Verrusio AC, Neidle EA. Self-reported percutaneous injuries in dentists: implications for HBV, HIV transmission risk. J Am Dent Assoc 1992;123:37-44.

16. Ahtone J, Goodman RA. Hepatitis B and dental personnel: transmission to patients and prevention issues. J Am Dent Assoc 1983;106:219-22.

17. Hadler SC, Sorley DL, Acree KH, et al. An outbreak of hepatitis B in a dental practice. Ann Intern Med 1981;5:133-8.

18. CDC. Hepatitis B among dental patients—Indiana. MMWR 1985; 34:73-5.

19. Levin ML, Maddrey WC, Wands JR, et al. Hepatitis B transmission by dentists. JAMA 1974;228:1139-40.

20. Rimland D, Parkin WE, Miller GB, et al. Hepatitis B outbreak traced to an oral surgeon. N Engl J Med 1977;296:95-38.

21. Goodwin D, Fannin SL, McCracken BB. An oral surgeon-related hepatitis B outbreak. Calif Morbid 1976;14.

22. Reingold AL, Kane MA, Murphy EL, et al. Transmission of hepatitis B by an oral surgeon. J Infect Dis 1982;145:262-8.

23. Goodman RA, Ahtone JL, Finton RJ. Hepatitis B transmission from dental personnel to patients: unfinished business. Ann Intern Med 1982;96:119.

24. Shaw FE, Barrett CL, Hamm R, et al. Lethal outbreak of hepatitis B in a dental practice. JAMA 1986;255:3261-4.

25. CDC. Outbreak of hepatitis B associated with an oral surgeon, New Hampshire. MMWR 1987;36:132-3.

26. Ciesielski C, Marianos D, Chin-Yih OU, et al. Transmission of human immunodeficiency virus in a dental practice. Ann Intern Med 1992;116:798-805.

27. CDC. Investigations of patients who have been treated by HIV-infected health-care workers United States. MMWR 1993;42:329-31, 337.

28. Gooch B, Marianos D, Ciesielski C, et al. Lack of evidence for patient-to-patient transmission of HIV in a dental practice. J Am Dent Assoc 1993;124:38-44.

29. Canter J, Mackey K, Good LS, et al. An outbreak of hepatitis B associated with jet injections in a weight reduction clinic. Arch Intern Med 1990;150:1923-7.

30. Kent GP, Brondum J, Keenlyside RA, LaFazia LM, Scott HD. A large outbreak of acupuncture-associated hepatitis B. Am J Epidemiol 1988;127:591-8.

31. Polish LB, Shapiro CN, Bauer F, et al. Nosocomial transmission of hepatitis B virus associated with the use of a spring-loaded finger-stick device. N Engl J Med 1992;326:721-5.

32. Siew C, Gruninger SE, Mitchell EW, Burrell KH. Survey of hepatitis B exposure and vaccination in volunteer dentists. J Am Dent Assoc 1987;114:457-9.

33. CDC. Immunization recommendations for health-care-workers. Atlanta, GA: CDC, Division of Immunization, Center for Prevention Services, 1989.

34. Petersen NJ, Bond WW, Favero MS. Air sampling for hepatitis B surface antigen in a dental operatory. J Am Dent Assoc 1979;99:465-7.

35. Bond WW, Petersen NJ, Favero MS, Ebert JW, Maynard JE. Transmission of type B viral hepatitis B via eye inoculation of a chimpanzee. J Clin Microbiol 1982;15:533-4.

36. CDC. Public Health Service statement on management of occupational exposure to human immunodeficiency virus, including considerations regarding zidovudine postexposure use. MMWR 1990;39(No. RR-1).

37. Miller CH, Palenik CJ. Sterilization, disinfection, and asepsis in dentistry. In: Block SS, ed. Disinfection, sterilization, and preservation, 4th ed. Philadelphia: Lea & Febiger, 1991:676-95.

38. Favero MS, Bond WW. Chemical disinfection of medical and surgical materials. In: Block SS, ed. Disinfection, sterilization, and preservation, 4th ed. Philadelphia: Lea & Febiger, 1991:617-41.

39. FDA, Office of Device Evaluation, Division of General and Restorative Devices, Infection Control Devices Branch. Guidance on the content and format of premarket notification [510 (k)] submissions for liquid chemical germicides. Rockville, MD: FDA, January 31, 1992:49.

40. Rutala WA. APIC guideline for selection and use of disinfectants. Am J Infect Control 1990;18:99117.

41. Proposed American National Standard/American Dental Association Specification No. 59 for portable steam sterilizers for use in dentistry. Chicago: ADA, April 1991.

42. CDC. Recommendations for preventing transmission of infection with human T-lymphotropic virus type III/lymphadenopathy-associated virus in the workplace. MMWR 1985;34:682-6,691-5.

43. Council on Dental Materials, Instruments, and Equipment; Dental Practice; and Dental Therapeutics. American Dental Association. Infection control recommendations for the dental office and the dental laboratory. J Am Dent Assoc 1988;1126:241-8.

44. Lewis DL, Boe RK. Cross infection risks associated with current procedures for using high-speed dental handpieces. J Clin Microbiol 1992;30:401-6.

45. Crawford JJ, Broderius RK. Control of cross infection risks in the dental operatory: prevention of water retraction by bur cooling spray systems. J Am Dent Assoc 1988;116:685-7.

46. Lewis DL, Arens M, Appleton SS, et al. Cross-contamination potential with dental equipment. Lancet 1992;340:1252-4.

47. Bagga BSR, Murphy RA, Anderson AW, Punwani I. Contamination of dental unit cooling water with oral microorganisms and its prevention. J Am Dent Assoc 1984;109:712-6.

48. Scheid RC, Kim CK, Bright JS, Whitely MS, Rosen S. Reduction of microbes in handpieces by flushing before use. J Am Dent Assoc 1982; 105:658-60.

49. Garner JS, Simmons BP. CDC guideline for isolation precautions in hospitals. Atlanta, GA: CDC, 1983; HHS publication no. (CDC)83-8314.

50. Tate WH, White RR. Disinfection of human teeth for educational purposes. J Dent Educ. 1991;55:583-5.

51. Favero MS, Bond WW. Sterilization, disinfection, and antisepsis in the hospital. In: Balows A, Hausler WJ, Herrmann KL, Isenberg HD, Shadomy HJ, eds. Manual of clinical microbiology, 5th ed. Washington, DC: American Society for Microbiology, 1991:183-200.

52. The Michigan Medical Waste Regulatory Act of 1990, Act No. 368 of the Public Health Acts of 1978, Part 138, Medical Waste, Section 13807—Definitions.

53. Oregon Health Division. Infectious waste disposal; questions and answers pertaining to the Administrative Rules 333-18-040 through 333-18-070. Portland, OR: Oregon Health Division, 1989.

54. Bell DM. Human immunodeficiency virus transmission in health care settings: risk and risk reduction. Am J Med 1991;91(suppl. 3B):294-300.

55. Bell DM, Shapiro CN, Gooch BF. Preventing HIV transmission to patients during invasive procedures: the CDC perspective. J Public Health Dent (in press).

The MMWR series of publications is published by the Epidemiology Program Office, Centers for Disease Control and Prevention (CDC), Public Health Service, U.S. Department of Health and Human Services, Atlanta, Georgia 30333.

Part Eight

Dental Emergencies

Chapter 62

Tooth Pain Guide

Momentary sensitivity to hot or cold foods.

If the discomfort lasts only moments, sensitivity to hot and cold foods generally does not signal a serious problem. The sensitivity may be caused by a loose filling or by minimal gum recession which exposes small areas of the root surface.

- Try using toothpastes made for sensitive teeth. Brush up and down with a soft brush; brushing sideways wears away exposed root surfaces.
- If this is unsuccessful, see your general dentist.

Sensitivity to hot or cold foods after dental treatment.

Dental work may inflame the pulp, or nerves, inside the tooth, causing temporary sensitivity.

- Wait four to six weeks. If the pain persists or worsens, see your general dentist.

Sharp pain when biting down on food.

There are several possible causes of this type of pain: decay, a loose filling or a crack in the tooth. There may also be damage to the pulp tissue inside the tooth.

©1993 American Association of Endodontists. Reprinted with Permission.

- See a dentist for evaluation. If the problem is pulp tissue damage, your dentist may send you to an endodontist. Endodontists are dentists who specialize in pulp-related procedures. Your endodontist will perform a procedure that cleans out the damaged pulp and fills and seals the remaining space. This procedure is commonly called a "root canal."

Lingering pain after eating hot or cold foods.

This probably means the pulp has been damaged by deep decay or physical trauma.

- See your endodontist to save the tooth with root canal treatment.

Constant and severe pain and pressure, swelling of gum and sensitivity to touch.

A tooth may have become abscessed, causing the surrounding gum and bone to become infected.

- See your endodontist for evaluation and treatment to relieve the pain and save the tooth.
- Take over-the-counter analgesics until you see the endodontist.

Dull ache and pressure in upper teeth and jaw.

The pain of a sinus headache is often felt in the face and teeth. Grinding of teeth, a condition known as bruxism, can also cause this type of ache.

- For sinus headache, try over-the-counter analgesic or sinus medicine. For bruxism, consult your dentist.
- If pain is severe and chronic, see your physician or endodontist for evaluation.

Chronic pain in head, neck or ear.

Sometimes pulp-damaged teeth cause pain in other parts of the head and neck, but other dental or medical problems may be responsible.

- See your endodontist for evaluation. If the problem is not related to the tooth, your endodontist will refer you to an appropriate dental specialist or a physician.

Chapter 63

Teeth Relief: A Guide for Minor Dental Emergencies

First Aid Procedures

What would you do if your child broke a tooth? What should you do? Parents and teachers are sometimes faced with dental emergencies ranging from toothaches to broken teeth to canker sores. The following is a guide of basic dental first aid procedures to follow until a dentist can be consulted. Although these first aid procedures should provide temporary relief, they cannot always cure the dental emergency. Please be sure to consult with a dentist as soon as possible when in doubt.

Toothache

If child has a toothache, rinse the mouth with warm water and floss teeth to remove food particles. If swelling occurs, apply cold packs to outside of face in area of swelling. DO NOT apply aspirin or other medications to aching tooth. Take child to dentist.

Bleeding Gums

Bleeding gums are usually the result of poor oral hygiene. By removing plaque daily from the teeth and gums with a soft-bristled toothbrush and dental floss, the gum tissue should return to normal. When red, swollen, or sore gums are present, rinse every two hours

1994 Maine Department of Human Services, Office of Dental Health.

with a mixture of equal parts of water and a 3 percent solution of hydrogen peroxide or with a warm, saltwater solution. If condition does not improve, a visit to the dentist is recommended.

Tooth Eruption Pain

Eruption of the permanent teeth is often accompanied by pain. Locate the eruption site and apply a cold pack to the exterior of the face for temporary relief. A topical anesthetic containing benzocaine or an aspirin substitute may also be beneficial. DO NOT apply aspirin to gums. If pain persists, contact a dentist.

Cold Sores, Canker Sores and Fever Blisters

Determine if there is a cause for the irritation. Is it a broken dental appliance? Braces? For temporary relief, apply a topical anesthetic containing benzocaine and avoid hot, spicy foods. An aspirin substitute may also be given for relief of pain or fever. DO NOT apply aspirin to sores. If sores are severe and not healed within 7-14 days and/ or signs of fever and pain persist, contact a dentist.

Knocked Out Tooth

If a tooth is knocked out, find it and place it in cold, whole milk or water. *Take the child and tooth to the dentist immediately! DO NOT CLEAN TOOTH!*

Broken Or Displaced Tooth

Clean injured area with warm water. If injured area begins to swell, apply cold packs to outside of face. *Take child to dentist immediately!*

Tongue or Lip Bite

If bleeding occurs, apply pressure with clean cloth. If injured area swells, apply cold packs. If bleeding does not stop or if bite is severe, take child to hospital emergency room.

Objects Wedged Between Teeth

Carefully remove object from between the teeth with dental floss. If unable to remove, see a dentist. *DO NOT remove sharp objects — see a dentist immediately.*

Possible Fractured Jaw

If jaw is broken or thought to be broken, do not move jaw. Wrap jaw with scarf, handkerchief, tie, towel, etc. to *immobilize the jaw and take child to hospital emergency room immediately.*

After-Hours Emergencies

Call family dentist or local hospital emergency room for names of dentists on call. Names of dentists who accept emergency patients can also be found in the yellow pages of the phone book.

Dental First Aid Supplies

The following should be added to your first aid kit, to be used for dental emergencies:

Medications

- Salt
- 3 percent Hydrogen peroxide
- *Aspirin or aspirin substitute
- *Oil of cloves
- *Orabase with Benzocaine

*Medications should not be used in schools without written approved protocol specific to each drug and signed by a physician or dentist. The protocol should include: name of drug, indications, contraindications, side effects, and dosage specific to age level.

Written permission from a parent or guardian should be provided for any medication given to a student in school. Aspirin should be avoided in children with influenza, chicken pox or other viral illnesses because of the possible association with Reye Syndrome.

Basic Supplies

- Cotton
- Cotton Swabs
- Sterile gauze squares (2 x 2)
- Sterile gauze pads
- Tea bags
- Toothbrushes
- Dental floss

- Stimudents or toothpicks
- Tweezers
- Paraffin, candle or dental wax
- Ice Pack or wet frozen washcloth

Mouth-Guards

Although this chapter is about treating minor dental emergencies a section on prevention is warranted. Mouth-guards prevent accidents such as broken or displaced teeth, traumatic avulsions of teeth, and a lacerated lip or tongue. These accidents occur very often in sports when the participants fail to wear protection. It only takes a single blow to the mouth area to create an emergency situation. Some excuses for not wearing mouth-guards are:

1. they are bulky;
2. they are uncomfortable;
3. they look funny;
4. others don't wear them.

Putting the excuses to the side, a custom made mouth-guard can be made at the dental office. By taking impressions of the teeth and then making the mouth-guard from these models, the fit is perfect, which alleviates any bulk or discomfort.

Another type of mouth-guard is pre-molded and can be purchased where sporting goods are sold. This type needs to be heated in boiling water to soften the plastic material. While the mouth-guard is warm and pliable, it needs to be placed in the mouth to get the shape of the teeth. The fit isn't as accurate because one size fits all, but it serves the purpose to protect the mouth area from injury.

Inflamed or Irritated Gum Tissue

Red, swollen or sore gums should be rinsed thoroughly with a warm salt water solution (1/2 teaspoon of salt in a glass of warm water). Another mouth rinse can be made by mixing equal parts of water and a 3 percent solution of hydrogen peroxide. Either of these mouth rinses should be swished around the entire mouth for 15 - 30 seconds twice a day, morning and evening.

Inflamed, bleeding gum tissue can be the result of poor oral hygiene. Diligent removal of plaque by brushing and flossing daily will allow the gums to regain healthy tissue and tone. Toothpaste does not have to be used to remove the plaque — baking soda, salt, or hydrogen peroxide (dilute 38 solution) can be used with a soft bristle toothbrush. Dental floss can be used to remove plaque and aid in maintaining healthy gums. The use of a toothbrush, coated only with saliva, has also been shown to be effective in plaque removal/control. Recommend to parent that a dentist be consulted.

Bleeding gums may also be caused by a Vitamin C deficiency or a systemic problem. If the condition does not improve with good oral hygiene (brushing 3-4 times a day and flossing at least once a day) a diet evaluation may be in order. Recommend to parent that a dentist be consulted.

A blow (trauma) to the mouth can cause the gum tissue to swell and bleed. The gums and teeth should be kept clean to decrease the chance of infection. A cold compress may be applied to the area from the outside of the cheek to help control swelling. Using a sterile 2 x 2 gauze square, apply direct pressure to the injured gum or cheek to control the bleeding.

Fever Blisters, Cold Sores and Canker Sores

- Apply Orabase with Benzocaine (in moderate amounts) for temporary relief of canker sores.

- Spicy and "acidy" foods should be avoided.

- Aspirin or aspirin substitute may be given for pain or fever (dosage according to child's weight and age). Never place the aspirin directly on the sore as this will cause a chemical burn to the tissue.

- A dentist should be consulted if pain or fever persists.

- Glyoxide or Listerine may be used to promote drying (fever blisters), avoid sun or wind exposure and "kissing" contact with others.

Toothache

1. Rinse the mouth vigorously with warm water to clean out any debris.

2. Use dental floss to remove any food trapped in the cavity.

3. If swelling is present, apply a cold compress to the outside of the cheek. **DO NOT USE HEAT.**

4. Aspirin or an aspirin substitute may be given to relieve pain (dosage according to child's weight and age). DO NOT place aspirin directly on the gum tissue or on the aching tooth as it will cause chemical burns.

5. Oil of cloves may be applied with a Q-tip or swab onto affected tooth.

IF A CHILD HAS A TOOTHACHE OR OTHER APPARENT DENTAL EMERGENCY, THE CHILD'S PARENTS SHOULD BE CONTACTED. IF THE CHILD HAS A PRIVATE DENTIST, HE OR SHE SHOULD BE REFERRED TO THAT DENTIST AS SOON AS POSSIBLE.

Note: The state dental association or local dental society can be contacted and through their referral service, the names of dentists who are willing to accept emergency patients and practice in the area can be given to the family.

Other resources: A dental school/university, hospitals with dental emergency facilities, public school dental clinics, local health departments with dental facilities and other community dental clinics.

Prolonged or Recurrent Bleeding after an Extraction

The child should be instructed not to rinse or swish at all for 24 hours after an extraction (having a tooth pulled), as this could wash out the blood clot forming at the extraction site. Normal drinking is permissible; however, straws should not be used for 24 hours because the suction created in the mouth could dislodge the blood clot.

DO NOT BE ALARMED IF THERE SEEMS TO A LOT OF BLOOD OOZING FROM THE EXTRACTION-SITE. REMEMBER THAT THE BLOOD IS MIXING WITH SALIVA AND, THEREFORE, IT MAY APPEAR THERE IS MORE BLEEDING THAN IS ACTUALLY THE CASE. IF THE BLEEDING IS DETERMINED TO BE MORE THAN OOZING (BRIGHT RED BLOOD) OR IS ALARMING THE CHILD, THE FOLLOWING IS RECOMMENDED:

1. Place a sterile folded gauze 2 x 2 on the extraction site, and have the child bite on it for about 30 minutes. Replace soaked gauze 2 x 2 pads with clean ones as necessary.

2. If the bleeding persists, wrap a moistened tea bag in a sterile gauze 2 x 2 and have the child bite on it for 30-45 minutes. Repeat this procedure if necessary.

3. An aspirin substitute may be given for pain (dosage according to child's weight and age). Avoid aspirin as it reduces the blood's ability to clot.

4. If bleeding cannot be controlled within an hour, contact the parent and recommend they consult a dentist or physician.

Broken or Displaced Teeth

1. Try to clean the soil, blood, and other debris from the injured area with a sterile gauze or cotton swab and warm water or 38 hydrogen peroxide.

2. Apply a cold compress on the outside of cheek next to the injured tooth to reduce swelling.

3. Have the child gently bite his teeth together. Check for displacement of teeth. If possible, gently move the displaced tooth or teeth into their correct position.

4. If the tooth has been pushed up into the socket or gum by the blow, do not attempt to pull it out into position. (It will re-erupt normally on its own.)

5. If the broken tooth has created a sharp edge, it may be covered with paraffin (wax) to prevent tissue lacerations.

6. An aspirin or aspirin substitute may be given for pain (dosage according to child's weight and age).

7. Contact the parent and arrange to have the child taken to the dentist AS SOON AS POSSIBLE for any of the above problems.

Traumatic Avulsion (Loss of) Permanent Tooth

1. Look in the accident area for the tooth that was knocked out.

2. If found, do not attempt to clean the tooth. Washing the tooth off could destroy the connective fibers which help anchor the tooth in the mouth.

3. If the tooth has been on the ground, wipe off tooth — do not wash. Place the tooth into the socket before a blood clot forms in the socket. Check on patient's medical/dental history to see if the tetanus immunization is current. If not current, the child should be taken to the family physician within 24 hours for a booster injection. Tetanus (lockjaw) can cause serious health problems. If the patient is not cooperative or if the school nurse or teacher is not comfortable with reinserting the tooth, place the tooth in a cup of milk (preferred storage medium) or wrap it in a clean wet cloth or gauze.

4. Contact the parent and arrange to have the child taken to the dentist IMMEDIATELY. Many times the tooth can be successfully re-implanted and saved, if accomplished within one hour.

5. An aspirin or aspirin substitute may be given for pain (dosage according to the child's weight and age).

Possible Jaw Dislocation or Fracture

If a jaw fracture or dislocation is suspected, immobilize the jaw by any means available. Place a scarf, handkerchief, tie, or towel under the chin and tie the ends on top of the child's head.

Contact the parent and arrange for child to be taken IMMEDIATELY to an oral surgeon or hospital emergency room. At the hospital the child should be seen by an oral, maxillofacial, orthopedic, or plastic surgeon, if available.

Orthodontic (Braces) Emergencies or Problems

FOR IRRITATION IN THE MOUTH CAUSED BY A PRO-TRUDING WIRE FROM ORTHODONTIC BANDS, THE FOL-LOWING PROCEDURES ARE RECOMMENDED:

- A blunt item (tongue depressor, cotton swab, or pencil eraser) may be used to gently bend the wire so it is no longer irritating to the soft oral tissues.

- When the protruding wire cannot be bent, simply cover the end of it with paraffin (wax), a piece of gauze, or a small cotton ball so it is no longer causing irritation.

- Do not attempt to remove any wire that is embedded in the cheeks, gum, or tongue. Contact the parents so that they can make an immediate appointment with the child's orthodontist.

- If a wire or appliance becomes loose or broken and cannot be removed easily, contact the parent to take the child and the wire to the orthodontist IMMEDIATELY.

- The placement and adjustment of orthodontic bands/wires can cause some discomfort for a few days. Some relief can be achieved by holding warm salt water (1/2 teaspoon of salt in a glass of warm water) in the mouth. Aspirin or aspirin substitute can give additional relief (dosage according to child's weight and age). A semi-solid diet is recommended until the mouth feels comfortable to resume normal chewing.

Tooth Eruption Pain

Try to determine if the pain is from a loose primary (baby) tooth pinching the gum tissue, or due to an erupting permanent tooth. Refer to the tooth eruption chart.

Prolonged pain (over one week) is unusual and may be caused by inflammation around an impacted or partially impacted tooth. This type of pain is usually intermittent and less painful than the type of pain associated with a badly decayed tooth. This periodic, prolonged pain is fairly common with eruption of first permanent molars and third molars or wisdom teeth. A dentist should be consulted.

An aspirin or aspirin substitute can be given for the temporary relief of pain (dosage according to child's weight and age). Never place the aspirin directly on the tissue in the area of pain as it can cause a tissue burn (chemical).

A cold compress or a piece of ice wrapped in a 2" x 2" gauze square can be directly applied to the eruption site. Due to the numbing effect of the cold, this method can provide temporary relief.

If the pain persists, contact the parent and tell them that a dentist should be consulted.

TOOTH ERUPTION CHART

REMEMBER THAT SOME CHILDREN'S TEETH ERUPT MUCH EARLIER AND SOME MUCH LATER THAN THE AVERAGE ERUPTION DATES GIVEN HERE. A YEAR ON EITHER SIDE OF THE AVERAGE ERUPTION TIMES IS NOT UNUSUAL.

ERUPTION AND SHEDDING OF THE PRIMARY TEETH (BABY TEETH)

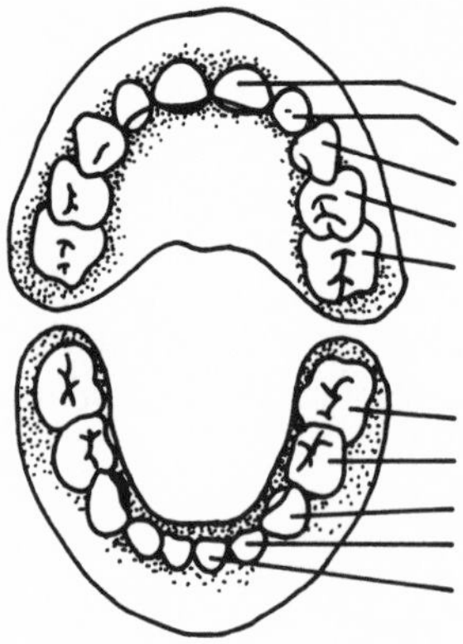

Upper Teeth	Eruption	Shedding
Central incisor	7½ mos.	7½ yrs.
Lateral incisor	9 mos.	8 yrs.
Cuspid	18 mos.	11½ yrs.
First molar	14 mos.	10½ yrs.
Second molar	24 mos.	10½ yrs.
Lower Teeth		
Second molar	20 mos.	11 yrs.
First molar	12 mos.	10 yrs.
Cuspid	16 mos.	9½ yrs.
Lateral incisor	7 mos.	7 yrs.
Central incisor	6 mos.	6 yrs.

ERUPTION OF THE PERMANENT TEETH

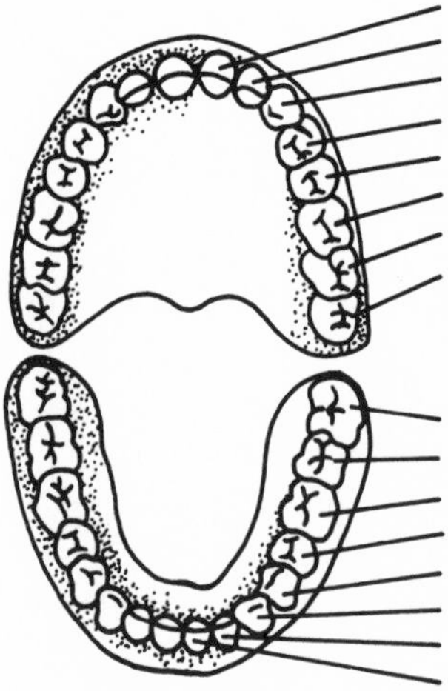

Upper Teeth	
Central incisor	7–8 yrs.
Lateral incisor	8–9 yrs.
Cuspid	11–12 yrs.
First bicuspid	10–11 yrs.
Second bicuspid	10–12 yrs.
First molar	6–7 yrs.
Second molar	12–13 yrs.
Third molar	17–21 yrs.
Lower Teeth	
Third molar	17–21 yrs.
Second molar	11–13 yrs.
First molar	6–7 yrs.
Second bicuspid	11–12 yrs.
First bicuspid	10–12 yrs.
Cuspid	9–10 yrs.
Lateral incisor	7–8 yrs.
Central incisor	6–7 yrs.

Figure 63.1.

Lacerated Lip or Tongue

1. Apply direct pressure to the bleeding area with a sterile 2 x 2 gauze square, for 15 to 30 minutes. Vigorous bleeding may be expected initially.

2. If swelling is present, apply a cold compress (lip injury).

3. Check for broken/fractured or avulsed teeth.

4. If the bleeding does not stop readily, or the injury is severe, contact the parent to take the child to a hospital emergency room.

Objects Wedged Between Teeth

*   Try to remove the object with a toothpick, tweezers or dental floss. Remember to guide the floss in gently (against teeth) so as not to injure the gum tissue.

*   Do not try to remove the object with a sharp or pointed tool/instrument, as injury may occur.

*   If unsuccessful, contact the parent to take the child to the dentist.

—by Michelle Carbone-Nadeau, R.D.H., B.S., Karen A. Hoague, and Bonny Myshrall, Maine Office of Dental Health.

Index

Index

Page numbers in *italics* refer to tables and illustrations; the letter "n" following a page number refers to a note.

A

AAID *see* American Academy of Implant Dentistry (AAID)
AAPD *see* American Academy of Pediatric Dentistry (AAPD)
abscesses 129
Academy of Osseointegration 392, 413
acidophilus 309
acinar cells 297
Acree, K. H. 508
acyclovir 292
  herpes simplex virus and 23
ADA *see* American Dental Association (ADA)
Adams, P. F. 101
addictions to tobacco 57–59
Addison's disease 22
adhesins and receptors 6
adhesive sealants 16
  see also dental sealants

adjuvant chemotherapy 268
adolescents
  caries (tooth decay) and 103, 104
  dental sealants and 173
  gum disease and 214
  oropharyngeal cancer and 77
  orthodontic treatments for 107
  periodontal disease and 106
  smokeless tobacco and 277
adults
  anesthesia and sedation 36
  braces for 384
  caries (tooth decay) and 17–19
  dental service use *93, 94*
  fluoridated water and 160–61
  fluoride and 53
  oral diseases and 72–79
Advisory Committee to the Surgeon General 278
African Americans
  cancers in *78*
  dental examinations and 89–90
  dental health status of 103
  oral disease and 72
age factor
  caries (tooth decay) and *74, 76,* 77
  dental examinations and 89
  dental treatment needs and 106
  dry mouth and 223

531

S

Safe Drinking Water Act 154
safety issues
  community water fluoridation and
    161
  dental sealants and 54–55, 174
  laser procedures and 208–9
  x-rays and 139–41
  see also risk assessments
saggital appliance 389
sailor's lip 254
saline sprays 231
saliva
  AIDS and 13–14
  caries (tooth decay) and 7
  composition of 8
  importance of 221–22
salivary enzymes 8
salivary flow
  pilocarphine and 9
salivary gland dysfunctions 224
  cystic fibrosis and 295–97
  oral tissues and 3
  taste cells and 8
salivary glands 247
  HIV and 14
  reasearch and 8–9
saliva stimulators 23
saliva subsitutes 23
saliva substitutes 226
salivation electrostimulator 237
salt water gargles 24
Samit, A. M. 275
Sande, M. A. 99
Sands, Barry E. 394, 396–97
San Francisco School of Dentistry
  210
Sant'Agnese, Paul di 296
Sargent, Larry A. 349, 359
Sass, Neil 156
scaling 190
scarlet fever 24
scatter radiation 141
Scheid, R. C. 510
Schluger, Saul 193
Schmitt, A. 420
Schnitman, P. 418

Schnitman, Paul A. 414
Schnurr, R. F. 101
schools
  dental sealants and 181
  first aid supplies for 519
  fluoride mouthrinse programs 149
Schottenfeld, D. 275
Schultz, Dodi 158
Schweitzer, S. 100
scleroderma 80, 241–44
Scott, H. D. 509
scurvy 22
sealed composite restorations
  as amalgam alternative 123–24
  caries (tooth decay) and 8
Seal of Acceptance 200
  see also American Dental Associa-
    tion (ADA)
Sears, Cathy 346
second-hand smoke 58
  see also tobacco
sedation, defined 35
sedative agents 33–42
Seifert, I. 419
self examinations, oral health and
  314–15
sensitive teeth 515–16
  care of 31
  toothpastes for 112
  see also receding gums
sensitivity to heat 129
septicemia, oral diseases and 81
Sertoma 375
Shadomy, H. J. 511
Shapiro, C. N. 509, 511
Shaw, F. E. 509
Sheiham, A. 100
Shepherd, Steven 201
shingles pain research 10
  see also herpes simplex virus
Shopland, D. R. 275
shortened limbs research 11
Shulman, L. 419
Shuman, S. K. 100
sialagogues 238–39, 293
sicca complex 227
  see also Sjögren's syndrome
Siegal, Mark 176